Cultural Competencies for Nurses

Impact on Health and Illness

The Pedagogy

Cultural Competencies for Nursing, Second Edition drives comprehension through various strategies that meet the learning needs of students, while also generating enthusiasm about the topic. This interactive approach addresses different learning styles, making this the ideal text to ensure mastery of key concepts. The pedagogical aids that appear in most chapters include the following:

Key Terms

Found in a list at the beginning of each chapter, these terms will create an expanded vocabulary. The "www" icon directs students to the text's online resources to explore these terms in an interactive glossary and to use flashcards and crosswords to master the definitions.

Objectives

These objectives provide instructors and students with a snapshot of the key information they will encounter in each chapter. The objectives are available in short-answer format within the text's online resources, allowing students to use them as a checklist to help guide and focus study.

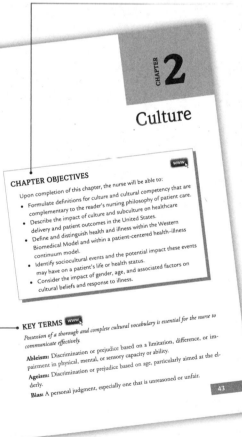

CHAPTER **2**

Culture

CHAPTER OBJECTIVES www
Upon completion of this chapter, the nurse will be able to:
- Formulate definitions for culture and cultural competency that are complementary to the reader's nursing philosophy of patient care.
- Describe the impact of culture and subculture on healthcare delivery and patient outcomes in the United States.
- Define and distinguish health and illness within the Western Biomedical Model and within a patient-centered health–illness continuum model.
- Identify sociocultural events and the potential impact these events may have on a patient's life or health status.
- Consider the impact of gender, age, and associated factors on cultural beliefs and response to illness.

KEY TERMS www
Possession of a thorough and complete cultural vocabulary is essential for the nurse to communicate effectively.

Ableism: Discrimination or prejudice based on a limitation, difference, or impairment in physical, mental, or sensory capacity or ability.
Ageism: Discrimination or prejudice based on age, particularly aimed at the elderly.
Bias: A personal judgment, especially one that is unreasoned or unfair.

43

Case Studies

Case studies allow students to read and analyze real-life situations and apply what they have learned. Additional case studies and accompanying critical thinking questions can be found in the text's online resources.

Review Questions

Students can work on these assignments individually or in a group after reading through the material. Students can delve deeper into concepts by completing and submitting these exercises online.

Redeem the access code at the front of your book at **www.jblearning .com.** If you do not have an access code, one can be purchased at the site.

---

hardship and political oppression, Native Americans continue to survive and to preserve their unique and valuable culture.

CASE STUDY 8–1

Kai is a 58-year-old Navajo (Native American) who has been severely immobile since suffering from a cerebral vascular accident nine months ago. She is cared for on a daily basis by a home health aide and is seen by the visiting nurse on a regular schedule. Kai has many other medical problems including some rather serious comorbidities, such as brittle DM and obesity. The nurse noticed that Kai was developing some contractures and arranged for a visiting physical therapist to come out to evaluate Kai.

When the visiting nurse returned for her next scheduled visit, Kai was not her usual mood. When the nurse asked Kai what was wrong, she was surprised to hear that the physical therapist had mentioned hospice care as a possibility in Kai's treatment plan. Kai told the nurse that she was extremely upset by this, that she "never wants to see that physical therapist again."

REVIEW QUESTIONS

1. If you were that visiting nurse, how would you respond?
2. In your response, make sure that you demonstrate your under Navajo culture.

Rationale: This case demonstrates the importance that all he members have knowledge of cultural beliefs of the patients for whos care. The nurse should acknowledge the PT's lack of knowledge cultural beliefs and the nurse's intention of advocating for the p should reach out to the PT to share the patient's concerns and to knowledge of cultural competency with the other healthcare t

CASE STUDY 8–2

Akule is a 24-year-old Native American male who identifi was diagnosed with HIV three years ago. Due to a lack of vation regarding his sexual orientation, which resulted physical attacks, he moved to the city of Phoenix at a home from time to time and seeks medical care at a

---

project funded by the Centers for Disease Control and Prevention and the National Institute of Diabetes and Digestive and Kidney Diseases, and is a 6-center prospective study of managed care and diabetes quality of care, costs, and outcomes in the United States.

The goal of this study was to determine if the utilization of clinical care strategies in managed care (diabetes registry, physician feedback, and physician reminders) is associated with attenuation of known racial/ethnic disparities in diabetic care. The study found that for the most part, high-intensity implementation of a diabetes registry, physician feedback, or physician reminders—three clinical care strategies similar to those used in many healthcare settings—are *not* associated with an attenuation of known disparities of diabetes care in managed care. The authors also reported that disparities in care do exist, particularly among the Black American population.

REVIEW QUESTIONS

1. Differentiate the terms *culture, cultural assessment,* and *cultural competency.*
2. List the six cultural phenomena of the Giger and Davidhizar model.
3. Purnell identifies the 12 domains of culture in his model. What are the similarities and differences between those 12 domains and the 6 cultural phenomena that are in the Giger and Davidhizar model?
4. Provide two nursing implications for a nurse administering antihypertensives or psychotropics to the non-White patient (ethnopharmacology principles).
5. What was the theoretical framework used to develop the 12 standards of culturally competent nursing care practice that were published in the *Journal of Transcultural Nursing* in 2009?
6. Describe the process to attain cultural competency.
7. Which nursing theorist gave birth to the transcultural nursing movement?
8. Identify and describe three potential areas of diversity.
9. Describe the potential consequences of culturally discordant care.
10. What can the nurse do to decease the likelihood of committing a cultural gaffe?

REFERENCES

Battalova, J., & Terrazas, A. (2010). Frequently requested statistics on immigrants and immigration in the United States. Retrieved from http://www.migrationinformation.org/feature/display.cfm?ID=818

SECOND EDITION

Cultural Competencies for Nurses

Impact on Health and Illness

Linda Dayer-Berenson, PhD, MSN, CRNP, CNE, FAANP

Assistant Clinical Professor
Drexel University
College of Nursing and Health Professions
Philadelphia, Pennsylvania

Assistant Professor
University of Medicine and Dentistry
School of Osteopathic Medicine, Neuromusculoskeletal Institute
Stratford, New Jersey

JONES & BARTLETT
LEARNING

World Headquarters
Jones & Bartlett Learning
5 Wall Street
Burlington, MA 01803
978-443-5000
info@jblearning.com
www.jblearning.com

Jones & Bartlett Learning books and products are available through most bookstores and online booksellers. To contact Jones & Bartlett Learning directly, call 800-832-0034, fax 978-443-8000, or visit our website, www.jblearning.com.

Substantial discounts on bulk quantities of Jones & Bartlett Learning publications are available to corporations, professional associations, and other qualified organizations. For details and specific discount information, contact the special sales department at Jones & Bartlett Learning via the above contact information or send an email to specialsales@jblearning.com.

Production Credits

Executive Publisher: Kevin Sullivan
Acquisitions Editor: Amanda Harvey
Editorial Assistant: Rebecca Myrick
Production Editor: Cindie Bryan
Senior Marketing Manager: Jennifer Stiles
Marketing Communications Manager: Katie Hennessy
V.P., Manufacturing and Inventory Control: Therese Connell
Composition: Publishers' Design and Production Services, Inc.

Cover Design: Michael O'Donnell
Rights & Photo Research Assistant: Joseph Veiga
Cover Image: © Jupiterimages/Comstock/ Thinkstock
Printing and Binding: Edwards Brothers Malloy
Cover Printing: Edwards Brothers Malloy

To order this product, use ISBN: 1-978-1-4496-8807-3

Library of Congress Cataloging-in-Publication Data
Dayer-Berenson, Linda.
    Cultural competencies for nurses : impact on health and illness / Linda Dayer-Berenson. — 2nd ed.
        p. ; cm.
    Includes bibliographical references and index.
    ISBN 978-1-4496-8765-6 — ISBN 1-4496-8765-2
    I. Title.
    [DNLM: 1. Transcultural Nursing—methods. 2. Cross-Cultural Comparison. 3. Cultural Competency. 4. Nurse–Patient Relations. 5. Nursing Care—methods. WY 107]
    362.17'3—dc23

                                                                        2012034071

6048

Printed in the United States of America
17 16   10 9 8 7 6 5 4

Dedication

To My Loving Family

This book is dedicated to my husband Richard and our sons, Justin and Jarret, with whom all things are possible. Thank you for forgiving the many hours spent away from you. Your support not only helped to minimize my guilt for taking time away from all of you, but it also kept me encouraged and motivated while writing both the first edition and the second edition of this text.

To My Parents

To my late father Robert and my mother Mary Ellen Dayer, who always encouraged my pursuit of higher education and the importance of being a caring member of society.

To My Current and Former Nursing Students

Your enthusiasm and desire to excel while providing nursing care is humbling and a great motivator to me. The future of nursing is in very good hands indeed.

To My Fellow Faculty and Nursing Colleagues

To all present and future nurses who desire to provide culturally appropriate nursing care during cross-cultural patient encounters: this book is for all of you.

Contents

Acknowledgments

The idea for this book was born while doing research for my doctoral dissertation so I must acknowledge and thank the members of my committee. Their commitment, unwavering support, and passion for the topic of cultural competency was contagious and resulted in a successful dissertation and textbook. Dr. Robin Eubanks, who was the chair of my dissertation, is an associate professor in the Department of Interdisciplinary Studies at the University of Medicine and Dentistry of New Jersey (UMDNJ), School of Health Related Professions, in Newark, New Jersey. I want to provide an extraspecial thank you to Dr. Richard Jermyn, a physiatrist/pain management specialist, who is an associate professor at the UMDNJ School of Osteopathic Medicine in Stratford, New Jersey. Dr. Jermyn, in addition to serving on my committee and providing the site for data collection for my study, is my collaborating physician for my pain management nurse practitioner practice at the UMDNJ, School of Osteopathic Medicine, Neuromusculoskeletal Institute. I am thrilled that Dr. Jermyn and I are continuing to collaborate on research and presentations related to the topic of cultural competency especially in those who suffer from the health disparity of chronic pain. The final committee member was Dr. Linda Wilson, who is an assistant professor at Drexel University, College of Nursing and Health Professions in Philadelphia, Pennsylvania. She is also a nursing colleague and fellow faculty member at Drexel University, College of Nursing and Health Professions. Special thanks to Dr. Robert Denmark who was the chair of my PhD program. Dr. Denmark was invaluable in providing feedback on my writing and editing of the dissertation. All of them have contributed to my professional development and expertise in cultural competency. They exemplify the principles of cultural competency and were wonderful and effective role models to me because they not only talked the talk but they walked the walk each and every day.

Preface

With each passing year, the United States is becoming more racially, ethnically, and culturally diverse. This growth in diversity is not occurring in our population of healthcare professionals, and this lack of parallel growth often results in the provision of culturally discordant care. While it is not in our power to change the demographic characteristics of our licensed nursing personnel, we can educate nurses to negotiate across cultural divides that may occur during our interactions with a patient whose cultural background is different from our own. It is from this perspective that my personal journey of striving to achieve cultural competency was born, and it is the motivating factor for writing this book. While there are several textbooks available on this topic, I have not found one book that can serve as a stand-alone resource for student nurses, practicing nurses, and advanced practice nurses. This book strives to be that stand-alone resource. By reading this book, nurses from all educational levels and backgrounds will be able to determine how to interact effectively and to provide care for patients whose ethnic or cultural background differs from their own.

An overview of the major transcultural and cultural competency models are provided in Unit 1. The original model that guides my nursing practice and provided the theoretical foundation for this textbook was originally Giger and Davidhizar's *Transcultural Nursing: Assessment and Intervention* (2004). Dr. Davidhizar is now deceased and the sixth edition is solely authored by Dr. Giger (2013).

The five chapters of Unit 2 on specific cultural groups are organized so that the six cultural phenomena that shape care, as identified by Giger (2013), are incorporated in such a way that the nurse will know how to proceed in situations where these phenomena provide a barrier to patient care delivery. Overall, the emphasis of the book is for the nurse to strive toward providing individualized care that considers and incorporates the cultural uniqueness of any given patient—a task that can be complicated by today's fast-paced, highly technical healthcare environment, with its emphasis on excessive documentation that takes time away from actual patient interactions and delivery of care. If the nurse can understand the patient's or family's motivation behind certain requests and behaviors, and if the nurse can feel comfortable that the inclusion of these requests or beliefs will not be harmful to the patient, then there can be no reason why the plan of care cannot be mutually defined in order to achieve our mutually established objectives for the patient encounter. As nurses, we are used to working with our patients to establish goals for nursing care; it should not require much of a stretch to extend this thinking, and spirit of inclusion, to pertain to the actual care delivery as well.

Overview of Cultural Foundations, Cultural Competency, and Transcultural Nursing/ Health Care

This textbook is intended to be a resource for practicing nurses, and for all types of nursing students (diploma, Associate's degree [AA], Bachelor of Science in Nursing [BSN], Master of Science in Nursing [MSN] and Doctor of Nursing Practice [DNP]) on cultural competency and its impact on health and illness. There has been an explosion in the allied health and nursing literature on cultural competency in the last few years, and a textbook of this kind is necessary to help the nurse, at all levels, navigate through the obstacles that culture can place on the patient experience. The textbook will provide a "one-stop shop" so the nurse can find the history and theory behind cultural competency in nursing as well as a resource for "pearls" regarding health beliefs and the impact of culture on health and illness.

This textbook is intended to serve as a resource and reference to be used by all nurses when they need to learn more about cultural competency and the health/illness beliefs of patients. Although providing information is an extremely important consideration, ideally, education is not just about information—it is also about knowledge. In order for information to become knowledge, it requires added context and interactivity. It is the intent that this textbook will transcend just being an information source to provide a framework and structure that permits the acquisition of knowledge by the reader. It is for this reason that this textbook will have the following pedagogic features: at the beginning of each chapter, objectives will be provided; inside each chapter that describes a particular racial/ethnic or cultural group there will be case studies that reinforce and highlight the essential facts regarding each group; key terms will be noted and definitions provided at the beginning of some chapters; pertinent research studies will be highlighted (this will be done for important or landmark research studies or findings); in addition, review questions of the key concepts will be provided at the end of each chapter. Unit One will provide the cultural foundation, with an overview of the important models of cultural competence included. The history and development of the transcultural nursing movement will be described. Unit One is entitled, "Overview of Cultural Foundations, Cultural Competency, and Transcultural Nursing/Health Care" and will consist of four chapters. The outline for each of the four chapters is as follows:

Chapter 1—Birth of Transcultural Nursing to Current Theories and Conceptual Models for Cultural Diversity

Theory of Culture Care Diversity and Universality (Sunrise Model) (Dr. Madeline Leininger—founder of the field of transcultural Nursing in the mid-1960s); Dr. Leininger's Sunrise Model was developed to help nurses manage when caring for diverse groups of patients in response to changing demographics in the United States, and due to the fact that the leadership in healthcare delivery in the United States led many people from other countries come to America for medical care. As a result, US nurses are often called upon to assess clinically, in a short period of time, individuals who, in many cases, are very different culturally, racially, and ethnically from themselves. *Culture Care Diversity and Universality* has been studied, praised, and criticized since it was first published in 1970.

Giger and Davidhizar's Transcultural Assessment Model (2008, 1988)

Purnell Model for Cultural Competence (2013, 1998)

Chapter 2—Culture

Appropriate terms defined: culture, ethnicity, acculturation, assimilation, health, health belief model, illness, sick role, healing, ethnocentrism, cultural diversity, cultural awareness, cultural sensitivity, cultural competency, stereotyping, generalizations

Chapter 3—Global Diversity

Multicultural populations

Census data

Cultural groupings/health disparities

Chapter 4—Organization of Healthcare Delivery in the 21st Century

Interdisciplinary healthcare delivery

Standards of Care: Institute of Medicine reports on unequal treatment

National Standards for Culturally and Linguistically Appropriate Services in Health Care, The Joint Commission

Shift from medical model (Western medicine) to health belief model

Barriers (communication issues, lack of access to preventive care, history of discrimination and abuse in some cultures, distrust of healthcare providers, noncompliance and/or refusal to enter the healthcare system at all).

Impact on Provision of Primary Care by nurse practitioners—The integration of cultural competency into primary care practice has been clarified in the National Organization of Nurse Practitioner Faculties document on cultural competency. It states that the nurse practitioner demonstrates cultural competence when she/he shows respect for the inherent dignity of every human being, whatever their age, gender, religion, socioeconomic class, sexual orientation, and ethnic or cultural group; accepts the rights of individuals to choose their care provider, participate in care, and refuse care; acknowledges personal biases and prevents these from interfering with the delivery of quality care to persons of other cultures; recognizes cultural issues and interacts with clients from other cultures in culturally sensitive ways and incorporates cultural preferences, health beliefs, and behaviors and traditional practices into the management plan; develops client-appropriate educational materials that address the language and cultural beliefs of the client and accesses culturally appropriate resources to deliver care to clients from other cultures; and assists clients to access quality care within a dominant culture.

Certification opportunities—Cultural Competence Certification for Clinicians is offered by the Center for Professional Development at the School of Nursing, University of Pennsylvania.

Unit Two will consist of chapters for different ethnic groups with an emphasis of the impact of health and illness on each group.

I do realize that it would be unreasonable to expect that any single textbook could satisfy all of the needs of a student/learner and that the same needs exist in all students/learners. This would dispute the importance of individuality which lies at the heart of the cultural competency movement. While writing this textbook, an attempt was made to consider the many different reasons, aims, and needs a student/learner has that led them on the journey of acquiring knowledge about cultural competency while also recognizing that different people with the same learning goal have different needs in this learning process. Each of us has individual learning styles, habits, abilities, and life and work circumstances. As a framing reference, this textbook will attempt to introduce cultural competency as a theoretical foundation; to explain the *why* and *how* when caring for patients from cultures that differ from our own; to teach the nurse how to use, implement, and utilize this new knowledge; to verify that this new knowledge has been acquired; and finally, to assist the nurse with the everyday application of this newly gained knowledge. To provide safe and effective nursing care in the 21st century, the nurse must not only have knowledge about our diverse society and the science of nursing, but also focus on the art of nursing care. This requires a global focus from the nurse, given the extensive cultural diversity that exists in the United States.

UNIT ONE OBJECTIVES

1. Differentiate among the various theories of cultural competency to select the model that will best support your nursing care delivery in the 21st century.
2. Know the history of the transcultural nursing movement from its birth (Dr. Madeline Leininger) to its present.
3. Distinguish among various ethnic/cultural groups as well as the primary and secondary characteristics of culture.
4. Describe the impact of global diversity on healthcare delivery in the United States.
5. Develop proficiency in cultural concepts and race categories and provide definitions for essential terminology.
6. Commit to providing culturally competent care to all patients.

Unit One provides the nurse with the theoretical foundation of the cultural competency movement. Various important cultural competency theories are described as well as the impact of diversity on cross-cultural exchanges and the impact that the Western biomedical model has on healthcare delivery in the United States. The Western Biomedical Model—with its emphasis on patient autonomy—often is in conflict with the health beliefs of many different racial and ethnic groups who enter the healthcare system and who require nursing care. In order to provide culturally aware nursing care, the nurse must not only understand where he/she comes from but also needs at a minimum a basic working understanding of the cultures of the patients for whom he or she delivers nursing care. This requires the nurse to be able to answer two questions: what is my culture, and what do I know/understand about my patient's culture? The overriding goal is for the nurse to develop a respect for cultural differences that will allow the nurse to demonstrate a genuine appreciation of different cultural values and views wherever they are encountered. Often, what we do not understand is viewed negatively. Cultural assessment is integral to understanding the meaning of patient behaviors so this does not occur. Nurses need to consider that each patient experience is likely to vary in many ways beyond just its medical presentation. The nurse needs to ask questions to determine the likely response, so that the appropriate interventions can be offered. For example, the nurse needs to consider if this is a patient who would respond positively to touch. Also, how should physical assessment be adjusted to provide for modesty, or to determine oxygen status of the tissues in a dark-skinned patient? The questions are many, but the answers are more likely to be determined when the nurse possesses a foundation of cultural awareness and has demonstrated a willingness to learn about, recognize, and most importantly, appreciate the individual differences of each and every patient in our care.

Unit Two provides cultural information on selected population groups in detail, with a focus on traditional health and illness beliefs, so that the nurse can determine if these beliefs are impacting the current healthcare issues. It is not possible to fully define or describe a cultural group, but the information provided can serve as a foundation to inform and sensitize the nurse as to the needs and beliefs of various cultural groups. The material is presented in a sensitive manner and is not intended to be viewed as stereotypical but to serve as a starting point for the nurse to seek clarification from the patient so that individual variation can be taken into account, and truly individualized patient care can be provided.

The journey begins by knowing ourselves and accepting our values; we possess the framework to accept the existence of values that differ from our own. This realization, and ultimately the acceptance of these differing values and needs, will permit the nurse to work collaboratively with patients in the provision of safe professional nursing care.

The book will also provide tips for effective cross-cultural communication as well as specific information to increase the chance that a cross-cultural patient encounter will be viewed as successful by both the patient and the nurse. Strategies on how to effectively use interpreters for communicating with patients with limited or no English speaking ability, and for integrating every patient's cultural beliefs and traditional health practices (whenever possible, considering safety) into the treatment plan will also be included.

DISCLAIMER

Membership in a particular culture does not mean that the person will necessarily reflect all of the customs, traditions, and beliefs that are associated with the culture. There are many other variables that impact all of us and contribute to who we are as people. These factors, including our place of birth, family background, socioeconomic status, educational level, urban versus rural geography, and level of acculturation attained, will also impact the degree to which we subscribe to the health and illness beliefs associated with that culture and our approach and preferences for health care. The material provided is meant as a guide; it is not a rule book. It provides information that the nurse can refer to and consider when providing individualized patient care and evaluating its response. The labels used in the book to classify or categorize various cultural groups are broad; it is important to remember that each group is comprised of different cultures, nationalities, histories, and heritages, and that the nurse must remember that individuals are unique and not all of the material will be pertinent to every person. Every effort was made to be as culturally sensitive in writing this book, but I do recognize that the information (based on an extensive review of the literature) may be interpreted differently from my intent, and offense may be taken by readers who are members of the cultural groups described in this book. Please know that the intent was to present factual information that is evidence-based, and stems from a true desire to improve nursing care delivery in the 21st century to be the best that it can be. Our patients do better when their needs are met and beliefs are understood.

Knowing about our patients' cultures and individual beliefs is as important as knowing about their physical problems, functional limitations, and response to illness in providing safe, competent, and comprehensive nursing care. Given the increasing diversity of patients and nurses, as well as other members of the healthcare team, cultural competence is an absolute necessity. It is hoped that this book will assist the nurse and nurse practitioner to provide the best nursing care possible and to confidently practice when in a cross-cultural patient encounter.

Birth of Transcultural Nursing to Current Theories and Conceptual Models for Cultural Diversity

CHAPTER OBJECTIVES

www

Upon completion of this chapter, the nurse will be able to:

- Provide working definitions for transcultural nursing, cultural competence, and diversity.
- Identify various areas of diversity that the nurse should assess for and be aware of in order to provide culturally appropriate care.
- Describe three nursing theories that promote the delivery of competent nursing care to culturally diverse patients.
- Select a theoretical model of cultural competency that is complementary to the reader's nursing philosophy of patient care.

KEY TERMS WWW

Cultural competency

Diversity

Giger and Davidhizar's Transcultural Assessment Model

Leininger's Culture Care, Diversity, and Universality Theory

Purnell Model for Cultural Competence

INTRODUCTION

Whether a nursing student in the clinical setting, a seasoned nurse, or nurse practitioner, you observe diversity within your patient population on a daily basis. Our patients come from many different races and ethnic groups, which means they often do not look, feel, or respond like we do. These differences result in a cultural mismatch. Helping you to develop a plan for proceeding in the face of a cultural mismatch is the guiding force behind this textbook. The Office of Minority Health in 2001 published recommendations for 14 national standards for culturally and linguistically appropriate services in health care to provide the knowledge necessary for nurses to work respectfully and effectively with patients and each other in a culturally diverse work environment. These standards are called CLAS for short and were revised in 2012. CLAS will be described and discussed in more detail in Chapter 4 of this book.

How have we come to this point where the federal government has provided mandates, guidelines, and recommendations? It would appear that all members of the healthcare team need to do a better job. The CLAS standards were developed with input from national leaders (including the American Nurses Association [ANA]) and are based on an analysis of current standards in use that are deemed essential and appropriate.

The members of the expert panel on cultural competence of the American Academy of Nursing (AAN) have developed recommendations (**Box 1–1**) to ensure that measurable outcomes be achieved to reduce or eliminate health disparities commonly found among racial, ethnic, uninsured, underserved, and/or underrepresented populations residing throughout the United States.

Achieving cultural competence suggests possession of the ability to respond effectively to the cultural needs of our patients. This view would be too narrow, however. We must recognize that diversity exists among patients but also within the members of the healthcare team (nurses, physicians, and other allied health professionals). As we continue to struggle with a nursing shortage, one ongoing

Box 1–1   Twelve Recommendations of the Expert Panel on Cultural Competence of the American Academy of Nursing

1. The AAN, through its publications, mission statements, and yearly conferences, must make an explicit commitment to quality, culturally competent care that is equitable and accessible by targeting four groups: healthcare customers, healthcare providers, healthcare systems, and communities.
2. The AAN will collaborate with other organizations and communities in developing guidelines.
3. The AAN shall develop mechanisms to synthesize existing theoretical and research knowledge concerning nursing care of ethnic/minorities and other vulnerable populations.
4. The AAN, through its expert panels and commissions, must create an interdisciplinary knowledge base that reflects healthcare practices within various cultural groups, along with human communication strategies that transcend interdisciplinary boundaries to provide a foundation for education, research, and action.
5. The AAN, through its expert panels and commissions, must identify, describe, and examine methods, theories, and frameworks appropriate for utilization in the development of knowledge related to health care of minority, stigmatized, and vulnerable populations.
6. The AAN shall seek resources to develop and sponsor studies to describe and identify principles used by organization magnets that provide an environment that enhances knowledge development related to cross-cultural, ethnic minority/stigmatized populations, and attract and retain minority and other vulnerable students, faculty, and clinicians.
7. The AAN, through its various structures, must identify healthcare system delivery models that are the most effective in the delivery of culturally competent care to vulnerable populations and develop mechanisms to promote the necessary changes in the United States healthcare delivery system toward the identified models.
8. The AAN must collaborate with other organizations in establishing ways to teach and guide faculty and nursing students to provide culturally competent nursing care practices to clients in diverse clinical settings in local, regional, national, and international settings.
9. The AAN must collaborate with racial/ethnic nursing organizations to develop models of recruitment, education, and retention of nurses from racial/ethnic minority groups.
10. The AAN will collaborate with other organizations in promoting the development of a document to support the regulation of content reflecting diversity in nursing curricula. In addressing regulations, specific attention needs to be given to the National Council Licensure Examinations, continuing education, and undergraduate curricula.
11. The AAN must take the lead in promulgating support of research funding for investigation with emphasis on interventions aimed at eliminating health disparities in culturally and racially diverse groups and other vulnerable

(Continues)

Box 1–1 *Continued*

populations in an effort to improve health outcomes. The AAN must take a more proactive stance to encourage policy makers to create policies that address the elimination of health disparities and ultimately improve health outcomes.

12. The AAN must encourage funding agencies' requests to solicit proposals focusing on culturally competent interventions designed to eliminate health disparities.

Source: Giger, J., Davidhizar, R. E., Purnell, L., Harden, J. T., Phillips, J., & Strickland, O. (2007). American Academy of Nursing Expert Panel Report: Developing cultural competence to eliminate health disparities in ethnic minorities and other vulnerable populations. *Journal of Transcultural Nursing, 18*(2), 95–102.

---

solution has been for large numbers of immigrant nurses to enter and work within the American healthcare system. Not only will the immigrant nurses have the challenge of adapting to our healthcare delivery system, but often their ethno-cultural background may be different than that of the dominant culture and of the patients to whom they are to deliver nursing care. Since the 1960s, the Philippines has been the number one source of foreign-trained nurses in the United States; this trend is continuing in the 21st century (Marquand, 2006). Cultural differences will not only impact the nursing care that is provided, but it also may negatively affect the ability of the immigrant nurse to assimilate effectively as an essential member of the healthcare team. The growing diversity that has been seen and that continues to widen in the U.S. population has not been seen within the population of healthcare professionals. This lack of parallel growth in diversity among healthcare professionals impacts healthcare delivery and suggests that many patients are receiving culturally discordant care. Culturally discordant care arises from unaddressed cultural differences between healthcare providers and patients. Research has shown that significant disparities exist in health status, treatment, and medical outcomes between groups of patients who differ on the basis of gender, race, or ethnicity. A provider's unconscious bias about a particular race, ethnicity, or culture, or his or her lack of effective cross-cultural communication skills, may contribute to discordant medical care and health disparities. This suggests that all healthcare providers should know how to interact effectively with and provide care for patients whose ethnic or cultural background differs from their own, and highlights the need for this text.

The population growth in the United States between 2000 and 2012 was almost entirely minority driven with more than one in three U.S. residents being a member of a minority group (U.S. Census Bureau, 2012). According to the most recent census, our country continues toward diversity, as demonstrated by significant increases in the numbers and proportion of populations such as Hispanics, Asians, and Pacific Islanders (U.S. Census Bureau, 2012). Data from the 2010 census released in 2011 reveals the Caucasian population (White or European American) of the United States is 223.5 million (72.4% of total population), 38.0 million Blacks (12.6% of total population), 14.6 million Asians (4.8%), and 50.5 million Latinos (16.4% of total population) (U.S. Census Bureau, 2010).

BICULTURAL/MULTICULTURAL

Another important consideration is that in contemporary U.S. society many individuals are bicultural (McGrath, 1998). Membership in more than one culture, being bicultural, is not the same as being biracial or multiracial. A bicultural person identifies with core elements of their culture of origin as well as those of the dominant culture. They self-identify with more than one cultural group, and the bicultural person sees both sides and can function in both worlds. The degree of biculturalism and acculturation that has occurred can influence intergenerational differences in health beliefs and behaviors for certain U.S. ethnic groups (English & Le, 1999). Bicultural individuals successfully integrate into and participate in important aspects of the values and belief systems of both cultures.

In today's increasingly diverse and mobile world, growing numbers of individuals have internalized more than one culture and can be described as bicultural or multicultural. In fact, 12.5% of U.S. residents are immigrants and have presumably internalized more than one culture (Battalova & Terrazas, 2010). We must also consider that U.S. born ethnic and cultural minorities (descendants of immigrants) identify with their ethnic culture and the mainstream culture of the United States. It is a process for the bicultural or multicultural person to navigate between these different cultural identities.

Biculturalism can be associated with feelings of pride, uniqueness, and a rich sense of community and history, while also bringing to mind identity confusion, dual expectations, and value clashes (Benet-Martínez & Haritatos, 2005).

ACCULTURATION

Acculturating immigrants and ethnic minorities have to deal with two central issues. The first issue is the extent to which they are motivated or permitted to retain their identification with their culture of origin (their ethnic culture), and the second is the extent to which they are motivated or are permitted to identify with the dominant mainstream American culture. The dominant mainstream American culture is usually defined as having a Northern European cultural tradition while utilizing the English language. As the immigrant wrestles and negotiates with this, he or she can end up in one of four identified acculturation positions. According to Berry (1990), the four distinct acculturation positions are assimilation (identification mostly with the dominant culture), integration (high identification with both cultures), separation (identification largely with the ethnic culture), or marginalization (low identification with both cultures). Acculturation is not a linear process—one does not move forward in a direct line from one position to the next. This is why individuals can simultaneously hold two or even more cultural orientations. People who are bicultural can move easily between their two cultural identities by engaging in cultural frame switching (Hong, Morris, Chiu, & Benet-Martínez, 2000). Cultural frame switching occurs in response to cultural cues. The important point is the individual response. There will be individual variation in the way the bicultural identity is negotiated and organized. Some bicultural individuals will find both cultural identities are compatible, integrated, and easy to negotiate. Others may struggle if they find the two cultures are oppositional or difficult to integrate or negotiate. Various terms for the acculturation process of biculturals have been developed by different theorists. Some examples of these terms are "fusion" (Chuang, 1999), "blendedness" (Padilla, 1994), and "alternating biculturalism" (Phinney & Devich-Navarro, 1997).

OTHER AREAS OF DIVERSITY

Although racial diversity is becoming more known, it is not the only potential area of diversity encountered by healthcare providers. Diversity can be categorized as dimensions of human diversity, dimensions of cultural diversity, or systems diversity dimensions. Examples of human diversity are race, gender, physical ability, marital status, family status, ethnicity, and age. A person's dimensions of cultural diversity are characterized by their beliefs, attitudes, values, personal characteristics, lifestyle, communication, and religion. There are also systems diversity dimensions, such as teamwork, empowerment, education, and strategic alliances (Guillory, 2001).

Healthcare providers increasingly have to care for and communicate with patients of varying backgrounds, preferences, and cultures. Diversity may even have an impact on treatment response. Some researchers suggest that there may be subtle differences in the way that members of different racial and ethnic groups respond to treatment, particularly with regard to some pharmaceutical interventions, suggesting that variations in some forms of treatment may be justified on the basis of patient race or ethnicity. Diversity may also impact rejection of treatment recommendations by patients. As an example, it was cited in the Institute of Medicine report (IOM, 2003) that a number of studies concluded that Black Americans are slightly more likely to reject medical recommendations for some treatments, but these differences in refusal rates are generally small (Black Americans are only 3 to 6% more likely to reject recommended treatments, according to these studies). The IOM report recommends that more research is needed to fully understand the reasons for the refusal of treatment, as this may lead to the development of different strategies to help patients make informed treatment decisions. The IOM report hypothesizes that stereotypes, bias, and clinical uncertainty may influence clinicians' diagnostic and treatment decisions; education may be one of the most important tools as part of an overall strategy to eliminate healthcare disparities. Clearly, there is much to consider, and we have much more that we need to learn.

OVERVIEW OF CONCEPTUAL MODELS FOR CULTURAL DIVERSITY

For more than five decades, nurses have recognized cultural diversity as an important variable and have attempted to provide culturally specific and appropriate care to a population that is continuing to become even more racially and ethnically diverse. This desire to provide appropriate care was based on the knowledge that people belonging to different cultures have different kinds of demands and needs in terms of health and illness. People having different cultural values should be respected, and the health care offered and provided should be inclusive of the patient's cultural values whenever possible. Transcultural nursing models provide the nurse with the foundation to become knowledgeable about the various cultures seen in their practice setting. Nurse scholars continue to develop and refine a vast number of cultural theories, models, and assessment guides that are used internationally. Dr. Madeline Leininger has provided the basic foundation for cultural competency in nursing practice. Today, arguably the most well-known and commonly used nursing cultural competency models are by Leininger (1991), Purnell (Purnell, 2013; Purnell & Paulanka, 1998) and Giger and Davidhizar (Giger, 2013; Giger et al., 2007). After the passing of Ruth

Davidhizar, Joyce Giger published the 6th edition of the textbook, *Transcultural Nursing: Assessment and Intervention* in 2013 (Giger, 2013). Each of these theories/models will be discussed in greater detail in this chapter because it is essential for the nurse to utilize the knowledge gained from these models to deliver culturally appropriate care. In today's diverse world, our nursing care must be grounded in the knowledge and science of transcultural nursing. Through these theories, nursing has made an important contribution to the provision of all health care by all types of practitioners.

Because of our global relationships and the leadership in the area of healthcare delivery in the United States, many people from other countries come to America for medical care. As a result, U.S. nurses are often called upon to assess clinically, in a short period of time, individuals who, in many cases, are very different culturally, racially, and ethnically from themselves. An area of formal study and practice developed in response to this fact; the knowledge and understanding of different cultures is called transcultural nursing (Leininger, 1995). Transcultural nursing is a learned branch of nursing that focuses on the comparative study and analysis of cultures as they apply to nursing and health/illness practices, beliefs, and values. Transcultural nursing was developed in the mid-1960s by Madeline Leininger, a nurse anthropologist. In the 1960s, the field received financial support for nurses who wished to obtain doctoral degrees and become nurse anthropologists. These nursing pioneers were convinced that an understanding of cultural diversity relative to health and illness was an essential component of nursing knowledge. The essential foundation of transcultural nursing is that cultures exhibit both diversity and universality.

The first course in transcultural nursing was offered by Dr. Leininger in 1966 at the University of Colorado (one year after she earned her PhD in anthropology from the University of Seattle). Dr. Leininger stated that transcultural nursing developed in response to nurses having increased exposure to diverse groups of patients. This increase was because of the changing demographics in the United States as well as the leadership of the United States in healthcare delivery, resulting in many people from other countries coming to America for medical care. Dr. Leininger and other transcultural nursing scholars refer to care as a universal phenomenon that transcends cultural boundaries. Because we provide direct patient care, it is critical for nurses to understand how to work effectively within a diverse cultural atmosphere.

Transcultural nursing, as defined by Leininger (1984), is a humanistic and scientific area of formal study and practice in nursing that is focused on the comparative study of cultures. Focusing on differences and similarities in care, health, and illness patterns based on cultural values, beliefs, and practices of different cultures in the world, transcultural nursing uses knowledge to provide culturally specific and universal nursing care to people. The goal of transcultural nursing is to provide care that is congruent with cultural values, beliefs, and practices— culturally specific care (Leininger, 1984). Today, transcultural nursing concepts are found in the curricula for nursing programs in the United States and Canada. This theory has provided the basic foundation for transcultural nursing practice.

The Transcultural Nursing Society was founded in 1974. It publishes a monthly journal (*The Journal of Transcultural Nursing*) and provides a certification process for transcultural nursing for nurses in the United States and Canada.

Although the importance of the work done by Dr. Leininger cannot be denied, there have been some problems identified in her transcultural nursing framework by nurse scholars. The major flaw, according to Tripp-Reimer and Fox (1990), is that it was based on the anthropological theory of functionalism. Dr. Leininger did, after all, receive her doctorate in anthropology. Functionalism in anthropology stresses understanding culture by emphasizing specific customs, folkways, and patterns such as diet preferences, religious practices, communication styles, and health beliefs and practices (Tripp-Reimer & Fox, 1990). Critics (Brink, 1990; Browning & Woods, 1993; Sprott, 1993; Tripp-Reimer & Fox, 1990) feel that this "narrow view" of people results in stereotyping. This is by no means a small concern. The fear of stereotyping is often cited as the major criticism of the cultural competency movement. It is important that this process of identifying the characteristics that may be associated with certain cultural groups be done with an extremely open mind, and for the nurse to realize that, just like in anything, exceptions can be found. It is important that we do not proceed with blinders on as the nurse must continually assess for affirmation or for exceptions.

Although the concern about stereotyping is an important one, there are other nurse scholars who argue that a reliance on generalizations about race, ethnicity, and culture are necessary to expand a nurse's knowledge about a particular patient population (Giger, 2013; McGoldrick, 1993; Valente, 1989). Looking at the situation from both sides, it is clear that it is important for the nurse to be cautious and to use these generalizations as a flexible guide that permits individualization of patient care at all times. We must strive to avoid stereotyping and oversimplification of the impact of culture (Betancourt, 2003) and the nurse must attempt to possess cultural humility, openness, and inquisitiveness toward each individual patient (Tervalon & Murray-Garcia, 1998).

In the 21st century, with the emergence of evidence-based medicine (EBM), a new challenge of integration with cultural competence has risen. There is some concern in the literature that cultural competence and evidence-based medicine can be contradictory goals. This is because the overriding goal of EBM is to provide quality health care through standardization of care, not individualized care. The overriding goal of cultural competence is the delivery of individualized health care that acknowledges and understands cultural diversity, with respect for individual health beliefs, values, and behaviors. Combining these approaches can result in optimal patient-centered care. Future research needs to focus on determining the best way to integrate EBM and cultural competence to ensure demonstrably improved patient outcomes. Nurses need to assess for a patient's explanatory model of the patient's health status (how they understand their illness) to avoid stereotyping and oversimplification of the impact of culture.

All of nursing's largest professional organizations—the ANA in 1991, the National League for Nursing in 1993, and the American Association of Colleges of Nursing in 1998—have cited the need for nurses to practice cultural competence.

The ANA established the American Academy of Nursing in 1973. Its purpose is to advance health policy and practice and it is often referred to as the think tank of nursing. The AAN has a number of expert panels including the Expert Panel on Cultural Competence. From 1991 to 1992, the Expert Panel on Cultural Competence proposed 10 recommendations in an attempt to address health disparities. This panel developed its most recent position paper in 2007 to help serve as a catalyst for substantive nursing action to promote outcomes that reduce or eliminate health disparities commonly found among racial, ethnic, uninsured, underserved, and underrepresented populations residing throughout the United States (Giger et al., 2007). Membership on any of the expert panels within the AAN are by invitation only to fellows of the AAN. Fellowship in the AAN is considered one of the highest honors a nurse can achieve. The members consist of major nursing theorists and scholars.

The Expert Panel on Cultural Competence developed a comprehensive list of 12 recommendations (Box 1–1) that can serve as a starting point for all health professionals who seek to address the problem of health disparities in the United States through cultural competency with the hope that measurable outcomes be achieved to reduce or eliminate health disparities commonly found among the minority and vulnerable populations in the United States (Giger et al., 2007).

Based on the work of the Expert Panel on Cultural Competence, a set of universally applicable standards of practice for culturally competent care were developed that nurses can use when providing care. The 12 standards were developed based on the social justice framework, which is the belief that each and every person is entitled to fair and equal rights and participation in healthcare opportunities (Douglas et al., 2009). The standards (**Box 1–2**) were collaboratively developed

---

Box 1–2   Standards of Practice for Culturally Competent Nursing Care

Standard	Description
1. Social Justice	Professional nurses shall promote social justice for all. The applied principles of social justice guide nurses' decisions related to the patient, family, community, and other healthcare professionals. Nurses will develop leadership skills to advocate for socially just policies.
2. Critical Reflection	Nurses shall engage in critical reflection of their own values, beliefs, and cultural heritage in order to have an awareness of how these qualities and issues can impact culturally congruent nursing care.
3. Transcultural Nursing Knowledge	Nurses shall gain an understanding of the perspectives, traditions, values, practices, and family systems of the culturally diverse individuals, families, communities and populations they care for, as well as a knowledge of the complex variables that affect the achievement of health and well-being.
4. Cross-Cultural Practice	Nurses shall utilize cross-cultural knowledge and culturally sensitive skills in implementing culturally congruent nursing care.
5. Healthcare Systems and Organizations	Healthcare organizations should provide the structure and resources necessary to evaluate and meet the cultural and language needs of their diverse clients.
6. Patient Advocacy and Empowerment	Nurses shall recognize the effect of healthcare policies, delivery systems, and resources on their patient populations, and shall empower and advocate for their patients as indicated. Nurses shall advocate for the inclusion of their patient's cultural beliefs and practices in all dimensions of their health care.
7. Multicultural Workforce	Nurses shall be activists in the global effort to ensure a more multicultural workforce in healthcare settings.
8. Education and Training	Nurses shall be educationally prepared to promote and provide culturally congruent health care. Knowledge and skills necessary for ensuring that nursing care is culturally congruent shall be included in global heathcare agendas that mandate formal education and clinical training, and ongoing, continuing education for all practicing nurses will be required.

(Continues)

Box 1–2 *Continued*

9. Cross-Cultural Communication	Nurses shall use effective, culturally competent communication with clients that takes into consideration the client's verbal and nonverbal language, cultural values and context, and unique healthcare needs and perceptions.
10. Cross-Cultural Leadership	Nurses shall have the ability to influence individuals, groups and systems to achieve outcomes of culturally competent care for diverse populations.
11. Policy Development	Nurses shall have the knowledge and skills to work with public and private organizations, professional associations, and communities to establish policies and standards for comprehensive implementation and evaluation of culturally competent care.
12. Evidence-Based Practice and Research	Nurses shall base their practice on interventions that have been systematically tested and shown to be the most effective for the culturally diverse populations that they serve. In areas where there is a lack of evidence of efficacy, nurse researchers shall investigate and test interventions that may be the most effective in reducing the racial and ethnic inequalities in health outcomes.

Adapted from: Douglas, M. K., Pierce, J. U., Rosenkoetter, M., Callister, L. C., Hattar-Pollara, M., Lauderdale, J., . . . Pacquiao, D. (2009). Standards of practice for culturally competent nursing care: A request for comments. *Journal of Transcultural Nursing, 20*(3), 257–269.

by Douglas et al. (2009), with participation from members of the Expert Panel on Cultural Competence, among others.

Nurses are ideally suited to strive toward cultural competence. When nurses consider the race, ethnicity, culture, and cultural heritage of their patients, they become more sensitive to each patient's individual needs. This is by no means an easy feat, as evidenced by the vast number of cultures and subcultures that exist on our planet (estimated to be more than 2,500 by Leininger), but a highly complex issue that requires a lifelong commitment (McGee, 2001).

It is important to learn from our mistakes, as each cultural gaffe provides the opportunity to learn, improve, and grow professionally. We must also realize that the practice of nursing should never be done by using a "cookbook approach." There is as much variation within certain races, cultures, or ethnic groups as there is across cultural groups. The informed nurse is being asked to consider the significance of culture to ensure that patients are then approached and cared for from a more informed perspective—this is the crux of transcultural nursing care delivery.

NONNURSING MODELS FOR CULTURAL ASSESSMENT

There are both nonnursing and nursing models for cultural assessment from which to choose. Arguably, the two most well-known nonnursing models are the *Outline of Cultural Materials* by Murdock (1971) and Brownlee's (1978) *Community, Culture and Care: A Cross-Cultural Guide for Health Workers*. The Murdock tool was designed for use by anthropologists and as such does not utilize the nursing process. The Brownlee tool is considered difficult by some and also is not a nursing tool. This lack of nursing focus has been a driving point behind the development of nursing-specific cultural assessment models.

SELECTED NURSING MODELS FOR CULTURAL ASSESSMENT

Culture Care, Diversity, and Universality: A Theory of Nursing

The first nursing cultural assessment model was developed by Dr. Madeline Leininger. She developed her theory—Culture Care, Diversity, and Universality—from both anthropology and nursing principles. She first published her theory in *Nursing Science Quarterly* in 1985. In 1988, the theory was further described in the same journal, and in 1991, she published her textbook, *Culture Care Diversity and Universality: A Theory of Nursing*. The theory states that nurses must take into account the cultural beliefs, caring behaviors, and values of individuals, families, and groups to provide effective, satisfying, and culturally congruent nursing care (Leininger, 1991). The central purpose of the theory is to discover and explain diverse and universal culturally based care factors influencing the health, well-being, illness, or death of individuals or groups. The goal is to identify ways to provide culturally congruent nursing care to people of diverse or similar cultures (Leininger, 2002). The foundation of the theory is that cultures exhibit both diversity and universality. Leininger (1985) defined diversity as perceiving, knowing, and practicing care in different ways, and defined universality as commonalities of care.

To fully understand any nursing theory or nursing care model, one must understand the operational definitions for key terms. Traditionally nursing has four metaparadigms: the concepts of person, environment, health, and nursing. Leininger feels that the paradigm of nursing is too limited in its definition, so that construct was replaced by caring. Caring, according to Leininger, has a better ability to explain nursing. She feels that the concept of *person* is too limiting and culture-bound to explain nursing, because the concept of *person* does not exist in every culture. The term *person* is often used globally to refer to families, groups, and communities. Leininger also views the paradigm of health as belonging to many other healthcare disciplines and as such it is not unique to nursing. The fourth paradigm is environment, which Leininger has replaced with environmental context. Environmental context includes events with meanings and interpretations given to them in particular physical, ecological, sociopolitical, and/or cultural settings (Leininger, 1995).

Leininger (1985) defines culture as a group's values, beliefs, norms, and life practices that are learned, shared, and handed down. Culture guides thinking, decision making, and our actions in specific ways. Culture is the framework people use to solve human problems. In that sense, culture is universal yet also diverse. Cultural values are usually long-term and are very stable. Caring is defined by Leininger (1985) as assisting, supporting, or enabling behaviors that ease or improve a patient's condition. Leininger (1985) states that the essence of nursing is caring; caring is unique to nursing. It is essential to life, survival, and human development. It is through caring that people can deal with life's events. Caring is the verb counterpart to the noun *care* and is a feeling of compassion, interest, and concern for people. Caring has different meanings in different cultures. Individual cultural definitions of caring can be discovered by examining the cultural group's view of the world, social structure, and language (Leininger, 1985). Culture care refers to the values and beliefs that assist, support, or enable another person or group to maintain well-being, improve personal condition, or face death or disability. Culture care, according to Leininger (1985), is universal, but the actions, expressions, patterns, lifestyles, and meanings of care may be different. A nurse cannot provide appropriate cultural care without having a knowledge and understanding of cultural diversity. Worldview is defined as the outlook a group or person has, based on their view of the world or universe. Worldview consists of both a social structure and environmental context. The social structure provides organization to a culture, and it can come from religion, education, or economics. The environmental context is any event or situation that gives meaning to human expressions. Folk health, or well-being systems, are care practices that have a special meaning within the culture. These practices are used to heal or assist people in their homes or within the community at large. Folk or well-being systems have the potential to supplement traditional healthcare delivery systems. Person is defined as a human being that is capable of being concerned about others. A key construct of all nursing theory is environment. Leininger did not specifically define environment in her theory other than providing an operational definition for environmental context. Health is viewed as a state of well-being. Most importantly though, health is culturally defined, valued, and practiced. Health is viewed as a universal concept across all cultures, but is defined differently by each to reflect its specific values and beliefs. Nursing is defined as a learned humanistic art and science that focuses on personalized behaviors, functions, and processes to promote and maintain health or recovery from illness. According to Leininger (1985), nursing uses three modes of action to deliver care: culture care preservation or maintenance, culture care accommodation or negotiation, and culture care restructuring or repatterning.

Leininger's Sunrise Model (1991) illustrates the major components and interrelationships of the culture care, diversity, and universality. Nurses can use the Sunrise Model when caring for patients to ensure that nursing actions are culture specific. It requires that the nurse understand the values, beliefs, and practices of the patient's culture. The Sunrise Model symbolizes the rising of the sun (the sun represents care). The model depicts a full sun with four foci. Within the circle in the upper portion of the model are components of the social structure and worldview factors that influence care and health.

When applying Leininger's model, it is important for the nurse to consider if there is a cultural mismatch present. A cultural mismatch is what occurs when people violate each other's cultural expectations. The healthcare provider needs to develop awareness into his or her personal style of interaction, because he or she may have a personal style of interaction that does not match the patient's. An example of a cultural mismatch would be the healthcare provider, attempting to keep to a tight schedule, interrupting the prayer session of a devoutly Muslim patient (Leininger, 1995). This interruption would definitely result in a cultural mismatch, but it could also result in causing cultural pain to the Muslim patient, which is a much more serious situation. Leininger (1997) states cultural pain occurs when hurtful, offensive, or inappropriate words are spoken to an individual or group. These spoken words are experienced by the receiver as being insulting, discomforting, or stressful. Cultural pain occurs because of a lack of awareness, sensitivity, and understanding by the offender of differences in the cultural values, beliefs, and meanings of the offended persons. When these types of events occur during a patient–provider encounter, they can result in significant consequences. It is essential that if a cultural mismatch or the infliction of cultural pain does occur, it be recognized, or we risk the development of consequences, one of which would be the inability to establish a therapeutic alliance with the patient. If a cultural mismatch or mistake is made, it is best for the healthcare provider to attempt to recover quickly from the mistake and to avoid becoming defensive. If the provider suspects that the mismatch has been serious enough to have caused cultural pain (as evidenced by seeing a sudden negative change in attitude), the health professional must act on this feeling and ask if they did or said anything offensive. Cultural pain occurs if the clinician inadvertently ignores an important cultural obligation or violates a cultural taboo. Making this type of adjustment requires cultural flexibility—this is only possible in those healthcare providers who have taken the time to develop self-awareness and who have examined their own cultural background and biases.

Leininger (2002) identified eight unique features of her model. The eight features include (1) the fact that it is one of the oldest nursing theories (1950s), (2) its focus is on the interrelationships of culture on health and illness, (3) its focus on comparative cultures, (4) it is holistic and multidimensional, (5) it was designed to discover global diversities (both differences and similarities), (6) it has its own associated research method (ethnonursing), (7) it consists of both abstract and practical modes for delivering culturally congruent care, and (8) it has a focus on ethnohistory for use in diverse environmental contexts (Leininger, 2002).

Leininger (2002) advocates the concurrent use of her theory and the Sunrise Model in order to discover factors that may impact the patient's response, such as cultural stresses and pain, and to reduce the incidence of anger and noncompliance.

The importance of Leininger's theory and Sunrise Model is substantial and invaluable as it has served as the prototype for the development of other culturally specific nursing models and tools.

Giger and Davidhizar's Transcultural Assessment Model

Giger and Davidhizar's model provides a framework for assessment that focuses on the six cultural phenomena that they believe shape care: communication, space, social organization, time, environmental control, and biologic variations (Giger, 2013). They also systematically explore the variations that exist in caregivers' responses and recipients' perspectives relative to the cultural diversity that is present in the United States. The model serves as a resource for healthcare professionals when they are called upon to provide culturally discordant care. The authors advocate that the model can and should be used in a variety of clinical settings (primary, secondary and tertiary) (Giger, 2013). The model was first developed in 1988 to help undergraduate nursing students assess and provide care for patients that were culturally diverse. Giger and Davidhizar state that although all cultures are not the same, they share the same basic organizational factors (Giger, 2013). In its present form, the model provides a framework to systematically assess the role of culture on health and illness and has been used extensively in a variety of settings and by diverse disciplines. In 1993, Spector combined this model with the Cultural Heritage Model, which appears in *Potter and Perry Fundamentals of Nursing*. Spector (1993) used the model's six phenomena, but placed them in a different hierarchical arrangement and then used this hierarchy as a guide for cultural assessment of people from a variety of racial and cultural groups. The model has been utilized in other healthcare disciplines such as medical imaging, dentistry, education, and administration. The model has also been the theoretical framework for dissertations and other research studies.

Giger (2013) provides the following definition of culture:

> Culture is a patterned behavioral response that develops over time as a result of imprinting the mind through social and religious structures and intellectual and artistic manifestations. Culture is also the result of acquired mechanisms that may have innate influences but are primarily affected by internal and external environmental stimuli. Culture is shaped by values, beliefs, norms and practices that are shared by members of the same ethnic group. Culture guides our thinking, doing and being and becomes patterned expressions of who we are. These patterned expressions are passed down from one generation to the next.... [Cultural values are] unique expressions of a particular culture that have been accepted as appropriate over time. (p. 2)

The model postulates that every individual is culturally unique and requires culturally competent care. Culturally competent care is defined by Giger (2013) as

> A dynamic, fluid, continuous process whereby an individual, system, or healthcare agency finds meaningful and useful care delivery strategies based on knowledge of the cultural heritage, beliefs, attitudes, and behaviors of those to whom they render care. Cultural competence connotes a higher, more sophisticated level of refinement of cognitive skills and psychomotor skills, attitudes, and personal beliefs. To develop cultural competency, it is essential for the healthcare professional to use knowledge gained from conceptual and theoretical models of culturally appropriate care. Attainment of cultural competence can assist the astute nurse in devising meaningful interventions to promote optimal health among individuals regardless of race, ethnicity, gender identity, sexual identity, or cultural heritage. (p. 8)

Patients should be assessed according to the six cultural phenomena. It is important to emphasize that the model does not presuppose that every person within an ethnic or cultural group will act or behave in a similar manner. In fact, Giger (2013) informs us that a culturally appropriate model must recognize differences in groups while also avoiding stereotypical approaches to client care. In addition, the six cultural phenomena described are not mutually exclusive but are related and often interacting. Whereas the phenomena vary with application across cultural groups, the six concepts of the model are evident in every cultural group. The six cultural phenomena will be discussed individually.

The Phenomena

Communication

The first phenomenon is communication. Communication embraces the entire world of human interaction and behavior and it is how we relate or connect to others. Communication is the way by which culture is transmitted and preserved. It is a continuous and complex process as it can be transmitted through written or oral language and nonverbal behaviors, such as gestures, facial expressions, body language, or the use of space. While the factors that influence communication are universal, they vary among culture-specific groups in terms of language spoken, voice quality, pronunciation, use of silence, and use of nonverbal communication (Giger, 2013). Effective communication is essential for effective healthcare delivery because it motivates both the patient and the nurse to work together to manage the patient's health because the patient is better informed and empowered to participate more fully. Motivating our patients to take action on behalf of their own health is one of the tenets of Healthy People 2020.

Communication can present a barrier between the nurse and the patient, as well as the patient's family, especially when the nurse and the patient are from different cultural backgrounds. This feeling of alienation or powerlessness can occur if the language spoken is the same or if it is different. Impaired communication can result in a poor outcome. There are many different types of communication differences that the nurse may experience. Even when the language is shared between patient and nurse, misunderstandings can occur because of cultural orientation. Even though people may speak the same language, word meanings may differ between the sender and the receiver. This is because vocabulary words have both a connotative and denotative meaning. A denotative meaning is the meaning that is used by most people who share that common language, but the connotative meaning comes from the person's personal experience. Differences in the meaning of words can cause numerous conflicts among various cultural groups. Overcoming language differences is probably the most difficult hurdle when attempting to provide cross-cultural health care. Clear and effective communication is essential. Nurses often become frustrated and find it difficult when faced with a language difference between patient and nurse. All parts of the nursing process are impacted negatively when we are unable to speak with our patients. When verbal communication is not possible, then we must rely instead on interpretation of the patient's nonverbal language. When patients are unable to communicate with us, they may withdraw or become hostile or uncooperative.

Both verbal and nonverbal communication is learned within one's culture. Communication and culture are intertwined. Our culture determines how our feelings are expressed and what is and is not appropriate. It is felt that cultural patterns of communication are firmly a part of us as early as age 5. Communication is essential to human interaction—it discloses information or provides a message. Through communication, we become aware of how another is feeling. Often, communication issues cause the most significant problems when working with people from a different culture. One of the most common barriers to communication is overcoming ethnocentrism (viewing one's culture as superior to another), particularly when assessing patients. An example of how to ensure that a patient's communication needs for patient education are met would be to provide oral instructions if the patient feels less comfortable with written materials. In contrast, when educating the Asian population, it is helpful to know that the majority of Asians prefer written materials over oral instructions.

Language differences need to be overcome with the use of competent interpreters. When caring for a patient who does not speak the dominant language, an interpreter is a must. In 1998, the National Council on Interpreting in Health Care was founded with the goal of promoting culturally competent healthcare interpretation. The Office of Minority Health recommends against the use of a patient's friends or family members as interpreters. One reason for this is that the patient may not be comfortable disclosing certain symptoms or behaviors to their friends or family. Other important considerations for the effective use of interpreters will appear later in the text.

Differences between patient and provider influence communication and clinical decision making. There is strong evidence that provider–patient communication is directly linked to patient satisfaction. When these differences are not acknowledged or explored, they result in poor patient satisfaction, poor adherence, and most alarmingly, a poor outcome (Betancourt, Green, Carrillo, &

Ananeh-Firempong, 2003). Failure to recognize the uniqueness of all of our patients can result in stereotyping and biased and discriminatory treatment.

Space

The second of the six phenomena is space. Space refers to the distance between people when they interact. Personal space is the area that surrounds the body. All communication occurs within the context of space. Rules concerning personal distance vary from culture to culture; therefore, views of appropriate spatial distance will vary between persons of different cultures. Discomfort occurs when one feels their personal space has been violated (Giger, 2013). Personal space is perceived through our biological senses, and the degree of comfort one feels in proximity to others, in body movement and perception of personal, intimate, and public space, is culturally based (Giger, 2013). European North Americans are aware of zones associated with personal space: the intimate zone, personal distance, social distance, and public distance. Other cultures may not be aware of these distinctions. Humans are similar to felines in that we wish to establish territoriality and we become uncomfortable when our territory is encroached upon. How large our territorial space is depends on individual and cultural preferences. Encroachment into one's intimate zone by another can cause many different types of reactions. One possible outcome is embarrassment and modesty. Modesty may pose a significant barrier that may be difficult to overcome when it is time to examine the patient.

Giger and Davidhizar identified four aspects of behavior patterns related to space that must be assessed to promote a healthy interaction: (1) proximity to others, (2) attachment with objects in the environment, (3) body posture, and (4) movement in the setting (Giger, 2013). These four concepts are particularly important during periods when family members are experiencing emotional chaos, such as during the grieving process. Although the desired degree of physical proximity between the client and provider is based on the degree of intimacy and the trust that has been mutually established, as a general rule, Hispanics and Asians tend to stand closer to each other than do Euro-Americans.

Social Organization

The third phenomenon is social organization. Cultural behavior, or how one acts in certain situations, is socially acquired, not genetically inherited. Patterns of cultural behavior are learned through a process called enculturation (also referred to as socialization), which involves acquiring knowledge and internalizing values (Giger, 2013). Most people achieve competence in their own culture through enculturation/socialization. Social organization refers to the manner in which a cultural group organizes itself around the family group. Family structure and organization, religious values and beliefs, and role assignments all relate to ethnicity and culture. Where we grow up and choose to live in adulthood plays an essential role in our socialization process. There is a strong need among many cultural groups to maintain social congruency. This need can negatively impact health care. Access to healthcare providers does not necessarily translate into positive lifestyle behaviors or risk-reduction activities as prescribed by the dominant society. People from some cultures may verbally agree with a treatment plan out of respect to the provider but then defer to folk remedies or alternative health practices upon discharge. Social organization consists of the family unit and the social organizations in which one may have membership. Social organizations are structured in a variety of groups, including family, religious, ethnic, racial, and special interest groupings. Membership in groups, except for ethnic or racial groups, is voluntary. Social barriers also exist and can impact access to health care as was pointed out in the IOM (2003) report. These social barriers include unemployment, socioeconomic status, and lack of health insurance.

Time

The fourth phenomenon of the Giger and Davidhizar model is time (Giger, 2013). Time has two meanings. The first is duration (interval of time) and the second is specified instances or points in time (Giger, 2013). Due to these two distinct meanings, time is very culture-bound, as it is perceived, measured, and valued differently across cultures (Giger, 2013). In essence, time is conceptualized in reference to our chronologic age, its perception in relation to events, and as an external entity that is outside of our control (Giger, 2013).

While it may not be readily apparent on the surface, time is an important aspect of interpersonal communication. The concept of time is not only based on clock hours and social influences (e.g., meals and holidays) but is culturally perceived. Clock time is frequently more highly valued by the majority of Western cultures, where appointments tend to be kept at the prescribed time. In a culture in which places and persons are more important than social time, activities start when a previous social event has been completed, and to be dominated by adherence to clock time is often considered rude. Persons in different cultures may have a time orientation that focuses on either the past, present, or future. This can impact tremendously on preventative health care because a patient must have at least a small degree of future time orientation to be motivated by a future-situated reward (improved health down the road, or a longer life). People who are future oriented are more likely to embrace preventive health measures as they are concerned about the onset of illness in the future. People who are present oriented are often late for medical appointments or may skip them entirely. Recognizing the patient's time orientation has value for the nurse. Considering the time orientation can provide a bridge to increase compliance with a medication regimen or with recommended health screenings.

Environmental Control

The fifth phenomenon is the environment and locus of control and refers to the ability of the person to control nature and to plan and direct factors in the environment that may affect them. Many Americans believe they have internal control over nature, which impacts the decision to seek out health care. If the patient comes from a culture in which there is less belief in internal control and more in external control, there may be a fatalistic view in which seeking health care is viewed as useless. Human attempts to control nature and the environment are as old as recorded history. At its most basic level, locus of control is a significant variable in how people react within the American healthcare system. In general, the willingness to accept responsibility for one's health is considered an internal locus of control. Persons who have an external locus of control believe the healthcare delivery system exists to provide essential care and can become especially frustrated with the complexities of health care in America and the myriad of options available.

The environment also encompasses a person's health and illness beliefs and whether they expand health delivery from that provided only from Western medicine with those of complementary or alternative practitioners. Understanding the patient's perspective on alternative therapies is essential when developing an optimal plan of care for our patients.

Biological Variations

The last of the six phenomena is biologic variations (Giger, 2013). Biologic differences, especially genetic variations, exist between individuals in different ethnic groups. Although there is as much difference within cultural and ethnic groups as there is across and among cultural and racial groups, knowledge of general baseline data relative to the specific cultural group is an excellent starting point to provide culturally appropriate care. This is also an important area when it comes to racial differences in how pharmaceuticals are metabolized and utilized (ethnopharmacology).

Ethnopharmacologic research has revealed that ethnicity significantly affects drug response. Genetic or cultural factors, or both, may influence a given drug's pharmacokinetics (its absorption, metabolism, distribution, and elimination) and pharmacodynamics (its mechanism of action and effects at the target site), as well as patient adherence and education. In addition, the tremendous variation within each of the broader racial and ethnic categories defined by the U.S. Census Bureau (categories often used by researchers) must be considered. For example, some researchers use the terms *race, ethnicity*, and *culture* synonymously, even though they each have distinct and unique definitions. Improper labeling can result in inaccuracies with data collection and the nurse should consider that when critically evaluating ethnopharmacologic research findings. In addition, most clinical drug trials are conducted on adult White males, with the results then generalized to all patients who might be prescribed and administered the drugs. Despite the growing evidence that ethnicity influences drug response, many nurses and healthcare providers still remain largely unaware of this. Research has shown that genetic variations in certain enzymes may cause differing drug responses (although the precise mechanisms are unknown); also, certain ethnic groups have more of these variations than others do. Individual factors, such as diet and alcohol and tobacco usage, can also influence gene expression, and therefore drug metabolism (Muñoz & Hilgenberg, 2005).

Nurses need to become knowledgeable about drugs that are likely to elicit varied responses in people with different ethnic backgrounds, as well as the potential for adverse effects. The existing ethnopharmacologic research focuses primarily on psychotropic and antihypertensive agents (Muñoz & Hilgenberg, 2005). The nurse should utilize caution and consider the possibility of biologic variations when administering antihypertensives and/or psychotropic drugs to culturally diverse patients. Some patients will have a therapeutic response at a lower dose than those typically recommended for a particular agent. The nurse must carefully monitor the patient to help prevent unnecessary increases in dosage, which will increase the likelihood of adverse events.

The nurse must also be on guard in the event a therapeutic substitution is required. Sometimes this is done to contain costs or because a drug is not on an institution's formulary. Drugs may vary in how they are metabolized, and substitution may be more clinically risky for patients from non-White racial and ethnic groups. While individual differences exist and should be considered, the nurse would be wise to be extra vigilant when drug substitutions occur in their non-White patients.

Healthcare providers must understand the biologic differences and suscepti-bility that exist in persons from different cultures. For example, Black Americans have a higher prevalence of cardiovascular disease, cancer, and diabetes than oth-ers. Cultural differences can also contribute to either noncompliance or poor compliance with therapy. Unfortunately, in many cases, lack of knowledge limits the ability of healthcare professionals to differentiate environmental, familial, and genetic predisposition to disease states. Although research is being conducted on biologic differences relating to ethnic groups, it lags behind the knowledge avail-able regarding other cultural phenomena. An important example of this is that the development of pain measurement instruments remains culturally centered, even though significant differences exist among members of different cultural groups in their perception and response to pain management.

There are several ways that people from one cultural group differ biologically from members of other cultural groups. These differences are called biologic vari-ants. They can include stature or size, skin color, genetic differences, disease sus-ceptibility, and nutritional variants. Asians traditionally are smaller in stature than other racial or ethnic groups. Skin color differences among races also impacts hair and nail texture. Genetic differences can result in enzyme deficiencies such as a lack of lactase, causing lactose intolerance. Certain ethnic groups, such as Hispanics and Black Americans, have higher morbidity rates than other groups because of differences in disease susceptibility. Even the diets that are followed by our patients can be culture-bound, such as a Jewish patient's kosher diet or balancing hot and cold foods, as is common in many Hispanic homes.

Another area that is under intense study is biocultural differences. This area of study is also known as biocultural ecology, and focuses on human adaptation and homeostasis (Giger, 2013). Biocultural ecology may help to lessen the frag-mentation that has occurred in the past where culture, biology, ecology, and the environment have been looked at separately or in isolation.

Clinical Application of the Model

It is essential for all healthcare professionals to be aware that not all patients with the same medical diagnosis are likely to have the same experience. Following this model permits the patient to be an equal partner with the nurse. A cultural assess-ment can be obtained by utilizing the questions posed by Giger and Davidhizar, which will provide a better understanding of patient behaviors that might, if not understood within the context of ethnic values, be regarded as puzzling or even negative (Giger, 2013). This approach is not meant to be stereotypical. If carefully listening and observing, and questioning appropriately, the nurse should be able to discover the health traditions or beliefs that belong to that individual patient. The recognition of the importance of providing culturally appropriate clinical approaches has developed in response to the easily discernible fact that the United States is rapidly becoming a multicultural, heterogeneous, pluralistic society. As the demographics of the population of the United States continues to expand, and especially when the demographics of the healthcare professional and the patient do not match, it is essential that the healthcare professional embark on a journey to develop sensitivity and cultural competence in order to provide safe and effective care. This can be achieved by performing cultural assessment according to the guidelines established by any transcultural nursing model.

See **Box 1–3** for examples of cultural gaffes that can occur within each aspect of the Giger and Davidhizar's Transcultural Assessment Model.

Purnell Model for Cultural Competence

One of the unique components of the Purnell (Purnell & Paulanka, 1998) Model for Cultural Competence is, as a holographic theory, it has applicability and can be used by all disciplines and healthcare team members. Nurses who are members of interdisciplinary teams may wish to use this model for this reason. Not only can this model be used by all team members, but it is also unique in that it includes the recognition of biocultural ecology and workforce issues and the impact of this on the culturally diverse patient. Often, team members can be from various cultures and this model can be helpful when trying to forge a greater understanding of what is similar and different among the various cultures that make up the healthcare team. Purnell (2013) identifies many benefits to the use of his model. First, the model provides a framework for all healthcare providers to utilize when learning about the inherent concepts and characteristics of new cultures.

The Purnell Model for Cultural Competence consists of a circle. The outermost rim represents the global society, the second rim represents community, and the third rim represents the family. The innermost rim represents the person. The interior of the circle is divided into 12 pie-shaped wedges. Each wedge depicts one of the 12 cultural domains. The dark center of the circle represents all unknown phenomena. There is a jagged line at the bottom that represents the concept of cultural consciousness, which is nonlinear (Purnell, 2013).

The model provides a link between historical perspectives and their impact on one's cultural worldview. It also provides a link for the central relationships of culture so that congruence can occur and to facilitate the delivery of consciously competent care.

Box 1–3   Six Phenomena of the Giger and Davidhizar Model and Examples of Cultural Gaffes

Phenomenon	Event	Response
Time	Visiting hours are not being respected.	Explain institution's time expectations.
Space	Poor eye contact on the part of your patient.	Make sure you are aware of the customs regarding contact, such as eye contact and touch, for many different cultural groups (optimally, all that you will come in contact with in practice). Poor eye contact is a sign of respect in some cultures (Vietnamese Americans, American Indian, Appalachians); excessive eye contact may be perceived as rude by Chinese Americans.
Communication	Family member is using a lot of hand gesturing when communicating.	Gestures do not have universal meaning; what is acceptable to one group may be taboo to another.
Social Organization	Prayer sessions in a hospital room by patient and family members.	Be aware of the expected rituals and how religious services are conducted for many different groups.
Biologic Variations	Family members repeatedly bring home-prepared meals for the patient with foods that are in violation of the prescribed diet plan.	Look for foods that are not in violation of the prescribed diet and encourage the family to only bring in foods from the approved list.
Environmental Control	Family members wish to bring in a folk medicine healer as a member of the healthcare team.	Advocate for the patient for inclusion of the complementary provider as a member of the team.

Adapted from: Giger, J. N. (2013). *Transcultural nursing: Assessment and intervention* (6th ed.). Philadelphia, PA: Elsevier.

Consciously competent care is an important concept because when we are conscious of the care we provide, we ensure that it is culturally competent and we can replicate that care delivery for this patient and for other patients in the future. The model also provides a framework that allows the nurse to reflect on and consider each patient's unique human characteristics such as motivation, intentionality, and meaning when planning for and providing patient care. The model provides a structure for analyzing cultural data, and it permits the nurse to view the individual, family, or group within its own unique and ethnocultural environment. The model encourages the nurse to consider communication strategies to overcome identified barriers. Effective communication depends not only on verbal language skills that include the dominant language, dialects, and the contextual use of the language, but also other important factors such as the paralanguage variations of voice volume, tone, intonations, reflections, as well as the openness of the patient (willingness to share their thoughts and feelings). Another important component is nonverbal communication. The varied and numerous components of nonverbal communication must also be considered. For example, the nurse must know whether to engage in the use of eye contact or to avoid it, depending on the cultural norms of the patient. This consideration must also be given to the type of facial expressions to utilize, as not all facial expressions will be acceptable to all patients. If or when to touch a patient is also culturally dependent, as is our use of and interpretation of the patient's body language. Even how close we are to our patients communicates information about us. Nurses must become aware of the spatial distancing practices and acceptable greetings associated with the various cultural groups who come under their care. The nurse's worldview in terms of whether the nurse or the patient utilizes a past, present, or future orientation must be considered and planned for. Does the patient place a focus on clock time (as is the case with the Western Biomedical Model) or is the focus on social time? Even consideration must be given on how to address our patient. Miscalculating the degree of formality in the use of names can result in breaking trust or blocking the establishment of a therapeutic alliance between nurse and patient. Communication styles may vary between insiders (family and close friends) and outsiders (strangers and unknown healthcare providers). Purnell (2013) reminds us that in regard to verbal and nonverbal communication, there is indeed much to consider.

The Purnell (2013) model has an organizing framework of 12 universal domains:

- Overview, inhabited localities, and topography
- Communication
- Family roles and organization
- Workforce issues
- Biocultural ecology

- High-risk health behaviors
- Nutrition
- Pregnancy and childbearing practices
- Death rituals
- Spirituality
- Healthcare practices
- Healthcare practitioners

An important consideration for the nurse to keep in mind is the higher level of regard or esteem that nurses are given in the United States compared to what is given to nurses in other parts of the world. This higher regard may be due to the amount of educational preparation required and the need to pass a licensing examination to become a nurse in the United States. In some ethnic or cultural groups, however, folk healers or other nonlicensed healthcare providers (e.g., shamans, medicine men, lay midwives) are held in higher regard than nurses who are educationally prepared and who practice within the Western Biomedical Model. When providing care to patients from a culture where this may be an issue, the nurse should spend time establishing a good interpersonal relationship in order to bridge the cultural gap and to improve the patient's outcome and the overall healthcare experience of the patient.

SUMMARY

By now, it should be clear that it is impossible to practice high-quality nursing to our culturally diverse patient population unless we gain knowledge in transcultural health care and cultural competency models. See **Table 1–1** for more information on cultural factors and **Table 1–2** for a process to follow to develop cultural competence. It is not enough to just gain this knowledge, however. In order to deliver high-quality culturally diverse nursing care, nurses need to utilize this unique nursing knowledge; it is not enough just to know, but we must also attempt to do. Utilizing any of the described nursing models allows the nurse to gain knowledge and to deliver culturally appropriate care. The use of transcultural models is beneficial for nurses to become knowledgeable about and for evaluating society in terms of culture, to find the cultural data in a more systematic and standardized way, and to improve the field of transcultural nursing. Having a greater knowledge of the cultures served by the nurse will play an important role in improving the quality of health care. It is well known that the meaning of health and illness is different for various cultural groups. Nurses who utilize

Table 1–1 Cultural Factors

Family structure and characteristics
Education levels
Family assets
Family in the community
Communication style
Health beliefs and practice
Help-seeking style
View of professional and family roles
View of early intervention
Knowledge of health and education system
Time orientation
Socioeconomic status

transcultural theories are in an ideal position to demonstrate how the provision of culturally competent care will shape health care in the future. These and other models provide a starting point for assessment of patients who are culturally diverse. The nurse just needs to select the one that fits him or her best. The key is to remember that patients' cultural behaviors are relevant to health assessment and should be considered when planning care for all patients. Nurses can be guided in this process by selecting and following one of the available nursing models. A description of three of these models was provided in this chapter—Leininger's Culture Care, Diversity and Universality Theory and the Sunrise Model; Giger and Davidhizar's Transcultural Assessment Model; and Purnell's Model for Cultural Competence—to help you select the model that is best for you. You are now ready to begin to develop your transcultural nursing practice.

Table 1–2 Process for Attaining Cultural Competence

Develop awareness of own cultural biases
Understand facets of culture
Acknowledge and honor range of diversity in families' values and beliefs
Develop cultural sensitivity
Develop collaborative partnerships with families
Develop methods of cross-cultural communication
Learn to collaborate with interpreters
Minimize cultural bias in assessments
Identify and address barriers to assessment and intervention

PERTINENT RESEARCH STUDIES OF SELECTED MEDICAL DISORDERS AND CULTURAL COMPETENCY

TUBERCULOSIS: Many studies have found that patients who stopped treatment worldwide for tuberculosis (TB) did so because they felt better, their symptoms abated, or they thought that they were cured. In addition, patient beliefs about TB may differ from the medical model, such as believing that the disease has a mystical, superstitious, or religious origin. Compliance can also be a factor, especially if a patient was a refugee, as the patient may perceive the healthcare worker as a government representative or as an oppressor. Various rumors have also spread among different cultures that TB is caused by smoking, pollution, or even hard labor.

VIETNAMESE PATIENTS

Hoa, N. P., Thorson, A. E. K., Long, N. H., & Diwan, V. K. (2003). Knowledge of tuberculosis and associated health-seeking behaviour among rural Vietnamese adults with a cough for at least three weeks. *Scandinavian Journal of Public Health, 31*(Suppl. 62), 59–65.

Houston, H. R., Herada, N., & Makinodan, T. (2002). Development of a culturally sensitive educational intervention program to reduce the high incidence of tuberculosis among foreign-born Vietnamese. *Ethnicity and Health, 7*(4), 255–265.

Johannson, E., Long, N. H., Diwan, V. K., & Winkvist, A. (1999). Attitudes to compliance with tuberculosis treatment among women and men in Vietnam. *International Journal Tuberculosis and Lung Disease, 3*(10), 862–868.

ASIAN INDIAN PATIENTS

Asghar, R. J., Pratt, R. H., Kammerer, J. S., Navin, T. R. (2008). Tuberculosis in South Asians living in the United States, 1993–2004. *Archives of Internal Medicine, 168*(9), 936–942.

Singh, V., Jaiswal, A., Porter, J. D., Ogden, J. A., Sarin, R., Sharma, P. P.,... Jain, R. C. (2002). TB control, poverty and vulnerability in Delhi, India. *Tropical Medicine & International Health, 7*(8), 693–700.

GAMBIA PATIENTS

Harper, M., Ahmadu, F. A., Ogden, J. A., McAdam, K. P., & Lienhardt, C. (2003). Identifying the determinants of tuberculosis control in resource poor countries: Insights from a qualitative study in The Gambia. *Transactions of the Royal Society of Tropical Medicine and Hygiene, 97*(5), 506–510.

DIABETES PATIENTS: According to the Centers for Disease Control and Prevention (CDC), there are 900,000 new cases of diabetes mellitus (DM) annually, which translates to more than 2,600 new cases each and every day. The worst-case scenario results when a strong genetic predisposition is combined with a poor lifestyle. When this occurs repeatedly, it results in escalating rates of type 2 diabetes. It is believed that this is one of the primary reasons why minority populations are experiencing such a high type 2 diabetes incidence. This is a worldwide problem because the burden of diabetes is growing even more rapidly in other countries than it is growing in the United States. This will result in a huge economic burden to some countries that are not in a financial position to handle it. Type 2 diabetes is becoming epidemic in areas with higher proportions of at-risk ethnic groups. In these areas, a child as young as 12 years old is more likely to have type 2 diabetes than type 1 diabetes (sometimes still referred to as juvenile diabetes).

Recognition that poor diabetes outcomes may be related to inadequate cultural competency could result in a reduction or elimination of poor outcomes in these high-risk ethnic groups. These poor outcomes can be eliminated or reduced by enhanced awareness and improved skills in cross-cultural encounters. This understanding needs to extend to the complications that can be associated with DM in minorities as well. The following contributing factors have been identified to explain the high incidence of long-term complications of diabetes in ethnic minorities: high prevalence rate of DM, earlier age of onset that results in a longer duration of diabetes, poor glycemic control, delayed diagnosis, limited access to health care, less intense or comprehensive healthcare encounters, and a genetic susceptibility to complications (IOM, 2001).

Type 2 diabetes affects different populations in different ways. The prevalence is significantly higher in minority groups in comparison to the White population. This important disparity is beginning to be shared with the public through public service announcements. The American Diabetes Association has used the public service campaign of "Diabetes Favors Minorities." These facts were included in that public service announcement: diabetes strikes 1 out of 3 Native Americans, 1 out of 7 Hispanics, and 1 out of 14 Blacks.

The Translating Research Into Action for Diabetes (TRIAD) study was published in *Medical Care* in December 2006 by Duru et al. TRIAD's overall goal is to understand and influence the quality of care (both processes and outcomes of care) for patients with diabetes in managed care settings. TRIAD is a 10-year project funded by the Centers for Disease Control and Prevention and the National Institute of Diabetes and Digestive and Kidney Diseases, and is a 6-center prospective study of managed care and diabetes quality of care, costs, and outcomes in the United States.

The goal of this study was to determine if the utilization of clinical care strategies in managed care (diabetes registry, physician feedback, and physician reminders) is associated with attenuation of known racial/ethnic disparities in diabetic care. The study found that for the most part, high-intensity implementation of a diabetes registry, physician feedback, or physician reminders—three clinical care strategies similar to those strategies that are used in many healthcare settings—are *not* associated with an attenuation of known disparities of diabetes care in managed care. The authors also reported that disparities in care do exist, particularly among the Black American population.

REVIEW QUESTIONS

1. Differentiate the terms *culture*, *cultural assessment*, and *cultural competency*.
2. List the six cultural phenomena of the Giger and Davidhizar model.
3. Purnell identifies the 12 domains of culture in his model. What are the similarities and differences between those 12 domains and the 6 cultural phenomena that are in the Giger and Davidhizar model?
4. Provide two nursing implications for a nurse administering antihypertensives or psychotropics to the non-White patient (ethnopharmacology principles).
5. What was the theoretical framework used to develop the 12 standards of culturally competent nursing care practice that were published in the *Journal of Transcultural Nursing* in 2009?
6. Describe the process to attain cultural competency.
7. Which nursing theorist gave birth to the transcultural nursing movement?
8. Identify and describe three potential areas of diversity.
9. Describe the potential consequences of culturally discordant care.
10. What can the nurse do to decease the likelihood of committing a cultural gaffe?

REFERENCES

Battalova, J., & Terrazas, A. (2010). Frequently requested statistics on immigrants and immigration in the United States. Retrieved from http://www.migrationinformation.org/feature/display.cfm?ID=818

Benet-Martínez, V., & Haritatos, J. (2005). Bicultural identity integration (BII): Components and psychosocial antecedents. *Journal of Personality, 73*(4), 1015–1049. Retrieved from University of California Postprints website: http://escholarship.org/uc/item/4vh6z3s2

Berry, J. W. (1990). Psychology of acculturation. In N. R. Goldberger & J. B. Veroff (Eds.), *The culture and psychology reader* (pp. 457–488). New York, NY: New York University Press. Reprinted from Nebraska symposium on motivation: Berman, J. J. (Ed.). (1989). *Cross-cultural perspectives.* Lincoln: University of Nebraska Press.

Betancourt, J. R. (2003). Cross-cultural medical education: Conceptual approaches and frameworks for evaluation. *Academic Medicine, 78*(6), 560–569.

Betancourt, J. R., Green, A. R., Carrillo, J. E., & Ananeh-Firempong, O. (2003). Defining cultural competence: A practical framework for addressing racial/ethnic disparities in health and health care. *Public Health Reports, 118*(4), 293–302.

Brink, P. J. (1990). *Transcultural nursing: A book of readings.* Prospect Heights, IL: Waveland Press.

Browning, M. A., & Woods, J. H. (1993). Cross-cultural family nurse partnerships. In S. I. Feetham, S. B. Meister, & J. M. Bell (Eds.), *The nursing of families: Theories, research, education, and practice.* Newbury Park, CA: Sage.

Brownlee, A. T. (1978). *Community, culture, and care: A cross-cultural guide for health workers.* St. Louis, MO: Mosby.

Chuang, Y. (1999). *Fusion: The primary model of bicultural competence and bicultural identity development in a Taiwanese-American family lineage.* Unpublished doctoral dissertation.

Douglas, M. K., Pierce, J. U., Rosenkoetter, M., Callister, L. C., Hattar-Pollara, M., Lauderdale, J., . . . Pacquiao, D. (2009). Standards of practice for culturally competent nursing care: A request for comments. *Journal of Transcultural Nursing, 20*(3), 257–269.

Duru, O. K., Mangione, C. M., Steers, N. W., Herman, W. H., Karter, A. J., Kountz, D., . . . Brown, A. F. (2006). The association between clinical care strategies and the attenuation of racial/ethnic disparities in diabetes care: The Translating Research Into Action for Diabetes (TRIAD) study. *Medical Care, 44*(12), 1121–1128.

English, J. G., & Le, A. (1999). Assessing needs and planning, implementing, and evaluating health promotion and disease prevention programs among Asian American population groups. In R. M. Huff & M. V. Klein (Eds.), *Promoting health in multicultural populations: A handbook for practitioners* (pp. 357–374). Thousand Oaks, CA: Sage.

Giger, J. N. (2013). *Transcultural nursing: Assessment and intervention* (6th ed). Philadelphia, PA: Elsevier.

Giger, J., Davidhizar, R. E., Purnell, L., Harden, J. T., Phillips, J., & Strickland, O. (2007). American Academy of Nursing Expert Panel report: Developing cultural competence to eliminate health disparities in ethnic minorities and other vulnerable populations. *Journal of Transcultural Nursing, 18*(2), 95–102.

Guillory, W. (2001). *Business of diversity: The case for action.* Salt Lake City, UT: Innovations International.

Healthy People 2020. Retrieved from http://www.healthypeople.gov/2020/default.aspx

Hong, Y. Y., Morris, M. W., Chiu, C. Y., & Benet-Martínez, V. (2000). Multicultural minds: A dynamic constructivist approach to culture and cognition. *American Psychologist, 55*(7), 709–720.

Institute of Medicine. (2001). *Exploring the biological contributions to human health: Does sex matter?* Washington, DC: The National Academies Press.

Institute of Medicine. (2003). *Patient safety: Achieving a new standard of care.* Washington, DC: The National Academies Press.

Leininger, M. M. (1984). Transcultural nursing: An overview. *Nursing Outlook, 32*(2), 72–73.

Leininger, M. M. (1985). Transcultural care, diversity, and universality: A theory of nursing. *Nursing & Health Care, 6*(4), 208–212.

Leininger, M. M. (1991). *Culture care diversity and universality: A theory of nursing.* New York, NY: National League for Nursing Press.

Leininger, M. M. (1995). Transcultural nursing: Concepts, theories, research and practices. (2nd ed.). New York, NY: McGraw-Hill.

Leininger, M. M. (1997). Understanding cultural pain for improved health care. *Journal of Transcultural Nursing, 9*(1), 32–35.

Leininger, M. (2002). Culture care theory: A major contribution to advance transcultural nursing knowledge and practices. *Journal of Transcultural Nursing, 13*(3), 189–192.

Leininger, M., & McFarland, M. (2002). *Transcultural nursing: Concepts, theories, research, and practice* (3rd ed.) Columbus, OH.

Marquand, B. (2006). Philippine nurses in the US—Yesterday and today. *Minority.* Retrieved from http://www.minoritynurse.com/filipino-philippine-nurses/philippine-nurses-us%E2%80%94yesterday-and-today

McGee, C. (2001). When the Golden Rule does not apply: Starting nurses on the journey toward cultural competence. *Journal for Nurses in Staff Development, 17*(3), 105–112.

McGoldrick, M. (1993). *Ethnicity, cultural diversity and normality.* New York, NY: Guilford Press.

McGrath, B. B. (1998). Illness as a problem of meaning: Moving culture from the classroom to the clinic. *Advances in Nursing Science, 21*(2), 17–29.

Muñoz, C., & Hilgenberg, C. (2005). Ethnopharmacology: Understanding how ethnicity can affect drug response is essential to providing culturally competent care. *American Journal of Nursing, 105*(8), 40–48.

Murdock, G. P. (1971). Ethnographic atlas. *Ethnology World Cultures, 19*(1), 24–136.

Office of Minority Health. (2000). *Assuring cultural competence in health care: Recommendations for national standards and an outcomes-focused research agenda.* Washington, DC: U.S. Department of Health and Human Services.

Padilla, A. M. (1994). *Bicultural development: A theoretical and empirical examination.* In R. Malgady & O. Rodriguez (Eds.), *Theoretical and conceptual issues in Hispanic mental health* (pp. 20–51). Melbourne, FL: Krieger.

Parsons, T. (1951). *The social system.* Glencoe, IL: The Free Press.

Phinney, J. S., & Devich-Navarro, M. (1997). Variations in bicultural identification among African American and Mexican American adolescents. *Journal of Research on Adolescence, 7*(1), 3–32.

Purnell, L. D. (Ed.). (2013). *Transcultural health care: A culturally competent approach* (4th ed.). Philadelphia, PA: F. A. Davis.

Purnell, L., & Paulanka, B. (1998). *Transcultural health care: A culturally competent approach.* Philadelphia, PA: F. A. Davis.

Spector, R. (1993). Culture, ethnicity and nursing. In P. Potter & A. Perry (Eds.), *Fundamentals of nursing: Concepts, process and practice.* St. Louis, MO: Mosby.

Sprott, J. E. (1993). The Black box in family assessment: Cultural diversity. In S. L. Feetham, S. B. Meister, J. M. Bell, & C. L. Gilliss (Eds.), *The nursing of families: Theory, research, education, & practice.* Thousand Oaks, CA: Sage.

Tervalon, M., & Murray-Garcia, J. (1998). Cultural humility versus cultural competence: A critical distinction in defining physician training outcomes in multicultural education. *Journal of Health Care for the Poor and Underserved, 9*(2), 117–125.

Tripp-Reimer, T., & Fox, S. (1990). *Beyond the concept of culture.* St. Louis, MO: Mosby.

U.S. Census Bureau. (2012). Census data. Retrieved from http://www.census.gov

U.S. Census Bureau. (2010). Fact finder. Retrieved from http://factfinder2.census.gov/faces/nav/jsf/pages/index.xhtml

Valente, S. M. (1989). Overcoming cultural barriers. *California Nurse, 85*(8), 4–5.

For a full suite of assignments and additional learning activities, see the access code at the front of your book.

Culture

KEY TERMS [www]

Possession of a thorough and complete cultural vocabulary is essential for the nurse to communicate effectively.

Ableism: Discrimination or prejudice based on a limitation, difference, or impairment in physical, mental, or sensory capacity or ability.

Ageism: Discrimination or prejudice based on age, particularly aimed at the elderly.

Bias: A personal judgment, especially one that is unreasoned or unfair.

Bicultural: Designed for or pertaining to two distinct cultures.

Biracial: Of two races; usually describing a person having parents of different races (not to be confused with bicultural).

Classism: Discrimination or prejudice based on socioeconomic status.

Cultural brokering: The act of bridging, linking, or mediating between groups or persons of differing cultural backgrounds; a cultural broker acts as a go-between, one who advocates on behalf of another individual or group (Jezewski & Sotnik, 2001).

Cultural dominance: The pervasiveness of one set of traditions, norms, customs, literature, art, and institutions, to the exclusion of all others.

Cultural group: A group of people who consciously or unconsciously share identifiable values, norms, symbols, and some ways of living that are repeated and transmitted from one generation to another.

Cultural humility: Incorporates a lifelong commitment to self-evaluation and self-critique, to redressing the power imbalances in the patient–clinician dynamic, and to developing mutually beneficial and advocacy partnerships with communities on behalf of individuals and defined populations. Cultural humility is proposed as a goal in healthcare education (Tervalon & Murray-García, 1998).

Cultural sensitivity: Experienced when neutral language, both verbal and nonverbal, is used in a way that reflects sensitivity and appreciation for the diversity of another. Cultural sensitivity may be conveyed through words, phrases, and categorizations that are intentionally avoided, especially when use of these may be interpreted as impolite or offensive (Giger et al., 2007).

Culturally appropriate: Demonstrating both sensitivity to cultural differences and similarities and effectiveness in communicating a message within and across cultures.

Culture: The shared values, traditions, norms, customs, arts, history, folklore, and institutions of a group of people who are unified by race, ethnicity, language, nationality, sexual orientation, and/or religion.

Differently abled: A limitation, difference, or impairment in a person's physical, mental, or sensory capacity or ability.

Discrimination: An act of prejudice or a manner of treating individuals differently due to their appearance, status, or membership in a particular group.

Diversity: The concept of diversity encompasses acceptance and respect. It means understanding that each individual is unique and recognizing our individual differences. Differences can be along the dimensions of race, ethnicity, gender, sexual orientation, socioeconomic status, age, physical abilities, religious beliefs, political beliefs, or other ideologies. It is the exploration of these differences in a safe, positive, and nurturing environment. It is about understanding each other and moving beyond simple tolerance to embracing and celebrating the rich dimensions of diversity contained within each individual. Also defined as the range of human variation, including age, race, gender, disability, ethnicity, nationality, religious and spiritual beliefs, sexual orientation, political beliefs, economic status, native language, and geographical background.

Dominant group/culture: The "mainstream" culture in a society, consisting of the people who hold the power and influence.

Ethnicity: The classification of a group of people who share common characteristics, such as language, race, tribe, or national origin.

Ethnocentrism: The attitude that one's own cultural group is superior.

Gender: A social or cultural category generally assigned based on a person's biological sex.

Gender identity: A person's sense of being masculine, feminine, or some combination thereof (not necessarily their biological sex).

Health literacy: The degree to which individuals have the capacity to obtain, process, and understand basic health information and services needed to make appropriate health decisions (U.S. Department of Health and Human Services, 2000).

Homophobia: Fear of, aversion to, or discrimination against homosexuality, homosexuals, or same-sex relationships.

Institutional racism: Biased policies and practices within an organization or system that perpetuate disadvantages for people of a certain race or ethnicity.

Language: The form or pattern of communication—spoken, written, or signed—used by residents or descendants of a particular nation or geographic area; language can be formal or informal, and includes dialect, idiomatic speech, and slang.

Minority: The smaller in number of at least two groups; can imply a lesser status or influence.

Multicultural: Designed for or pertaining to two or more distinct cultures.

Multiracial: Describing a person, community, organization, and so on composed of many races.

National origin: The country or region where a person was born.

Person of color: Usually used to define a person who is not a descendant of people from European countries; individuals can choose whether or not to self-identify as a person of color.

Prejudice: Overgeneralized, oversimplified, or exaggerated beliefs associated with a category or group of people, which are not changed even in the face of contrary evidence.

Race: A socially defined population characterized by distinguishable physical characteristics, usually skin color.

Racism: The belief that some racial groups are inherently superior or inferior to others; discrimination, prejudice, or a system of advantage and/or oppression based on race.

Sexism: Discrimination or prejudice based on gender or gender identity.

Sexual orientation: Describes the gender(s) of people to whom a person feels romantically and/or sexually attracted.

Socioeconomic status: Individuals' economic class (e.g., poor, working class, middle class, wealthy) or position in society based on their financial situation or background.

Stereotype: A highly simplified preconception or belief about a person, place, or thing, based on limited information.

Transgender: Describes a person whose gender identity differs from his/her assigned gender and/or biological sex.

Values: What a person believes to be important and accepts as an integral part of who he/she is.

Vulnerable populations: Refers to social groups with increased relative risk (i.e., exposure to risk factors) or susceptibility to health-related problems. The vulnerability is evidenced in higher comparative mortality rates, lower life expectancy, reduced access to care, and diminished quality of life (Center for Vulnerable Populations Research, UCLA School of Nursing, 2008).

Xenophobia: A fear of all that is foreign, or a fear of people believed to be "foreigners."

INTRODUCTION

Our patients come from many different races and ethnic groups, which means they often do not look, feel, or respond like we do. According to the U.S. Census Bureau (2010), Black Americans, Hispanics, Asian Americans, Pacific Islanders, and Native Americans currently account for 34.8% of the U.S. population. In addition, there has been a significant increase in the number of people (2.9% of the total U.S. population) who belong to two or more races (an increase of 32% from the 2000 census data). Clearly, the color of America is continuously changing. There is and will continue to be an explosion in population growth in the United States and globally. Nurses and other healthcare providers have to increasingly care for and communicate with patients of varying backgrounds, preferences, and cultures. This change has resulted in cross-cultural encounters and the development of the cultural competency movement. The cultural competency movement is here to stay, so as nurses, we need to get on board the train so that we have a say in the destination and how we plan to get there.

No single definition of cultural competency is universally accepted, yet all of the definitions share the requirement that healthcare professionals adjust and recognize their own culture in order to understand the culture of the patient (Johnson, Roter, Powe, & Cooper, 2004). This provides the foundation for the expansion of one's understanding of other cultures. When the nurse is a member of the dominant culture, it is even more important that he or she develops cultural awareness. This is because failing to recognize that one's values, behaviors, and traditions are cultural may result in the person thinking that their view is the "norm" for all. Cultural competence begins with an understanding and appreciation for your own identity. You are a culturally rich individual with your own blend of culture, ethnicity, race, gender, class, sexual orientation, age, religion or spirituality, geographic location, and physical and mental abilities, as are all of your patients.

So what is culture? Culture, according to Locke (1992, p. 3), is "socially acquired and socially transmitted by means of symbols, including customs, techniques, beliefs, institutions and material objects." According to this definition, culture is learned, not predetermined or genetic. Our culture determines our way of life and our worldview. It is important to remember that members of a particular racial group may not share the same cultural experiences. It is for this reason that one must assess for variances from the group's norm in each individual's experiences. This is an extremely important point that must be recognized. Additionally, culture helps to determine our innermost feelings and our response to illness or physical symptoms such as pain (Andrews & Boyle, 2008).

Many definitions exist for culture. In essence, our culture sets the guidelines and standards for how we exist in society. Not everyone in society agrees with or follows the same guidelines and standards, and this is true for culture. It would be incorrect to believe or even to expect that all members of a cultural group follow the expected guidelines and standards ascribed to by the majority. This intracultural variation increases the difficulty of providing culturally appropriate or competent nursing care. For this reason, the nurse must perform a thorough cultural assessment prior to planning nursing care delivery. People from a given racial group may, but do not necessarily, share a common culture. Culture also can be influenced by the context or the setting we find ourselves in and must also be considered. Culture is not something that the individual is often consciously aware of, despite its powerful influence on our health and response to illness. How symptoms are described and perceived is also affected by the culture of the patient. This can have a tremendous impact on disease processes or conditions (such as chronic pain) in which patient history is the primary means of diagnosis. Culture shapes the ways in which patients express, experience, and cope with their feelings of distress and, therefore, how they describe and explain their symptoms. Social and cultural factors include the ease with taking on the sick role, the consistency of the individual's beliefs with the main cultural environment, and the consistency of the individual's beliefs with those of the healthcare provider in determining which symptoms will be reported, and the expectations for treatment.

Culture influences our health status and it shapes our concept of health, illness, and health practices. This is a dynamic process for, as we grow and develop, we become exposed to more cultural variables. In childhood, we are molded very much by our family and community. Our family and community are influenced by history, ethnicity, religion, and socioeconomic situation. As we leave childhood and enter adulthood, we may become more educated, we may change our geographic location and political perspectives, and we may even change how we define family as we begin to build our own family. These cultural variables influence our understanding of how to maintain health and health behaviors related to the development of illness in ourselves and in our loved ones.

THE FUNCTION OF CULTURE

Culture exists to distinguish one society from another. It provides a framework or structure for the content and interpretation of the values of its members in a systematic manner that distinguishes its members from nonmembers. Culture provides a universal ideation—it uses ideas and symbols to give meaning to environment and life experiences. These ideas are shared and transmitted from person to person and generation to generation. The feeling of belonging to a culture results in "social solidarity." Social solidarity is how people come together as a coherent and united force; it inspires loyalty and devotion to a common cause (Crow, 2002). The culture of a society establishes rules or norms to follow in social situations. Ultimately, it is our culture that provides a meaning for our existence and helps to guide the life direction that we chose to follow.

THE SICK ROLE AND THE NEED FOR CULTURAL SENSITIVITY

Our culture provides the framework for how we strive to attain health, how we recognize when we are ill, and how we act in the sick role, because health and illness are defined and interpreted by our personal experiences and the context of our worldview. The impact or meaning that is attached to the alteration in health is also culture-bound. This means that the impact and meaning ascribed to an illness by a patient could be in conflict with the meaning ascribed by the nurse. This different view can result in cultural misunderstandings that can negatively impact the process and outcome for the patient. This is why all nurses must develop cultural sensitivity, so that they can be the bridge between the patient and the healthcare system. To determine if a cross-cultural encounter was culturally sensitive, look for signs that the patient has the feeling of being understood, the feeling of being respected, and the feeling of being supported.

The decision of if or when to enter the healthcare system as a patient also has cultural implications. With the onset of illness or when an alteration in health occurs, the individual asks himself or herself many questions such as: What is the meaning of this? Is it serious? Does it require medical attention? They may seek assistance from their family or community to aid in the decision process. How each of these questions is answered and how the patient chooses to proceed is based on the person's cultural beliefs, values, and practices, as well as social factors (e.g., money, employment, availability of health insurance). The decision of if or when to enter the healthcare system is also culturally determined. Many people with medical illness or health problems never enter the healthcare delivery system; if they do, they may be nonadherent to the recommendations provided. The decision of if or when to seek medical care is a complex one with social- and symptom-related determinants. Culturally different populations have varying determinants of when, or if, the transition from person to patient occurs (i.e., the decision to seek medical care for their symptoms). The consequence of this is serious in that patients from racial and ethnic minority groups use fewer healthcare services and are less satisfied with their care than patients from the majority White population (Saha, Komaromy, Koepsell, & Bindman, 1999).

PRIMARY AND SECONDARY CHARACTERISTICS OF CULTURE

Culture can be further defined and described by its characteristics. The primary characteristics of culture are generally unchangeable and begin to shape our worldview beginning at a very early age. The primary characteristics of culture are what one commonly thinks of when considering culture: nationality, race, color, gender, age, and religious affiliation (the only primary characteristic that has the potential for change).

The secondary characteristics of culture come from life circumstance and life experience and, as such, can and often do change over time. There are many secondary characteristics of culture, including educational level, socioeconomic status, occupation, political beliefs, and marital/parental status, to name a few (**Box 2–1**). Changes in secondary characteristics over time leads to variations within one's culture. Members of a culture who share secondary characteristics form a

---

Box 2–1 Primary and Secondary Characteristics of Culture

Primary Characteristics	**Secondary Characteristics**
Nationality	Educational status
Race	Socioeconomic status
Color	Occupation
Gender	Military experience
Age	Political beliefs
Religious affiliation	Place of residence (urban vs. rural)
(potential to be changed)	Marital/parental status
	Physical characteristics
	Sexual orientation
	Gender issues
	Reason for migration to the United States
	Length of time away from country of origin

Adapted from: Purnell, L. D. (Ed.). (2013). *Transcultural health care: A culturally competent approach* (4th ed.). Philadelphia, PA: F. A. Davis.

subculture that shares the same worldview, whereas members of a cultural group with differing secondary characteristics would have a very different worldview.

People belonging to a specific racial group may, but do not necessarily, share a common culture. There is great confusion among definitions for many terms such as *race* and *ethnicity*.

SUBCULTURES

As mentioned previously, not all members of a cultural group may hold all of the same values, which results in the formation of a subculture. A subculture consists of groups of people who don't think or behave like the members of the core cultural group. There may be some overlap with the values and beliefs of the main cultural group, but changes are made so that the beliefs, desires, and needs more closely match those of the members of the subculture. **Box 2–2** describes important features of a subculture.

Subcultures have different experiences than those of the dominant culture. A subculture differs from the dominant group. An example of a subculture that holds differing views from the dominant culture would be second-generation Asian Indian immigrants compared to first-generation (recent) immigrants to the United States. Although both groups share the primary characteristic of culture of nationality, they differ in time away from the country of origin (a secondary characteristic of culture). Members of subcultures are often unified by commonalities.

Box 2–2   Important Features of a Subculture

Identification with a subculture can result in the following benefits:

1. Providing a more descriptive and comprehensive group identity.
2. An evolution and adaptation of member characteristics over time.
3. A blueprint on how to interact with members and nonmembers of the subculture and the larger cultural group.
4. A greater sense of community and belongingness within a narrower context.
5. Knowledge of and the ability to recognize other subculture members through the use of social behaviors. These social behaviors can include the use of unique or colloquial language, wearing certain clothing styles, and providing appropriate methods of greeting.
6. Establishes an us-against-them paradigm to its members.

Adapted from: Boisinier, A., & Chatman, J. A. (2002). The role of subcultures in agile organizations. Retrieved from http://www.hbs.edu/research/facpubs/workingpapers/papers2/0102/02-091.pdf

The Professional Subculture and the U.S. Biomedical Model of Health

All nurses, as well as other members of the healthcare team, belong to the professional subculture. As we become educated as nurses and members of the healthcare team, we are socialized into this professional subculture (Clark, 2004; Helman, 2000). This professional subculture not only has its own unique vocabulary, but it also possesses a perspective on health and illness (the U.S. Biomedical Model of health care, or Western medicine) with its emphasis on patient autonomy. This can also result in a block or barrier when the philosophy of the healthcare professional and the patient are not congruent. A common mistake made by Western-trained healthcare providers is the assumption that the U.S. Biomedical Model for diagnosis, healing, and prevention is common to all cultures, which is not the case. We must always strive to remember that as nurses, when we interact with patients, we come to the encounter with two cultures: our personal culture and our professional subculture.

Even when a nurse has the same culture as his or her patient, there can be cultural gaffes because the nurse belongs to the professional subculture. This can be even more complicated when the nurse is also a member of a different culture than the patient. Unfortunately, this is a very likely occurrence, because the racial and ethnic profile of the registered nurse (RN) population is substantially different from that of the U.S. population (Health Resources and Services Administration [HRSA], 2010). While the overall U.S. population of White, non-Hispanics makes up 65.6% of the total U.S. population, the nursing workforce is made up predominately of White, non-Hispanics (83.2% of RNs) (HRSA, 2010).

According to the 2008 national sample survey of registered professional nurses, there are 3,063,162 RNs in the United States. There are 250,527 RNs who are prepared as an APRN in one or more advanced specialties or fields (HRSA, 2010). The vast majority of RNs are White (83.2%); male nurses only account for 9.6% of all RNs (HRSA, 2010). The likelihood of a patient of color being cared for by a White nurse is extremely high. While the population of Black Americans in the United States is in the double digits (12.2%), this is not true of the nursing workforce. As of 2008, Black American nurses were only 5.4% of the nursing workforce. For other cultural groups, the numbers of RNs are even lower. Asians/ Native Hawaiian and Pacific Islanders make up 5.8%, while Hispanic/Latinos make up 3.6% of the RN workforce (HRSA, 2010). Historically there has been a substantial number of RNs who are educated in countries other than the United States, and who have been recruited from the Philippines or India. This has made

Table 2–1 Population Characteristics of the RN Workforce

Percentage of U.S. Population	Percentage of RN Workforce
White, Non-Hispanic 65.6%	83.2%
Black American 12.2%	5.4%
Hispanic/Latino 15.4%	3.6%
Asian/Native Hawaiian/Pacific Islander 4.5%	5.8%
American Indian/Alaskan Native 0.8%	0.3%

Source: Health Resources and Services Administration. (2010). *The registered nurse population: Findings from the 2008 National Sample Survey of Registered Nurses.* Retrieved from http://bhpr.hrsa .gov/healthworkforce/rnsurveys/rnsurveyfinal.pdf

a positive contribution to the higher number of Asians compared to other racial/ethnic groups among RNs (HRSA, 2010). See **Table 2–1** for population characteristics of the RN workforce compared with the total U.S. population.

IMPACT OF CULTURE AND ETHICS

In addition to our professional culture being based on the U.S. Biomedical Health Belief Model, it is also based on Western ethical principles. These ethical principles, such as do no harm, patient autonomy, and self-determination, are not shared by all. Relying on these ethical principles without considering a patient's culture may result in a cultural gaffe. One area where this can have important consequences is with advance directives. Advance directives are based on the ethical principle of patient self-determination, a principle that is not followed or valued in all cultures.

There are two types of organizing cultures: collectivist or individualist. In a collectivist society, groups or the government take priority over individuals. When a patient has roots in a collectivist society, the nurse should expect that medical decisions are not patient determined, but family determined. Whether people function more fundamentally as an individual (autonomous) or as part of a group (collectivist) has a very specific impact on communication and other factors that will impact healthcare outcomes (**Table 2–2**). The underlying principle is that an individual must be subjugated to the group and do what is good for the majority (i.e., the common good).

In a collectivist culture such as Latino and many Asian cultures, communication is indirect. This is important for the nurse to consider when planning for patient education, as the use of direct and specific information may not be effective

Table 2–2 Characteristics of Individualistic Cultural Values Versus Collectivistic Cultural Values

Individualism—The Individual	Collectivism—The Group
Privacy	Company
Time over human interaction	Human interaction over time
Precise time	Loose time
Future oriented	Past oriented
Task related	Nontask related
Appreciates competition	Appreciates cooperation
Human equality	Hierarchy/rank/status
Autonomy	The group
Independence	Interdependence
Assigns individual credit and blame	Group shares credit and blame
Common sense and change	Order and tradition

Adapted from: Leake, D., & Black, R. (2005). *Essential tools: Cultural and linguistic diversity: Implications for transition personnel*. Minneapolis, MN: University of Minnesota, Institute on Community Integration, National Center on Secondary Education and Transition.

(Theisen, 2004). When dealing with patients from collectivist societies, such as Asian Indians, the nurse practitioner (NP) should consider including the family when discussing advance directives or when considering do not resuscitate (DNR) orders with the patient. To be respectful of culture and ethics, the NP may wish to permit both the patient and a family member to sign informed consents for any procedures the patient requires. For Japanese patients, the selected family member may be the eldest son instead of a spouse. The NP can and should advocate for this type of inclusion to occur on the patient's behalf.

CULTURE AND MENTAL HEALTH

Mental health concerns human behavior and interaction; cultural understanding is especially important. Culture determines the behaviors that are considered normal or abnormal, the beliefs and values deemed important, and the rules that direct human interaction. Not only are behaviors important, but so too are their situational contexts, along with a host of other practices, such as personal hygiene, dress, hairstyle, and religious beliefs and values. When caring for patients, nurses need to be aware of cultural variations in what is deemed appropriate or inappropriate, as well as understand how patients from particular cultures may display mental distress. See **Box 2–3** for information on culture-bound syndromes.

RACE AND ETHNICITY

Race and ethnicity (and culture) are important to comprehend. These terms are not interchangeable. The nurse needs to have an accurate understanding of each term to ensure that a proper distinction regarding these terms is maintained. Lack of understanding and poor term definition has contributed to confusion and some controversy in this area. Race and ethnicity have their roots in multiple venues including environmental, socioeconomic, ancestral/geographic origins, education, and socioeconomic status, which all influence health. Race is a social construct that is used to categorize and divide people based on physical characteristics, which often leads to conflict and oppression. A person's race is externally decided and has nothing to do with culture, intellect, ability, or personality. It is easy to find examples throughout history where a racial categorization has resulted in oppression or conflict (Kean, 2011). Ethnicity is made up of many more internal attributes, such as one's cultural traditions, religion, ancestry, beliefs, and even communication (including language) (Rubenstein, 2011). This is complex and often results in confusion because members of one racial group can have varying ethnicities and possess many different cultures among them, just as people of the same culture can have many different races among them (Kean, 2011).

Emerging genetic knowledge may transform the current notions attached to race and ethnicity. Genomic researchers have found that any two human individuals are approximately 99.9% the same genetically, and it is hypothesized that the most important genetic material for human functioning is encompassed in that shared set. The 0.1% difference, although comparatively small, represents about 3 million differences between individuals' DNA. Whereas most of those differences probably have no effect on phenotype, a small fraction (perhaps about 200,000 common variants) is responsible for the genetic component of the differences in health, behavior, and other human traits. As we learn more, we can expect racial differences to become better understood.

Race

Race is generally considered genetic in origin because it includes physical characteristics (skin color, blood type, hair and eye color) as well as biologic variations such as predisposition to certain disease processes and differences in drug metabolism. The U.S. government uses the classification of race, not ethnicity, for data collection.

The classification of humans by race is extremely problematic. Newer research highlights the limitations and dangers inherent in biologic explanations of group differences in health and disease. An emphasis on biologic sources of "racial" variations in health obscures the social origins of disease, while reinforcing group stereotypes. The placement of human beings into racial categories is complicated even further when the person is multiracial. The inclusion of a multiracial demographic racial category would further undermine the concept of race as an irreducible difference between people while highlighting the arbitrariness of racial categorization in the first place (Taylor, 2008). There is a paradigm shift occurring in research related to the label of race. The dominant perspective in the social sciences views race as socially constructed through political, legal, economic, and scientific institutions. From this perspective, the meaning of race finds its origins in social practices and a system of social relations that signify social conflict and group interests. Race is a societal construct as it is not individuals who create racial categories, but macrolevel social processes and institutions (Taylor, 2008).

Despite its lack of usefulness as a biologic determinant, the use of race as an organizing principle is prevalent in society. Race is a major source of personal and collective identity as it is a central category of social recognition. The United States is a society where race is deeply fused with power and cultural patterns; it provides a social organization (Taylor, 2008). In striving toward cultural competency, the nurse should revise the definition of race to minimize or even exclude biology and consider race as a marker for historical, social, and cultural experiences and conditions. Consider that race informs and influences our perceptions, behaviors, and attitudes.

Ethnicity

Ethnicity is a cultural construct and refers to membership in a particular cultural group. It is defined by shared cultural practices, such as food, holidays, language, and customs. The perceived cultural distinctiveness creates the ethnic group. Eller (1999) states that ethnicity is fundamentally about symbolism, group cohesion, and personal identity. Rubenstein (2011, p. 208) defines ethnicity as "identity with a group of people who share the cultural traditions of a particular homeland or hearth." Therefore, ethnicity is a cultural process through which individuals affiliate themselves within and around a group. First, a person must be conscious of a difference between himself or herself and others. This difference must then be seen as being both important and relevant, and finally the difference must cause the individual to mobilize around that difference (Eller, 1999). According to Eller (1999), ethnicity is no mere reflection of culture, but a complex reworking, remembering, and reinvention of culture. While a unifying difference has to be identified, resulting in affiliation, for ethnic group development, any differences noted within the group must be overlooked in order to ensure group cohesion. This embracing and overlooking of differences can result in ethnic group inconsistencies. For example, the Hispanic ethnic group is distinguished by a tremendous variation among its people (Puerto Rican, Cuban, Mexican, etc.) unified by a common language and geography from which they or their ancestors descend. Ethnicity requires a consensus of group belonging and a differentiation from others that has its roots in a shared past and a perceived future interest. Unifying differences of ethnicity include religion, socioeconomic class, geographic background of the family, and cultural experiences.

Limitations Associated with the Labels of Race and Ethnicity

It is clear that there are limitations associated with the labels of race and ethnicity. The current use of federal definitions for race may not adequately address the individual's ancestry of origin/ethnicity. The National Healthcare Disparities report (U.S. Department of Health and Human Services, 2008) defines race as White, Black, American Indian, Asian, Native Hawaiian, or Pacific Islander, and ethnicity is limited to only two categories: "Hispanic" or "not Hispanic." It is also important to remember that terms such as *African American* are census terms and may not be considered appropriately descriptive of many Blacks in America who hail from other areas throughout the world and who have maintained their unique cultural heritage and, in some cases, their specific genotypes from their original geographical location (e.g., immigrants from Haiti, Jamaica, or Uganda).

ETHNOCENTRISM

Ethnocentrism can be a barrier to the delivery of culturally competent nursing care. Ethnocentrism is the belief that one ethnic group is superior to all others. The word *ethnocentrism* derives from the Greek word *ethnos*, meaning "nation" or "people," and the English word *center*. *Ethnic* refers to cultural heritage and *centrism* refers to a central starting point. Therefore, ethnocentrism refers to judging other groups from our own cultural point of view. We are all ethnocentric—how can we not be? We need to recognize this fact because problems occur when we are placed in a situation where we have limited (or no) information about another group. This can result in the nurse making a false assumption or assumptions based on limited experience. The root of the issue and the inherent danger is that we do not know what we do not know and cannot understand what we do not understand. An ethnocentric nurse feels that those whose beliefs are different from their own are strange or bizarre, or most alarmingly, totally wrong.

Unfortunately, ethnocentrism is a universal tendency of all human beings; it is natural to think that their way of thinking, acting, and believing is the only right, proper, and natural way. The nurse must avoid being ethnocentric and recognize that patients and their families feel that their values and principles are just as valid as the nurse feels her own values and principles to be.

In an attempt to avoid ethnocentricity in our nursing practice, we must learn more about the cultures of the patients for whom we provide care. See **Table 2–3** for information on several cultural variations as well as associated nursing interventions. Even learning about cultural competency in and of itself does not guarantee success or smooth sailing. There are inherent barriers, some that are obvious and visible and others that are yet to be identified or viewed. One barrier that is known is the impact of whether verb tenses exist or not in the language spoken. The English language does have verb tenses that result in a time orientation (the importance of time is highly valued and demonstrated by statements such as "time is money," "it is important to be punctual," or "if it was important you would make the time"). The Algonquian Indian language, in contrast, does not have tenses but has animate or inanimate verb forms. If a Native American who speaks the Algonquian language (e.g., Chippewa tribe) does not show or is late for a medical appointment, the nurse may make the assumption that the patient has a present time orientation (a concept frequently highlighted in the cultural competency literature). Cultural groups are often identified as having a present or future time orientation. The nurse's assumption would be incorrect in this particular situation because the nurse would be imposing a time frame where none exists.

Assumptions can result in either false-negative or false-positive judgments. An example of a false-negative judgment would be the nurse who views the taking of a siesta by the Mexican American patient as being lazy. Because Western culture (and the professional healthcare subculture) values being industrious, being lazy is a very negative attribute. This view does not permit the nurse to recognize the positive impact a rest or a nap can have on the health of the patient. An example of a false-positive judgment would be for the nurse who, as a member of an industrial society, views an Amish patient living in Lancaster County, Pennsylvania, as being free of the stress of a modern society. In reality, the patient may be experiencing a significant amount of stress caused by bad weather that is impacting the ability to work the land or harvest the crops.

The nurse needs to be on guard and recognize that our limited experience will result in the making of false assumptions. What we have already experienced is the basis for our reality. Our perceptions on all things, such as time orientation, social roles, and even life and the universe, work for us, or else we would not have

Table 2–3 Cultural Variations and Associated Nursing Implications

Cultural Groups	Cultural Variations	Nursing Implications
Black Americans	Language—slang terms may have opposite meanings. Example: "bad" can actually mean "good."	Ensure understanding through careful questioning and seeking clarification.
Mexican Americans	Touch—when interacting with or admiring children, it is important to touch the child. Not doing so is giving the "evil eye." The male head of the family is the healthcare decision maker.	During encounters with children, it is important to associate touch. The nurse should include the entire family, both immediate and extended, in all aspects of nursing care delivery. Ultimately, it is the male head of the family who will make healthcare decision.
Vietnamese Americans	The head is considered sacred and should not be touched. An upturned palm is an offensive gesture.	The nurse should only touch the head if it is absolutely essential to do so. If it is essential, then the nurse should explain the reasons for the need to touch the head and to seek permission before proceeding. The nurse should be aware of nonverbal communication and should avoid hand gesturing in order to prevent a cultural gaffe.
American Eskimos	It is not considered polite to disagree publicly.	The nurse should always clarify patient intent. A patient may nod their head yes to be polite and to avoid public disagreement, even though they actually mean no.
Orthodox Jewish Americans	Excessive touching by members of the opposite sex is offensive.	Consider ways to minimize touching the patient and only do so if absolutely necessary and only after permission from the patient has been received. If possible, male nurses should be assigned to male Orthodox patients and female nurses to female Orthodox patients.

Sources: Giger, J. N. (2013). *Transcultural nursing: Assessment and intervention* (6th ed.). Philadelphia, PA: Elsevier; and Purnell, L. (Ed.). (2013). *Transcultural health care: A culturally competent approach* (4th ed.). Philadelphia, PA: F. A. Davis.

those perceptions. These perceptions help us to organize our life experience and to provide meaning to events as we live our daily lives. Our experiences provide the basis for interpreting others' behaviors. This ethnocentric view can lead to misunderstanding because we see their ways in terms of our life experiences, not their context. An ethnocentric view causes us to not understand that the ways of others have their own meanings and functions, just as our ways have for us.

Carrying on in an ethnocentric manner can have serious consequences. We can unintentionally offend others, generate ill will, and even contribute to a harmful situation—the last thing that an ethical nurse would ever wish to occur. So, what should we do? We need to remove the blinders and recognize that we are all ethnocentric (we can never experience every life situation of everyone in the world). When we are being ethnocentric, we need to identify that we are, attempt to control for any bias, and strive to develop a better understanding of the other person and the situation at hand. We should strive for a grounded understanding that can only occur from the recognition and control of bias. We need to open ourselves up to the reactions or cues from our patients and ourselves that let us know that our assumptions are wrong or are not working.

When we experience a negative reaction to a situation (such as the patient acting offended or confused), this is a clue that our assumptions are not working in this situation. Also, recognizing that our patient is not responding in the way that we would is also an important clue that our assumptions are not working in this situation. Once we recognize that we do not understand the patient or the situation, we can be in a better position to control any biases and to strive to develop a more valid understanding of the patient and the situation.

Ask questions and seek information. Ask for an explanation, in a respectful manner, for what they say or do. An open "can you help me understand this better?" will often result in willingness of the other person to help us in our understanding. Avoid asking questions that impose your own reality and negate their reality, and be aware that not all patients may wish to answer your question as they may feel it is personal or even sacred. Anthropologists would suggest using an *emic* and *etic* approach to questioning our patients to provide more insight into the patient's life experiences within their context. The nurse would utilize the emic approach when trying to determine the meanings about the behavior and the situation to the patient. Questioning what are the adaptive functions of the behavior and the situation utilized by the patient would be to utilize the etic approach. "What are the adaptive functions?" is the question that is generally *not* asked, but that could lead to the greatest insight as we come to realize that there are many valid ways in which human beings can live and experience life.

The development of a functional understanding (as opposed to the development of a true and deep understanding) is possible and important for the nurse to strive for. Practice at every opportunity to develop proficiency—just like any other nursing skill. Cross-cultural patient encounters reveal more about our own perspectives and values, and as such they provide us with unique opportunities to truly learn more about ourselves.

GENERALIZATIONS AND STEREOTYPING

Any generalizations made by the nurse about the behaviors of patients or large groups of people are almost certain to be an oversimplification. When faced with the overwhelming amount of diversity present in the United States, it is easy to generalize about people. A question the nurse should ask himself or herself is: Is my generalization based on the actual observed behavior or is it based on motives I think underlie the behavior? If he or she answers yes to the second part of the question, he or she is probably oversimplifying.

The consequence of generalization is stereotyping. Stereotyping is an oversimplified opinion or belief about a group of people. This is where nursing walks a fine line. Generalizations have value for nurses because they help to guide the questioning process. It provides a starting point only—it is not the ending point. The nurse gains information, compares it with the information known about the cultural group, and then makes assessments based on prior knowledge and current findings.

The nurse must not forget to consider intraethnic differences in cultural diversity. Despite the variation that exists among all cultural groups, there is the tendency to assume that all members of the group are the same. One must consider that much variation within cultural groups exists, just as there is variation between cultural groups. Ultimately we are a unique blend of the diversity found within our culture of origin, combined with the uniqueness of our life experience, as well as the degree of acculturation that has occurred during our life.

A large body of research in psychology has explored how stereotypes evolve, persist, shape expectations, and affect interpersonal interactions. Stereotyping can be defined as the process by which people use social categories (e.g., race, sex) in acquiring, processing, and recalling information about others. The beliefs (stereotypes) and general orientations (attitudes) that people bring to their interactions help organize and simplify complex or uncertain situations and give perceivers greater confidence in their ability to understand a situation and respond in efficient and effective ways. There is considerable empirical evidence that even well-intentioned Whites who are not overtly biased and who do not believe that they are prejudiced typically demonstrate unconscious implicit negative racial attitudes and stereotypes. Stereotypes significantly shape interpersonal interactions, influencing how information is recalled and guiding expectations and inferences in systematic ways. They can also produce self-fulfilling prophecies in social interaction, in that the stereotypes of the perceiver influence the interaction with others in ways that conform to stereotypical expectations. This can also be true of healthcare professionals. According to the Institute of Medicine (IOM) report on unequal treatment (2002), although there is no direct evidence that provider biases affect the quality of care for minority patients, research suggests that healthcare providers' diagnostic and treatment decisions, as well as their feelings about patients, are influenced by the patients' race or ethnicity. Research findings suggest that the relationship between race or ethnicity and treatment decisions is complex and can be influenced by many different factors. It may be influenced by gender of the patient or provider, the providers' perceptions and attitudes toward their patient, as well as by the patient's race or ethnicity. So subtle are these influences that often the provider is not even aware that the influence is even being exerted (IOM, 2002).

Nurses and NPs may often make stereotypes or assumptions about patients based on limited or inaccurate information. These rushed judgments are often constructed of negative biases, assumptions, and stereotypes made in the hurry to complete the clinical encounter in the required limited time. This rushed approach does not permit the recognition of the inherent diversity and preferences that may be present in each individual patient. The nurse works to foster an attitude that incorporates and validates the cultures of those we treat.

CULTURAL MISMATCH AND CULTURAL PAIN

The nurse also needs to develop awareness into his or her personal style of interaction because he or she may have a personal style of interaction that does not match the patient. A cultural mismatch is what occurs when people violate each other's cultural expectations (Leininger, 1995). An example of a cultural mismatch would be the nurse, attempting to keep to a tight schedule, interrupting the prayer session of a devoutly Muslim patient. This interruption would definitely result in a cultural mismatch, but it could also result in causing cultural pain to the Muslim patient, which is a much more serious situation. Cultural pain occurs when hurtful, offensive, or inappropriate words are spoken to an individual or group. These spoken words are experienced by the receiver as being insulting, discomforting, or stressful. Cultural pain occurs because of a lack of awareness, sensitivity, and understanding by the offender of differences in the cultural values, beliefs, and meanings of the offended persons. When these types of events occur during a patient–provider encounter, they can result in significant consequences. If cultural mismatch or cultural pain occurs, it is essential that that it be recognized and corrected. If this does not occur then we risk the development of consequences, one of which would be the inability to establish a therapeutic alliance with the patient. It is recommended that, if a cultural mismatch or mistake is made for the healthcare provider to attempt to recover quickly from the mistake and to avoid becoming defensive. If the provider suspects that the mismatch has been serious enough to have caused cultural pain (as evidenced by seeing a sudden negative change in attitude), the health professional must act on this feeling and ask if they did or said anything offensive. Cultural pain occurs if the clinician inadvertently ignores an important cultural obligation or violates a cultural taboo. Making this type of adjustment requires cultural flexibility—this is only possible for those healthcare providers who have taken the time to develop self-awareness and who have examined their own cultural background and biases.

CULTURE AND ITS IMPACT ON THE PATIENT ROLE

Many people with medical illness or health problems never enter the healthcare delivery system, or if they do, they are often nonadherent to the recommendations provided. The decision of if or when to seek medical care is a complex one with many social- and symptom-related determinants. Culturally different populations have varying determinants of when, or if, the transition from person to patient occurs (i.e., the decision to seek medical care for their symptoms). It has been reported that patients from racial and ethnic minority groups use fewer healthcare services and are less satisfied with their care than patients from the majority White population (Saha et al., 1999). In fact, the White population receives better and more aggressive health care than minorities, with associated improved patient outcomes (IOM, 2002).

CULTURAL FORMULATION AND CULTURE-BOUND SYNDROMES

The area of psychiatry permits healthcare providers, including psychiatric NPs and clinical nurse specialists, a comprehensive means of achieving culturally competent care through the use of cultural formulations. It is essential to consider

Box 2–3 Culture-Bound Syndromes

For many years anthropologists and providers have used the *Diagnostic and Statistical Manual of Mental Disorders* (DSM-IV) to provide information to assist with the diagnosis of disorders that may have variations in presentation due to the impact of culture (as well as developmental stage/age and gender). Specific identified factors are described when providing information regarding every psychiatric diagnosis in DSM-IV-tr. For example, when considering communication disorders it would be unfair to consider the impact of culture on language development, especially in a bilingual home, as this may dramatically impact the context of language (DSM-IV-tr). Culture bound syndromes is the newer term for "folk illness." These disorders are made up of a combination of somatic and psychiatric symptoms (which explains the placement in the DSM-IV manuals). There are no discrete objective findings to support the diagnosis and the syndrome must not be found in any other culture to fit the diagnostic criteria. All identified culture-bound syndromes that may be seen by the nurse in clinical practice are included in the DSM-IV. It may be helpful for the nurse to be aware that this information is also readily available on the internet, at websites including Wikipedia and http://rjg42. tripod.com/culturebound_syndromes.htm. Some of the more prevalent culture-bound syndromes have been placed in this table.

Amok (Malaysia) Cafard or Cathard (Laos, Polynesia, the Philippines) Mal de pelea (Puerto Rico) Iich'aa (Navajo)	A predominately male disorder characterized by episodes of extreme violence that is triggered by an event where the patient feels he (or she) has been negated or insulted. The violent episode is often followed by symptoms such as exhaustion, and often the patient may have no memory of the violent episode at all. Today this is considered a rare occurrence confined to rural areas in Southeast Asia. Age of occurrence is typically between the ages of 20 and 45.
Ataque de nervios (Latin America, Latin Mediterranean, Caribbean)	This disorder is typically triggered by pent-up anger over time. The patient erupts and feels out of control, often following a stressful episode or event. Symptoms can range from crying and anger with the use of a raised voice and can extend to acts of both verbal and physical violence. Suicide and suicide attempts have been reported. Often amnesia follows the event as the patient returns to their baseline mood.
Bilis or Cólera or Muina (Latinos)	This disorder is attributed to anger or rage that results in both physical symptoms such as HA and GI upset and emotional symptoms. Patients often experience significant fatigue after an episode.
Ghost sickness (Navajo)	This emotional disorder is associated with multiple physical complaints accompanied by a fixation on death and dying.

Box 2–3 *Continued*

Rootwork (southern United States, Caribbean) Mal puesto or Brujeria (Latino societies)	The etiology for this disorder is ascribed to supernatural origins. The patient may experience anxiety, GI upset, and be overwhelmed with the fear of death or injury, often by poisoning.
Hwa-byung or Ul-hwa-byeong or Wool-hwa-byung (Korea)	This diagnosis is frequently used by Korean psychiatrists. It is accepted as a part of traditional Korean culture as the manifestation of an imbalance in life. Patients may, among many other symptoms, complain of feeling a mass in the stomach area. Patients tend to be middle-aged or elderly females who live in rural areas and who come from a lower socioeconomic status.
Boufée delirante (West Africa, Haiti)	This disorder is characterized by a sudden onset of agitation and aggression that can be associated with confusion, paranoia, and hallucinations.
Brain fag or brain fog (West Africa) Studiation madness (Trinidad)	This disorder is associated in students following periods requiring academic rigor. Most of the complaints are associated with anxiety or panic such as rapid heartbeat, difficulty concentrating, shaky hands, dizziness, and difficulty with sleeping. Other symptoms include blurry vision and/or watery eyes and pressure in the head or neck.

Source: American Psychiatric Association. (2000). *Diagnostic and statistical manual of mental disorders* (4th ed.). Arlington, VA: Author.

and examine the impact of cultural factors on psychiatric illness, including on symptom presentation and help-seeking behavior. To ensure that an accurate diagnosis is made across cultural boundaries and that the formulated treatment plan is acceptable to the patient, clinicians need a reliable method to determine and evaluate the cultural information discovered during the clinical encounter. The Cultural Formulation Model has been advocated as an effective model to meet this purpose and has been used internationally (Lewis-Fernández & Díaz, 2002). It consists of five components: assessing cultural identity, cultural explanations of the illness, cultural factors related to the psychosocial environment and levels of functioning, cultural elements of the clinician–patient relationship, and the overall impact of culture on diagnosis and care. This assessment and diagnosis of diverse individuals, the cultural formulation, has been incorporated into the *DSM-IV-Text Revision*. The cultural identity of the individual is determined for reference. Immigrant status and the degree of involvement in the host or culture of origin are evaluated. Language abilities and preferences are noted. Cultural explanation of the individual's illness is assessed to look for culture-bound syndromes (such as posttraumatic slavery syndrome), culture-specific meanings of symptoms, and how the individual interprets disease and behaves toward health and healing within and outside of his or her cultural reference group. Cultural factors related to psychosocial environment and level of functioning put the family and social context of the patient's functioning into perspective and examine support networks. Cultural elements of the relationship between the individual and healthcare provider are determined. Overall cultural assessment for diagnosis and care is formulated, along with consideration of how the identified factors may influence the patient's diagnosis, management, and functioning.

CULTURAL DIFFERENCES IN MORTALITY AND MORBIDITY

It is also important to be aware of cultural differences because of their effect on mortality and morbidity. For example, American Indian and Alaska Native populations have patterns of mortality that differ from the general population. Mortality data reveal excess overall mortality for American Indians and Alaska Natives. American Indians and Alaska Natives have a higher incidence of accidents, diabetes, liver disease, pneumonia, influenza, suicide, homicide, and tuberculosis, whereas a relative deficit of deaths has been noted from heart disease, cancer, and human immunodeficiency virus infection. As another example, lung cancer is the second most commonly diagnosed cancer among males and females in the United States (Centers for Disease Control and Prevention [CDC], 2010). Lung cancer does not impact all races equally, however. Blacks have a higher incidence and mortality rate than whites (CDC, 2010).

Knowledge of distinctive mortality patterns among populations will help healthcare providers recognize the unique needs of their patients. Just as disease entities can vary from population to population, so can the response to an illness. Remission of symptoms may be considered to be a cure by people in some ethnic groups, such as Latinos. Black Americans understand and subscribe to the U.S. Biomedical Health Belief Model and, with little variation, hold mainstream cultural views about health and management of illness. Older Latinos (older than age 50) do not hold these mainstream cultural views of health and disease management; in fact, they do not perceive themselves as responsible for changing aspects of their lifestyle, such as diet and exercise, nor do they develop self-care practices. This lack of self-care can result in a serious lack of illness management when younger family members are unavailable to take on this responsibility for the patient. Mexican Americans emphasize respect, caring, understanding, and patience in healthcare encounters or a personal process in health care. Filipino Americans' views about health, while grounded in different cultural traditions, are complementary to mainstream U.S. cultural views of health and illness. Filipino Americans ascribe to the concept of responsibility for maintaining good health; however, this is not viewed as an individual responsibility, but as a responsibility to the family and social group. Filipino Americans, like other Asians, diminish the importance of their illness and place a strong emphasis on appearing healthy and active, which in that culture is referred to as the maintenance of "face." Inquiring about the patient's preferences and practices with the goal to incorporate and negotiate acceptable approaches to healthcare delivery will serve both the patient and provider best.

IMPACT OF GENDER

Culture determines our understanding and behaviors associated with our gender role. Because gender roles are determined by role models, how a male or female functions is ingrained in him or her from a very early age. The value of our gender and whether one gender is considered more valuable than another is clearly known within a culture and communicated to all of its members. How a girl should act is learned by observing her female relatives, whereas boys look to the males in the family for guidance. Body image is also culturally driven and can have a tremendous impact on health. In some cultures, weight is an important consideration. In some cultures, obesity is so revered, as in the Mauritania's White Moor Arab population in Africa, that young girls are sometimes force-fed until extremely obese. Being extremely overweight or obese is considered highly valued for a female to achieve, as it makes her much more attractive as a potential mate. In other cultures, such as the dominant American culture, thinness is valued, sometimes to an obsessive level that has resulted in the onslaught of eating disorders in both females and males.

In some cultures, the female is viewed by the children as the primary caretaker, not only for their family but for the community. Children observe if it is the mother's role to offer treatment remedies, which may include tea, herbal concoctions, soup, prescribed medications, or a combination of treatment modalities. They also observe who is contacted when someone is ill—do the mothers take their children to folk healers, herbalists, older members of the community, physicians, or a combination of care providers? Children soon find out if the females or males are viewed as healers by witnessing who is consulted within the community during periods of illness.

During puberty and the onset of sexual development, different cultures react in very different ways. In some cultures (e.g., Navajo), the onset of menstruation (menarche) is cause for celebration; this is not the case in other cultures. In both Iranian and Orthodox Jewish cultures, menstruation is a period of uncleanness. Iranian tradition also holds that menstrual blood can pollute the body unless discharged each month, a belief also held by many African Americans.

Islamic tradition emphasizes that Allah values people who are clean and pure, because jinn (predatory evil spirits) may be strongly attracted to blood and the unclean (Jones, 2003). In some Islamic traditions it is believed that anyone who sees or touches "unclean" menstrual blood becomes impure and vulnerable to dire consequences (Jones, 2003).

During menstruation, Muslim females have many rules to follow, including not touching any holy objects, not entering a mosque, and abstaining from sexual intercourse. In fact, if menstruation begins during intercourse, the male must immediately withdraw from the female. Sexual activity cannot begin again until after the cessation of menstruation and cleansing (*ghusl*) has occurred (Al-Islam Org, 2010). There are two types of ghusl—*ghusl tartibi* and *ghusl irtimasi*. Ghusl tartibi is the preferred method according to Al-Islam.org (2010). This cleansing consists of washing the body in three stages: first the head and neck, then the right side of the body from shoulders to foot, and finally the left side of the body. The application of henna may also be a part of the cleansing ritual. According to Jones (2003), henna applied to the feet, hands, and hair, which remains visible for several weeks, shows that the body has been purified and is worthy in the eyes of God. Different sects and tribes use different techniques and rituals reflecting local culture (Jones, 2003). In addition, because women are considered to be in a fragile condition during menstruation, showers and strenuous exercise are also restricted (Purnell, 2013).

Nurses must always keep in mind that adherence to any of the highlighted menstrual traditions is not consistent throughout a culture and therefore does not hold for every patient associated with a specific culture. There are many factors impacting this process, including the degree of assimilation that has occurred to the dominant mainstream culture, the degree of family and religious ties, and educational level, among others. Because of the variety of cultural traditions that surround menstruation and the social and physical activities proscribed during this period, nurses need to question each patient about her personal beliefs and practices before offering any education or advice. Failure to do so may produce care based on cultural stereotypes, which can have significant negative consequences. It is important for the nurse to recognize that education may not change these beliefs and the patient and her family should be reassured that her beliefs will be respected and incorporated into the plan of care as long as they are neutral or beneficial to the patient. The nurse's duty to do no harm would need to be considered and disclosed to the patient in the event that patient education is necessary regarding a cultural belief that is deemed potentially harmful to the patient.

Culture prescribes and determines sexual conduct, including what sexual acts are allowed, what type of marriage is permitted (one partner or many), and what the rules are regarding sexual activity outside of marriage, as well as the rules and beliefs about cleanliness and the genitalia.

The transition to motherhood is also culture-bound as it impacts the existence or lack of prenatal care, types of birth, and postnatal care. The decision to breast-feed or bottle feed is also impacted by culture.

The movement through menopause also varies based on the culture of the patient. Western women suffer with greater menopause symptoms than other women globally (Mills, 2011). In a study by Zeserson (2001), it was determined that the menopause experience for Japanese women was different than for White women. White women complained of hot flashes quite frequently, whereas the Japanese women did not. The Japanese women's main complaint was of stiff neck and shoulder discomfort. One possible explanation for this difference may be diet. Japanese women ingest a diet high in soy protein, and soy has estrogenic properties (Hamilton-Reeves, Rebello, Thomas, Slaton, & Kurzer, 2007). In fact, the low frequency of hot flashes in Japan (less than 25%) meant there was not a word in the Japanese language to describe this phenomenon. Only recently have Japanese words been adopted for menopausal symptoms such as hot flash (*hotto furasshur*) and hormone balance (*horumon baransu*). This was not a result of an increased incidence of hot flashes in Japan, but was instead due to the desire to maintain an updated, globally oriented language (Mills, 2011).

Culture also impacts health promotion and screening initiatives. No matter the age or number of children, the nurse should not assume that the female patient has had a gynecological exam, a Pap smear, and/or a mammogram. There are three beliefs in the Korean culture that make it less likely that Korean American women will get a Pap smear: (1) the belief that once a women reaches menopause she no longer needs a Pap smear as frequently, (2) the belief that after women stop having children they no longer need a Pap smear, and (3) that there is a significant feeling of embarrassment associated with having a Pap smear (Theisen, 2004). Many elderly Korean Americans are of the belief that having one Pap smear is all that is needed in a lifetime; of course the more acculturated the Korean American, the more likely preventive measures will occur (Theisen, 2004).

Culture plays a major role in screenings for breast cancer as well. Underutilization of mammography screening by Hispanic American women has resulted in poorer survival rates and increased likelihood of death (Palmer, Fernandez, Tortolero-Luna, Gonzales, & Mullen, 2005). There seems to be a difference in subgroups of Hispanics that the nurse should also be aware of. For example, Mexicans have the lowest mammography utilization rates of all Hispanics; higher levels of acculturation may positively impact the use of preventive services (Palmer et al., 2005). A study by Lannin et al. (1998) found that psychosocial, cultural, and socioeconomic variables explained the difference between late-stage presentation of breast cancer between Black American and White women. Another investigation found that Hispanic women had poorer outcomes with breast cancer, despite a lower incidence, regardless of the fact that they may have been taught breast self-examination. Women with breast tumors in this study presented later to their healthcare providers because of cultural influences (Coe et al., 1994).

In addition to changes associated with sexuality and reproductive ability, both genders experience changes associated with aging that have cultural implications. Cultural beliefs affect attitudes about whether families should care for dying women at home or whether they should be cared for in hospitals or nursing homes. Some members of Arab, Black American, and Chinese cultures prefer to die in hospitals to avoid the bad luck of dying in the home. Members of other groups, such as some Southeast Asian cultures, care for dying relatives in the home because not doing so may be viewed as shirking family duty.

IMPACT OF CULTURE ON END-OF-LIFE CARE

Culture also influences attitudes toward life support and DNR orders. For example, some older Korean Americans support the use of advance directives and not using life-supportive measures, but worry about family conflict if the eldest son disapproves (Phipps, True, & Pomerantz, 2000). For Muslims, futile treatment is not deemed mandatory (Lawrence & Rozmus, 2001). Cultural traditions that place a high value on karma are often at odds with the use of advance directives (Braun, Pietsch, & Blanchette, 1999). People from cultures that ascribe to ancestor worship or believe that children are the reincarnation of dead ancestors may refuse to consent to turning off the life support of an infant or adult for fear of retaliation. Patient autonomy, which is an ethical principle associated with nursing and medicine, may conflict with the patient's culture.

Sharing the prognosis with the patient also has cultural implications and the wishes vary by culture. In many cultures, the family does not wish to inform the patient about a negative prognosis or to discuss how to proceed in advance in the event of any mental or physical incapacity, and they do not wish to be told of an impending death. In many Asian cultures it is perceived as cruel to directly inform a patient of a cancer diagnosis. Even among people of a European background this can be true. Bosnian Americans and Italian Americans perceive direct disclosure of illness as disrespectful, and in some extreme cases, even inhumane. Many cultures also expect that the words used to communicate diagnosis or prognosis be extremely well thought out by the nurse or NP. Native Americans (including the Navajo), Bosnians, Chinese, and Filipinos feel that once the words are spoken they may become reality. There is significant reluctance among Chinese patients and their families to discuss end-of-life care or the possibility of death due to the concern that the direct acknowledgment of mortality will result in death (Searight & Gafford, 2005).

See **Box 2–4** for important points related to the tremendous areas of diversity that may occur within cultural groups the NP and nurse should consider when planning for end-of-life care.

IMPACT OF LESBIAN, GAY, BISEXUAL, AND TRANSGENDER

The definition of culture over the years has been expanded to ensure inclusivity for all people. This expansion has resulted in the recent call for the inclusion of lesbian, gay, bisexual, and transgender (LGBT) people as a cultural group (McManus, 2008). Like the general United States population, LGBT people are diverse in terms of cultural background, ethnic or racial identity, age, education, income, and place of residence. The degree to which sexual orientation or gender identity is central to one's self-definition, the level of affiliation with other LGBT people, and the rejection or acceptance of societal stereotypes and prejudice vary greatly among individuals. These differences parallel the diversity among members of other minority groups.

Nurses and advance practice nurses are ethically required to provide competent and compassionate care to all members of society. This is only the minimum standard, however. There are unique challenges all LGBT patients face when seeking health care, and there can be devastating consequences if a cultural gaffe

---

Box 2–4   Key Aspects of Cultural Diversity in End-of-Life Health Care for the Nurse to Consider

1. Does the patient exhibit individualism or collectivism?
2. How does the patient define family (nuclear, extended, non-blood-related members)?
3. What is the patient's view on gender roles?
4. What is the patient's worldview on marital relationships and the role of the family (patriarchal worldview)?
5. What is the patient's communication pattern (direct versus indirect, reliance on nonverbal versus verbal communication)?
6. What are the patient's spiritual beliefs? Is there membership in a religious organization? Does he or she believe in an afterlife?
7. What is the patient's view of the healthcare system (role of physician/provider in making medical decisions)?
8. What is the patient's view on suffering or use of palliative measures?

Adapted from: Searight, H. R., & Gafford, J. (2005). Cultural diversity at the end of life: Issues and guidelines for family physicians. *American Family Physician, 71*(3), 515–522.

---

occurs. It is for this reason that all nurses must learn more about this population in order to provide appropriate, culturally competent care. There are many situations described in the literature where even the minimum ethical standard, the provision of competent and compassionate care, was not achieved. For example, there was a transgender patient, who ultimately expired from ovarian cancer, who was refused health care by 20 healthcare providers in the state of Georgia. In New Jersey, a transgender female was denied care at several emergency departments despite having a fever of 104 degrees and an eventual diagnosis of bacterial endocarditis (Jillson, 2002).

Nurses who do not recognize the qualities and beliefs of any given culture, including LGBT patients, risk losing patient trust and having poor outcomes. LGBTs are at high risk for disenfranchisement from society as a whole and enter the healthcare arena with a high degree of fear and anxiety. If they experience an uncomfortable medical or nursing encounter, often it results in the patient choosing to stop seeking medical care all together (McManus, 2008).

Basic Lesbian, Gay, Bisexual, and Transgender Definitions

It is important for the nurse to be aware of the correct definitions that can be associated with this population as well as the difference between sexual identity and gender identity. Homosexuality is a type of sexual identity and refers to a sexual, affectional, or emotional attraction toward persons of the same sex (Gay and Lesbian Medical Association, 2005). The above definition is expanded to include both males and females when describing bisexuals (Gay and Lesbian Medical Association, 2005). Sexual preference is not the same as gender identity. Gender identity refers to the perception of oneself as male or female, neither, or both and, as such, may have unique associated concerns. The label *transgender* is used as a global term to describe people who do not conform to typical accepted gender roles and the label *transsexual* to people who identify with the gender that is opposite to the gender identity that was assigned at birth. The person who has sex chromosomes, genitalia, and/or secondary sex characteristics that are neither exclusively male nor exclusively female are labeled *intersex* (Gay and Lesbian Medical Association, 2005).

Homophobia and Incidence of Discrimination

The consequence of homophobia is discrimination. Discrimination can be overt or subtle, intended or inadvertent. Nurses often unknowingly contribute to subtle inadvertent incidences of discrimination. An example of this is when the nurse or NP, while performing a history, asks the lesbian patient about the type of birth control she is using. Our workplace can be the culprit as well. Intake forms that only list the default gender identities of male and female or that only include heterosexual couplings as options (single, married, divorced) can be offensive to the LGBT population.

Many lesbian people avoid seeking health care because of past negative experiences with homophobic practitioners. These experiences have been well documented within the medical literature and may include patronizing treatment, intimidation, attempts to change the patient's sexual orientation, hostility toward the patient or his/her partner(s), breach of confidentiality, invasive and inappropriate personal questioning, neglect, denial of care, undue roughness in the physical exam, and even reported cases of sexual assault (Rankow, 1995). The incidence of screening for cervical cancer and breast cancer is much lower in lesbians than what is found in the general female population. Even if the lesbian female goes for routine gynecological care, the provider may be under the false impression that lesbians do not need Pap smears (Rankow, 1995). The consequences of healthcare avoidance, including health screening activities, can run the gamut from minor to lethal.

It is difficult to truly gauge the number of LGBT people in the United States because of fear of reprisal of respondents to surveys, even when anonymity is ensured. The U.S. Census Bureau (2011) estimates that there are 131,729 same-sex "married couple households," and 514,735 same-sex unmarried partner households in the U.S. for a total of 646,464 same-sex households. Approximately

25% of same-sex households are raising children (U.S. Census Bureau, 2011). Often, nurses and physicians are unaware of or are in denial about their patient's sexuality. A study of gynecologists conducted by Lehmann, Lehmann, and Kelly (1998) reported that half of the respondents did not believe they had ever seen a lesbian in their practice. Unfortunately, this myopic view is not just confined to physicians.

It is essential that nurses have knowledge of their patient's sexual behavior because it can alert the nurse or NP to potential conditions that may not be considered if that knowledge is lacking.

The Importance of Acceptance

The nurse must recognize the impact of attitudes on patient interaction and clinical judgment and strive to develop a nonhomophobic attitude when caring for patients who are LGBT. The process of achieving cultural competency with this population is the same as for any other. The nurse must first recognize that they have a knowledge deficit as they do not possess the necessary skills or information to provide competent care for this population. They should seek out opportunities to learn more and expand their knowledge base. In the case of the NP, the patient should be referred to providers who are culturally competent regarding the LGBT community. Achieving cultural competency in caring for any cultural group, including LGBT, begins first with introspection, followed by the challenging of core beliefs, followed by the making of adjustments as to how these patients are approached and managed by the nurse. Once the NP feels that competency with this group has been achieved, it is recommended that a welcoming environment be created. Many LGBT persons respond to symbols that indicate openness on the provider's part to caring for this group. These symbols, including displaying artwork with same sex couples, pamphlets that are inclusive, or the posting of a nondiscrimination statement that is easily visible in the waiting room, have been identified by LGBT patients as effective welcoming interventions (Saulnier, 2002). The process of striving toward a nonhomophobic environment can be prolonged, but it will result in improved health outcomes for the LGBT population.

SUMMARY

Culture consists of primary and secondary characteristics. Culture is an important component of any healthcare encounter as it impacts communication between patient and nurse, traditional health beliefs versus those of Western modern medicine, and the health practices that the patient will agree to follow. Subcultures influence cultural understanding and experiences. The nurse must not only consider the patient's cultural background when planning care, but also any subculture influences that may impact the patient as well. Once cultural data are analyzed, the nurse can adopt, modify, or reject interventions and treatments in a manner that respects the patient's cultural differences. Providing this adaptation will not only improve the quality of patient care but also the patient's life. Becoming culturally competent is not easy, but it is a rewarding and necessary endeavor. Patients do better when their needs are understood and met. Embarking on this journey requires the nurse to learn culture-specific behavior. Cross-cultural patient encounters reveal more about our own perspectives and values and as such they provide us with unique opportunities to truly learn more about ourselves. Competence requires the recognition that there are exceptions to every rule and uniqueness in all people so that the best nursing care can be provided to that patient.

REVIEW QUESTIONS

1. Differentiate between the primary and secondary characteristics of culture.
2. Describe the impact that various subculture membership may have on both the nurse and patient.
3. Define ethnicity and race.
4. Explore the relationship of culture bound syndromes to mental health diagnoses.
5. What is the consequence of homophobia to the LGBT population? What is the potential impact of the nurse's attitude to providing culturally competent nursing care to the LGBT population?

REFERENCES

Al-Islam.org. (2010). *The ritual ablutions for women*. Retrieved from http://www.al-islam.org/taharah_women/2.htm

American Psychiatric Association. (1994). *Diagnostic and statistical manual of mental disorders* (4th ed.). Arlington, VA: Author.

Andrews, M. M., & Boyle, J. S. (2008). *Transcultural concepts in nursing care* (5th ed.). Philadelphia, PA: Lippincott Williams & Wilkins.

Braun, K. L., Pietsch, J. H., & Blanchette, P. L. (1999). *Cultural issues in end of life decision making*. Thousand Oaks, CA: Sage.

Centers for Disease Control and Prevention (CDC). (2010). Racial/ethnic disparities and geographic differences in lung cancer incidence—38 States and the District of Columbia, 1998–2006. *Morbidity and Mortality Weekly Report, 59*(44), 1434–1438.

Clark, C. L. (2004). The professional socialization of graduating students in generic and two-plus-two baccalaureate completion nursing programs. *Journal of Nursing Education, 43*(8), 346–351.

Coe, K., Harmon, M. P., Castro, F. G., Campbell, N., Mayer, J. A., & Elder, J. P. (1994). Breast self-examination: Knowledge and practices of Hispanic women in two southwestern metropolitan areas. *Journal of Community Health, 19*(6), 433–448.

Crow, G. (2002). *Social solidarities: Theories, identities and social change.* Philadelphia, PA: Open University Press.

Eller, J. D. (1999). *From culture to ethnicity to conflict: An anthropological perspective on international ethnic conflict.* Ann Arbor: University of Michigan Press.

Gay and Lesbian Medical Association. (2005). *Guidelines for care of lesbian, gay, bisexual and transgender patients.* San Francisco, CA: Author.

Giger, J., Davidhizar, R. E., Purnell, L., Harden, J. T., Phillips, J., & Strickland, O. (2007). American Academy of Nursing Expert Panel report: Developing cultural competence to eliminate health disparities in ethnic minorities and other vulnerable populations. *Journal of Transcultural Nursing 18*(2), 95–102.

Giger, J. N. (2013). *Transcultural nursing: Assessment and intervention* (6th ed.). Philadelphia, PA: Elsevier.

Hamilton-Reeves, J. M., Rebello, S. A., Thomas, W., Slaton, J. W., & Kurzer, M. S. (2007). Soy protein isolate increases urinary estrogens and the ratio of 2:16alphahydroxyestrone in men at high risk of prostate cancer. *Journal of Nutrition, 137*(10), 2258–2263.

Health Resources and Services Administration (HRSA). (2010). *The registered nurse population: Findings from the 2008 National Sample Survey of Registered Nurses.* Retrieved from http://bhpr.hrsa.gov/healthworkforce/rnsurveys/rnsurveyfinal.pdf

Helman, C. G. (2000). *Culture, health and illness* (4th ed.). Oxford, UK: Butterworth-Heinemann.

Institute of Medicine, Committee on Understanding and Eliminating Racial and Ethnic Disparities in Health Care. (2002). *Unequal treatment: Confronting racial and ethnic disparities in health care.* Washington, DC: National Academies Press.

Jezewski, M. A., & Sotnik, P. (2001). *Culture brokering: Providing culturally competent rehabilitation services to foreign-born persons.* Buffalo, NY: Center for International Rehabilitation Research Information and Exchange. Retrieved from http://cirrie.buffalo.edu/monographs/cb.pdf

Jillson, I. A. (2002). Opening closed doors: Improving access to quality health services for LGBT populations. *Clinical Research and Regulatory Affairs, 19*(2–3), 153–190.

Johnson, R. L., Roter, D., Powe, N. R., & Cooper, L. A. (2004). Patient race/ethnicity and quality of patient-physician communication during medical visits. *American Journal of Public Health, 94*(12), 2084–2090.

Jones, C. C. (2003). Menstruation and henna: Pollution and purification. Retrieved from http://www.tapdancinglizard.com/mens/mens1.html

Kean, M. (2011). The difference between race, ethnicity, and culture. *Progressive Scholar* [blog]. Retrieved from http://progressivescholar.wordpress.com/?p=615

Lannin, D. R., Mathews, H. F., Mitchell, J., Swanson, M. S., Swanson, F. H., & Edwards, M. S. (1998). Influence of socioeconomic and cultural factors on racial differences in late-stage presentation of breast cancer. *Journal of the American Medical Association, 279*(22), 1801–1807.

Lawrence, P., & Rozmus, C. (2001). Culturally sensitive care of the Muslim patient. *Journal of Transcultural Nursing, 12*(3), 228–233.

Lehmann, J. B., Lehmann, C. U., & Kelly, P. J. (1998). Development and health care needs of lesbians. *Journal of Women's Health, 7*(3), 379–387.

Leininger, M. (1995). *Transcultural nursing: Concepts, theories, research, and practice.* Columbus, OH: McGraw-Hill College Custom Series.

Lewis-Fernández, R., & Díaz, N. (2002). The cultural formulation: A method for assessing cultural factors affecting the clinical encounter. *The Psychiatric Quarterly, 73*(4), 271–295.

Locke, D. C. (1992). *Increasing multicultural understanding: A comprehensive model.* Newbury Park, CA: Sage.

McManus, A. J. (2008). Creating an LGBT-friendly practice: Practical implications for NPs. *The American Journal for Nurse Practitioners, 12*(4), 29–38.

Mills, D. (2011). *Menopause and perimenopause: A look at menopause across cultures.* Retrieved from http://www.womentowomen.com/menopause/menopauseacrosscultures.aspx

Palmer, R. C., Fernandez, M. E., Tortolero-Luna, G., Gonzales, A., & Mullen, P. D. (2005). Acculturation and mammography screening among Hispanic women living in farmworker communities. *Cancer Control: Cancer, Culture and Literary Supplement,* 21–27.

Phipps, E., True, G., & Pomerantz, S. (2000). *Approaches to End of Life Care in Culturally Diverse Communities.* [On-line]. Available: http://www.lastacts.org/scripts).

Purnell, L. D. (Ed.). (2013). *Transcultural health care: A culturally competent approach* (4th ed.). Philadelphia, PA: F. A. Davis.

Rankow, E. J. (1995). Breast and cervical cancer among lesbians. *Women's Health Issues, 5*(3), 123–129.

Rubenstein, J. M. (2011). *The cultural landscape: An introduction to human geography* (10th ed.). Upper Saddle River, NJ: Prentice Hall.

Saha, S., Komaromy, M., Koepsell, T. D., & Bindman, A. B. (1999). Patient–physician racial concordance and the perceived quality and use of health care. *Archives of Internal Medicine, 159*(9), 997–1004.

Saulnier, C. F. (2002). Deciding who to see: Lesbians discuss their preferences in health and mental health care providers. *Social Work, 47*(4), 355–365.

Searight, H. R., & Gafford, J. (2005). Cultural diversity at the end of life: Issues and guidelines for family physicians. *American Family Physician, 71*(3), 515–522.

Taylor, R. L. (2008, September). *The changing meaning of race in the social sciences: Some implications for research and social policy.* Keynote address presented at the 2nd Statewide Meeting on Health Disparities—Monitoring Health Disparities: Creating Data Collection Policies That Work, Hartford, CT. Retrieved from http://www.ct.gov/dph/lib/dph/hisr/pdf/taylor_remarks.pdf

Tervalon, M., & Murray-García, J. (1998). Cultural humility versus cultural competence: A critical distinction in defining physician training outcomes in multicultural education. *Journal of Health Care for the Poor and Underserved, 9*(2), 117–125.

Theisen, C. (2004). In different cultures, cancer screening presents a challenge. *Journal of the National Cancer Institute, 96*(1), 10–12.

U.S. Census Bureau. (2010). 2010 census data. Retrieved from http://2010.census.gov/2010census/

U.S. Census Bureau. (2011). Census Bureau releases estimates of same-sex married couples. http://2010.census.gov/news/releases/operations/cb11-cn181.html

U.S. Department of Health and Human Services, Agency for Healthcare Research and Quality. (2008). *2007 National healthcare disparities report.* Rockville, MD: Author. Retrieved from http://www.ahrq.gov/qual/nhdr07/nhdr07.pdf

Zeserson, J. M. (2001). How Japanese women talk about hot flashes: Implications for menopause research. *Medical Anthropology Quarterly, 15*(2), 189–205.

For a full suite of assignments and additional learning activities, see the access code at the front of your book.

3

Global Diversity

KEY TERMS www

Bicultural

Diversity

Health disparities

INTRODUCTION

The movement toward cultural competency is in no small part a response to the growing diversity occurring in the United States. The population of the United States is extremely diverse and becoming even more so with each passing year. Depending on what Congress decides to do about immigration—curtail it, expand it, and so forth—the United States is facing a future population just 40 years away that could vary by more than 135 million residents. Our population is going to be growing in any case, largely because of immigrants who have arrived in the past few generations, but that growth could be limited to about 72 million persons (a 24.6% increase) if illegal immigration is significantly curtailed (Martin

& Fogel, 2006). Alternatively, if current proposals of immigration reform, such as giving legal status to those currently here illegally, and the creation of a new guest worker program were adopted, we will likely be facing the prospect of a population in 2050 of half a billion people. That would be about 200 million more persons than live here today (a 67% increase) (Martin & Fogel, 2006). What is known from the 2010 census data is that the U.S. population grew by 9.7% since the year 2000. There was growth seen in the Latino population, but overall immigration to the United States has slowed, reversing a trend of steady growth over the past 30 years (U.S. Census Bureau, 2010a).

What is the cultural makeup of our current and projected population? For the first time, racial and ethnic minorities make up more than half the children born in the United States At the same time the Hispanic/Latino population boom appears to have peaked due to the overall decline in immigration (Census 2012 estimates). Minorities increased 1.9% to 114.1 million (36.9%) of the total U.S. population. The recent slowdown in the growth of the Hispanic/Latino and Asian populations has resulted in a change to the projection on when the true tipping point in diversity will arrive—the time when non-Hispanic Whites become the minority. Initial review of the 2010 census data (U.S. Census Bureau, 2010a) suggested that this tipping point may occur as early as 2040, but now experts believe this date needs to be pushed back several more years. In 2011, non-White babies outnumbered non-Hispanic White babies for the first time (Pew Research Center, 2012).

Hispanic/Latinos and Asians remain the fastest growing minority groups. Hispanic/Latinos make up approximately 16.7 % of the U.S. population and Asians account for 4.8% of the total U.S. population. Blacks, who compose about 12.3% of the population, have maintained a population increase rate of about 1% annually, while the proportion of Whites in the United States has increased very little in recent years (U.S. Census Bureau, 2010a).

In 1970, about 83% of the 203 million U.S. residents were non-Hispanic Whites and only 6% were either Hispanic/Latino or Asian. In 2010, the United States had 310 million residents, of which 66% were non-Hispanic White, 13% were Black, 16% were Hispanic/Latino, 4% were Asian, and 2% were identified as "other" (U.S. Census Bureau, 2010a).

Recent immigration patterns and policies show both continuity and change. Continuity is reflected in the arrival to the United States of an average of 104,000 foreigners per day. This group includes 3,100 persons who have received immigrant visas that allow them to settle and become naturalized citizens after five years, and 99,200 others who are made up of tourists and those with either a business or student visa. On average, approximately 2,000 people enter the United States without authorization per day. Over half of these come from Mexico. The other half initially enter the country legally but then violate the terms of their visa by either going to work illegally or by failing to depart the country when their visa expires (Passel & Taylor, 2010). From 2005 to 2009, the number of people entering the United States illegally declined by nearly 67%, according to the Pew Hispanic Center, from 850,000 yearly average in the early 2000s to 300,000 (Passel & Taylor, 2010).

Immigration, legal and otherwise, impacts not only the United States, but also impacts the country from which the immigrants come. Previously, Mexico was the primary source of immigration into the United States—both legal and illegal. Mexico accounted for approximately 18% of legal immigration admissions between 1993 and 2002. Net migration from Mexico to the United States, both legal and illegal, now stands at zero—or less. In other words, the number of migrants coming here from Mexico is equal to, or less than, the number of migrants leaving or being deported from the United States and returning to Mexico (Passel & Taylor, 2010).

Racial and ethnic minorities, especially those with low incomes and limited English proficiency, experience multiple barriers to health care, encounter lower access to and availability of health care, and experience less favorable health outcomes according to the groundbreaking Institute of Medicine report (IOM, 2003), *Patient Safety: Achieving a New Standard of Care*. There is also evidence that stereotypes associated with sex, age, diagnosis, sexual orientation, socioeconomic status, obesity, and race/ethnicity influence providers' beliefs about and expectations of patients.

CULTURAL DIVERSITY DEFINED

The very nature of nursing encompasses the need to be aware of cultural diversity. The culture of the United States is made up of cultures from throughout the world. This complexity of cultural diversity within the healthcare system requires dedication and an ongoing commitment by the nurse to master—it cannot be achieved overnight, and in reality should be a career-long endeavor (Lowe & Archibald, 2009). The continuing and ongoing changes of the cultural makeup of patients within the U.S. healthcare delivery system results in a daily challenge for the nurse to not only recognize the diverse needs of each and every patient, but also incorporate their needs into the quality nursing care that needs to be provided. The prevalence of cultural diversity requires the nurse to strive for cultural competence, so he or she may meet society's expectations regarding nursing care delivery. The cultural makeup of the nursing workforce indicates that nursing does not have sufficient numbers of minority nurses. The minority nursing workforce totals only 16.8% of the total RN workforce. The registered nurse (RN) minority workforce is made up of 5.4% Black American, 3.6% Hispanic/Latino, 5.8% Asian/Native Hawaiian, and 0.3% American Indian and Alaska Native. The remaining 1.7% identified as multiracial (National Sample Survey of Registered Nurses [NSSRN], 2008).

Healthcare disparities persist for the millions of Americans who are members of minority groups because they are not attaining patient outcomes that reflect the progress in medical technology and medical research. Just how different are minority patient outcomes? Members of ethnic minority groups (even those who are well educated, well insured, and who possess adequate financial means) have a shorter lifespan and die faster from every type of disease or illness—with the exception of suicide (Lowe & Archibald, 2009). To combat this phenomenon, it is therefore essential that every nurse is prepared to meet the unique healthcare needs for each and every culturally diverse patient who enters his or her care. The nurse must not lose site of the risk of falling prey to stereotyping. Each patient must be individually assessed to see which (if any) cultural beliefs they possess that differ from the nurse's beliefs (Lowe & Archibald, 2009). The nurse must also avoid being ethnocentric. The avoidance of ethnocentrism means that you view yourself as being different rather than the "others" as being different, and to give value to each culture for its unique contributions to society and to the world at large.

CULTURAL FACTORS IMPACTING THE CLINICAL RELATIONSHIP

An awareness of a person's cultural frame of reference is essential. Cultural frame of reference is defined as those elements that cause a cultural group to interpret the world in a particular manner. This can also be described as the filter through which perceptions of, encounters with, and understandings of the outside world are ordered and made meaningful. Culture can be assessed according to four specific areas: cultural identity of the individual, cultural explanations of the individual, cultural factors regarding social environment, and lifestyle and cultural factors affecting relationships with others.

Unaddressed cultural differences between the nurse and the patient can result in difficulties with diagnosis, nonadherence, and mutual frustration when the patient or the nurse does not meet the implicit, culturally determined expectations of the other. There can, in some circumstances, be a benefit when there are cultural differences between nurse and patient. For example, some patients may report symptoms and more readily accept treatment from an empathetic nurse who is not of the same culture as the patient, because they may believe that confidentiality will be maintained and the stigma will be lessened (Rubio-Stipec, Hsiao-Rei Hicks, & Tsuang, 2000).

The nurse should be aware that no one is culture-free in their assessments. The encounter between the patient and the nurse is an interaction between two explanatory models of illness. This is true even when both are from the same cultural background because intracultural differences in how sickness and the healthcare system are viewed can be as great as any existing intercultural differences. To avoid any misunderstandings, the nurse must be aware of his or her own belief system and take care not to stereotype or make assumptions about the patient.

The physician's model, which is the Western Biomedical Model, is disease oriented, with the goal of determining the biologic or pathologic cause and executing a cure for that disease process. Nurses, by virtue of working in the healthcare system and following medical orders, often share this disease-oriented view. Many nurse practitioner programs educate using this model for diagnosis and treatment as well. Not only is the biomedical model in contrast to the illness model of the patient, it is also flawed because medicine is commonly viewed as a reductionist science. Medicine is considered to be objective and neutral, dealing only in the truth or facts. In reality, medicine is grounded in social and cultural behaviors. Therefore, the nurse, to be truly culturally sensitive, must be aware of assumptions about medical systems and recognize that other systems may be considered equally valid for patients. The patient's explanatory model will be illness oriented. This model is culturally determined and provides the meaning of the sickness for the individual: how they decide that they are ill, what they believe is the reason for the illness, how they cope, and when or if they decide they are no longer ill.

Although the patient's explanatory model is culturally determined, it may differ in the same individual with different illnesses or different stages of illness. Therefore, the nurse must determine the model for each illness episode for each patient. For instance, a patient may have a relatively biomedical approach to a sickness episode until the stress of end-of-life issues results in a reversion to original values and traditions.

It is also important to consider whether the explanatory framework is a physical or psychosocial one. Utilizing a physical explanatory framework (illness is a result of a disruption of a bodily or physiologic process) instead of a psychosocial explanatory framework (illness is a response to thoughts or emotions that are a result of social factors) results in a very different view of the illness itself. This can be problematic when the nurse's and patient's explanatory frameworks are different.

An attempt should be made to determine how culture-bound the patient may be for each illness, and again periodically throughout a prolonged illness. The nurse should ask for an explanation, as a part of the history of present illness, as to what the patient believes caused the illness, the expected course, and expectations of treatment. Determining the patient's explanatory model should be a routine part of taking a patient's history (Kleinman, 1988). See **Table 3–1** for questions the nurse can ask to determine the patient's explanatory model for illness.

If necessary, ask for clarifications of the patient's illness along the way. If you feel the explanation is unusual or unfamiliar, consider that it may have a cultural explanation, rather than being indicative of or a result of a psychiatric disorder (e.g., the African patient who feels he may have a spell cast on him). It is also important not to automatically use culture as the sole explanation—striking a balance is the key. Culture can be a red herring, which means it can be overattributed as the cause or reason for symptoms to be present. This can result in mistakes in diagnosis and treatment (Stein, 1985).

The questions associated with the patient's explanatory model of illness address the major issues of concern to the nurse and nurse practitioner: etiology, pathophysiologic alteration, usual or expected course, and treatment. Neither the medical nor the patient's model is sufficient alone. Both approaches are needed for the provision of culturally sensitive, patient-centered care. Once the nurse has a working knowledge of the patient's model, the nurse can determine if treatments

---

Table 3–1 Questions the Nurse Can Ask to Determine a Patient's Explanatory Model of Illness

1. What do you call this illness? Does it have a name?
2. What do you think caused it?
3. Why did it happen at this time?
4. How does the illness affect you?
5. What does it do to you?
6. How bad is it?
7. How long do you think it will last?
8. Do you think treatment will work for it?
9. What kind of treatment do you think you should have?
10. Have you tried any other treatments already?

Source: Hanson, M., Russel, L., Robb, A., & Tabak, D. (1996). *Cross-cultural interviewing: A guide for teaching and evaluation.* Toronto, Ontario: University of Toronto.

(such as herbal or alternative therapies) are previously or concurrently being used by the patient and if they are beneficial, harmful, or neutral. If a treatment is determined to be beneficial or neutral, it is recommended to incorporate the patient's intervention into the plan of care. If an intervention is deemed harmful, it requires that the nurse develop a teaching plan that is culturally competent, and must ensure that the patient is fully informed as to the danger, or potential risk for danger, the intervention poses. The nurse's view of illness can be shared with the patient, and then a negotiation must take place to achieve a shared understanding of the illness so that a treatment plan can be put in place.

THE IMPORTANCE OF STRIVING FOR UNDERSTANDING

The progression toward cultural understanding, and ultimately to competency, is vital to be an effective nurse in the multicultural 21st century. The impact of global health work can only be as strong as its cultural relevance. As much as we would like to jump in and begin the encounter, there are many various cultural nuances and ethnic differences that are not readily apparent. Success of the nursing interaction rests on the nurse's ability to work with the patient within their cultural context. The successful nurse today must be able to function in cross-cultural patient encounters. Developing this ability begins with first having the willingness to learn as much as possible, maintaining cultural humility, and taking the time for self-reflection to evaluate your progress along the way.

The degree of family involvement in patient illness is also culturally driven. Many patients come from cultures in which the family and community involvement in the individual's illness episode is much more than occurs in other cultures, such as those from countries in Europe and North America. This has implications for how the nurse approaches important issues such as consent, patient confidentiality, and controversy over how to proceed with treatment and ethical dilemmas (e.g., do not resuscitate orders, transplantation, organ donation, assisted suicide). Obtaining information regarding the family structure is a good starting point: Who is the head of the family? Is this the same person who will be making the medical decisions? Is this the same person as the patient? Another important consideration is what community resources are available, and if the patient utilizes those services, whether confidentiality be maintained (this may be more of an issue in small geographic areas or if limited resources or agencies are available). Other relevant questions include the patient and medical decision maker's educational backgrounds, as well as the patient's health literacy level. It is important that these factors be assessed prior to planning any educational interventions.

LANGUAGE BARRIERS

The nurse needs to assess the patient's fluency in English if the patient is communicating without an interpreter and he or she speaks English as a second language. Do not automatically assume that a patient with a heavy accent is not fluent or that just because it appears a patient is fluent that they comprehend the conversation. The easiest and quickest way to assess comprehension is to ask the patient to repeat back an explanation or instruction.

Do not rely on nonverbal cues for comprehension, as many patients will nod or indicate agreement out of respect or embarrassment, even when they do not understand. Even the apparent proper use of language in seemingly fluent individuals can result in misunderstandings. In addition, violations in the rules of grammar may make a person seem vague and indecisive. The nurse should consciously avoid the use of idioms when speaking with patients and especially when providing patient education. The use of idiomatic expressions may baffle a person not well versed in English (e.g., quitting "cold turkey" when discussing smoking cessation).

PROPER USE OF INTERPRETERS

Because it is essential that the nurse and patient be fully able to communicate effectively with each other, if it is determined that an interpreter is needed, request one. It is essential that all medical and cultural issues be fully explored, which cannot occur if there is a language barrier not bridged by the use of a qualified professional interpreter. If an interpreter is used, he or she becomes a critical component of the encounter. It is highly recommended to use only professional interpreters who are culturally competent in the patient's culture. This is so important that it is recommended that if the medical situation is not urgent, and it is safe to do so, it is preferable to postpone the interview until the services of a cultural or professional interpreter can be obtained. This is often very time consuming and frustrating, but it will be well worth the effort because of the quality of information that will be obtained. Often, because of time constraints or other variables, this may not be possible and poor choices can be made.

The use of or reliance on family members to serve as translators should be avoided unless absolutely necessary. This is very important to emphasize because there can be serious negative consequences if family members are used as translators/interpreters. The family member or the patient may editorialize extensively, and the nurse would have no way of knowing this was occurring. Editing questions and responses greatly reduces the amount and accuracy of the information transmitted from and to the patient. Role strain can be another serious consequence resulting from this practice. Both editorializing and role strain can occur if a child is asked to translate sensitive issues regarding his parents (e.g., a male child translating for his mother who is having a gynecological issue such as extensive vaginal bleeding).

Access to a professional interpreter does not mean adequate communication is guaranteed. There are some skills associated with the effective use of interpreters that the nurse should be aware of. Ascertain the interpreter's qualifications. If a trained professional interpreter is available, they probably need no instructions or reminders about confidentiality or the process of triadic interviewing. A professional interpreter will be capable of culturally interpreting the patient's meaning, which saves time. If there is no professional interpreter available and you must use a nonprofessional who speaks the same language, such as a hospital employee, you will need to spend time explaining the process in much more detail and emphasizing the interpreter's responsibility to maintain confidentiality and not to editorialize. Brief the interpreter by informing them about the situation and the need for interpreter services. Let them know how you wish to proceed. Just because the interpreter may work in the hospital does not mean they are familiar with or comfortable dealing with a patient encounter, especially if it is an acute or urgent situation. Let the interpreter know that you expect and need them to translate exactly what is said by both parties. Assure them that you will use brief sentences to allow the interview to proceed more quickly and to increase accuracy. Let the interpreter know that you will be looking at and speaking to the patient and that you will be seated in a triad during the interview process. Be alert for signs that all of the information is not being translated accurately (e.g., a long conversation in the patient's language, followed by a short translation to you, or vice versa).

CULTURAL HUMILITY

A nurse who possesses cultural humility recognizes the limitations of his or her cultural perspective and works toward overcoming this perspective in order to provide better nursing care to all patients. It is an acknowledgment that you are aware of the inherent barriers that exist from your own culture—that indeed your own perspective is limited. Having this focus makes it much easier for the nurse to be reflective and proactive about any prejudices or assumptions they have, so that they are less likely to have an impact on a cross-cultural nursing interaction. This is not the whole description, however. The nurse must also not assume that all members of a certain culture conform to a certain stereotype and acknowledge that each patient is a unique individual and deserves to be treated as such.

The nurse who has cultural humility will be less likely to act in an authoritarian way or assume a power position over the patient. Cultural humility is seen as an important step in redressing the power imbalance between provider and patient, because the nurse who recognizes that his or her own perspective is full of assumptions is more likely to maintain an open mind, be respectful of all people, and not act as if his or her way is the only or best way to proceed. Cultural humility should always be practiced, even if a nurse feels they have worked and developed true cultural competency. This is necessary because even though the nurse may have extensive knowledge of a culture, he or she is not "living" that culture, which means there will still be differences between the nurse's perspectives and those of the actual members of the learned culture.

IMPACT OF DIVERSITY

The data presented here is to provide you with an overview of demographic data from the 2010 U.S. census and other government agencies (U.S. Census Bureau, 2010a). There is no doubt that the population of the United States is extremely diverse and becoming even more so with each passing year.

According to the U.S. Census Bureau estimates from 2011, the minority population now accounts for 36.9% of the total U.S. population. This means one in three U.S. residents is a minority (U.S. Census Bureau, 2010a). The nation's Black population is 12.8% of the total U.S. population, a 12.3% increase from the 2000 census data (U.S. Census Bureau, 2010a).

According to the 2012 estimate from the U.S. Census Bureau (2010a), the current population of the United States is 314,454,829. Of that number, 72.4% are considered White (non-Hispanic). Hispanic/Latinos make up 16.3% (a 43% increase from the 2000 census data) of the population, African Americans 12.8% (an increase of 12.3% from the 2000 census data), Asians 4.8% (an increase of 43.3%), American Indian and Alaska Native 0.9% (an increase of 18.4%), Native Hawaiian/Pacific Islander 0.2% (an increase of 35.4%), and 2.9% of our population was identified as belonging to two or more races (an increase of 32%) (U.S. Census Bureau, 2010a). Our country continues toward even more diversity, as demonstrated by significant increases in the numbers and proportion of minority populations.

Another key consideration in attempting to understand diversity is that in contemporary U.S. society, many individuals, probably the majority, are or consider themselves to be bicultural. Membership in more than one culture is not the same as being biracial or multiracial (McGrath, 1998). A person may self-identify with more than one cultural group and that bicultural person sees both sides and can function in both worlds (McGrath, 1998).

There is a correlation among race, economic status, and poor health (**Boxes 3–1** and **3–2**): 12% of nonelderly (age 65 or younger) Whites (non-Hispanics) are considered poor, as they fall below the federal poverty level, and 8% self-rated their health as fair or poor; 29% of nonelderly Hispanic/Latinos are considered poor and 13% have fair or poor health; 33% of nonelderly Black Americans are considered poor and 15% have fair or poor health; 17% of nonelderly Asians are considered poor and 9% have fair or poor health; 34% of nonelderly American Indians are considered poor and 17% have fair or poor health; and 21% of the nonelderly members of two or more races are considered poor and 13% have fair or poor

---

Box 3–1 Nonelderly Population by Race/Ethnicity as of 2005

White	African American	Hispanic	Asian	American Indian/ Alaska Native	Two or More Races
166.6 million	32.6 million	40.8 million	11.8 million	1.5 million	4.2 million

Source: U.S. Census Bureau, 2005.

Box 3–2 Poverty Status of the Nonelderly Population by Race/Ethnicity as of 2005

White	African American	Hispanic	Asian	American Indian/ Alaska Native	Two or More Races
74% Nonpoor (200% + FPL)	46% Nonpoor (200% + FPL)	42% Nonpoor (200% + FPL)	68% Nonpoor (200% + FPL)	43% Nonpoor (200% + FPL)	59% Nonpoor (200% + FPL)

Source: U.S. Census Bureau, 2005.

health (Urban Institute and Kaiser Commission, 2006). The federal poverty level was set by the government as income below $19,971 for a family of four.

Diversity also impacts health insurance coverage (**Box 3–3** and **Box 3–4**). The racial group with the highest percentage of people lacking health insurance is the nonelderly American Indian/Alaska Native population at 32.9%. Whites, at 14.3%, have the lowest percentage of people lacking health insurance coverage (Institute of Medicine, 2009). Lack of health insurance coverage is a significant barrier and clearly this burden is felt more severely by minority patients. The Institute of Medicine (2004, p. 11) states in its report, *Insuring America's Health*, that "health insurance contributes essentially to obtaining the kind and quality of health care that can express the equality and dignity of every person." Clearly, the lack of health insurance is an important barrier to the elimination of healthcare disparities.

Historically, our culture diversity has identified, separated, bound, and evolved us. The implication is that some cultural features are not only different from others but are better than others. This is supported by the fact that all people have repeatedly chosen to abandon some feature of their own culture in order to replace it with something from another culture, because the replacement feature is deemed more effective. Some examples of this are the switch from Roman numerals (even

Box 3–3 Uninsured (Health Insurance) Percentage of the Nonelderly by Race/Ethnicity as of 2007

White	African American	Hispanic	Asian	American Indian/ Alaska Native	Two or More Races
14.3%	19.2%	32.1%	16.8%	32.9%	19.5%

Source: The Institute of Medicine (2009). America's uninsured crisis: Consequences for health and health care. Washington, D.C.: The National Academies Press.

Box 3–4 Percentage of Adults (Age 18–64) without a Usual Source of Health Care by Race/Ethnicity as of 2005

White	African American	Hispanic/ Latino	Asian	American Indian/ Alaska Native	Two or More Races
15%	18%	31%	19%	21%	18%

Source: U.S. Census Bureau, 2005.

in countries whose own cultures derived from Rome) to Arabic numerals and the fact that produce indigenous to one area of a country is now being produced and exported from a different country (most rice is now grown in Africa but originated in Asia). One should view cultural diversity both internationally and historically as a dynamic competition in which what serves humankind survives, and what does not disappears (Sowell, 1991). The will to survive is a common link as exemplified by the explorers that moved throughout the globe to explore "new" worlds and lands. Just as the colonists in America learned survival skills from Native Americans, the first Europeans who entered Australia with its rough terrain learned from the Australian aborigines. The goal was survival, and meeting that objective often required change and adaptation. A given culture may not be superior in all settings and at all times, but certain cultural features of that specific culture may be superior for certain purposes and at certain times.

Certain countries and civilizations have experienced different levels of cultural leadership over time (Sowell, 1991). There have been rises and falls of nations and empires throughout history: the Roman Empire, the Golden Age of Spain, the technology explosion in Japan, and the West of today. Certain cultural groups have been associated with certain skills or talents and occupations. Italians are known for wine production, Germans for beer making, and Jews in the apparel industry (Sowell, 1991). Geography has a role to play not only through the provision of or lack of natural resources, but also because geography permits or limits opportunity for cultural interaction among different groups. The more isolated the geography, the more isolated the culture associated with that area. Access to water (either the sea at a port on the coastline or a river near or in a city) is another very important geographical determinant associated with sustaining life. Positive geographical features permit humans to interact with each other and with others, sharing their culture. Culture can exist in isolation as well. Culture dictates how we do all of the things that have to be done to live life where we are living it. Culture exists to serve the practical requirements of life: to structure society, to perpetuate life, to pass on hard-earned knowledge and skills, and to spare the next generation the trial and error of learning how to live life.

How much culture a person chooses to retain is a personal decision. Every culture makes changes over time—how much of the old to retain and how much of the new to embrace—and as such culture is dynamic.

CULTURALLY DISCORDANT CARE

Although this growing diversity has been seen and continues to widen within the American population, the same cannot be said for our country's population of healthcare professionals. This lack of a parallel growth in the diversity among healthcare professionals impacts healthcare delivery and suggests that many patients are receiving culturally discordant medical care. Culturally discordant care arises from unaddressed cultural differences between healthcare providers and their patients. Research has shown that significant disparities in health status, treatment, and medical outcomes between groups of patients who differ on the basis of gender, race, or ethnicity exist. A provider's unconscious bias about a particular race, ethnicity, or culture, or a lack of effective cross-cultural communication skills may contribute to discordant medical care and health disparities. Racial discordance in medical encounters is prevalent and often inevitable due to the lack of diversity in the healthcare workforce in the United States. A relatively small percentage of minority patients are likely to have access to health professionals that are from the same race or ethnic group (only 23% of Black Americans, 26% of Hispanic/Latinos, and 39% of Asian Americans). This is a significantly lower percentage than the 82% of White patients who have a physician from the same racial or ethnic group (Collins et al., 2002). Although research supports the desire for patients to have a provider from their racial/ethnic group, the lack of workforce diversity makes this very difficult, if not impossible, for everyone except White patients. To compensate for the lack of diversity, all healthcare providers should know how to interact effectively with and provide care for patients whose ethnic or cultural background differs from their own to lessen the impact of culturally discordant care on health disparities.

HEALTH DISPARITIES

It is also important to recognize that perception can impact our understanding of health disparities. Two studies conducted by the Kaiser Family Foundation (2004) are revelatory when physician and patient perceptions are compared to each other (**Box 3–5**). There was no significant difference found between physicians and the public in the perception of how often they thought our healthcare system treats people unfairly based on whether a patient had insurance (72% doctors and 70% patients).

Healthcare disparities refer to differences in access to or availability of facilities and services (National Library of Medicine, 2012). Health status disparities refer to the variation in rates of disease occurrence and disabilities between socioeconomic or geographically defined population groups, and differences in the incidence, prevalence, mortality, and burden of diseases and other adverse health conditions that exist among specific population groups (National Library of Medicine, 2012). Despite scientific medical advances, the poor and non-White ethnic minorities are

---

Box 3–5 Physician Versus Public Perceptions of Disparities in Health Care

Question: Generally speaking, how often do you think our healthcare system treats people unfairly based on:

	(Percentage stating very/ somewhat often)
What their race or ethnic background is?	29% physicians 47% patients
Whether they are male or female?	15% physicians 27% patients
How well they speak English?	43% physicians 58% patients

---

ranked lower in health status on numerous measures. The literature reveals that the reasons for the lower health status rankings are potentially many: genetic differences, gender differences, stereotyping, perceived discrimination, mistrust of the medical community, ineffective or poor communication, economic differences, clinical uncertainty by provider, biologic treatment variations, and lack of access. This problem is so significant, that in 2010 the National Institutes of Health (NIH) transitioned the National Center on Minority Health and Health Disparities to the National Institute on Minority Health and Health Disparities, because an institute can have a more defined research agenda within the NIH than a center.

IMPACT OF DIVERSITY ON DIAGNOSIS AND TREATMENT

At no time in the history of the United States has the health status of minority populations—Black Americans, Native Americans, Hispanic/Latinos, and some Asian subgroups—equaled or even approximated that of White Americans (Geiger, 2003). Despite the medical and scientific advances that occurred in the 20th century, the excess morbidity and decreased life expectancy for people of color have persisted. In 1995, the overall Black American mortality rate was 60% higher than that of Whites—precisely what it had been in 1950. Black Americans today continue to die disproportionately from chronic disease (Geronimus, Bound, & Colen, 2011). Despite steady improvement in the overall health of Americans, racial and ethnic minorities, with few exceptions, experience higher rates of morbidity and mortality than nonminorities. **Table 3–2** lists barriers to cross-cultural communication that can impact the advance practice nurse or

Table 3–2 Barriers to Cross-Cultural Communication That Can Impact Diagnosis and Treatment

1. Belief that cross-cultural communication entails learning the details of every existing cultural belief system.
2. Belief that such skills are impractical in that it is too time consuming.
3. Belief that the Western Biomedical Model is the only valid model of health care.
4. Physician/nurse lack of experience.

Source: Hanson, M., Russel, L., Robb, A., & Tabak, D. (1996). *Cross-cultural interviewing: A guide for teaching and evaluation.* Toronto, Ontario: University of Toronto.

Table 3–3 Strategies to Improve Cross-Cultural Communication

1. Do not rush through the encounter; take time to establish a human connection.
2. Use plain language whenever possible (avoid medical jargon and never assume the patient understands any medical terminology).
3. Use pictures (show them or draw them) to better illustrate the content.
4. Provide just enough information; do not overload the patient with too much information.
5. Use the "teach back" technique (in a nonthreatening way, have the patient repeat back what was discussed during the encounter).
6. Encourage questions through the provision of a comfortable and open environment.

Adapted from: Mandell, B. F. (2012) Talking to patients: Barriers to overcome. *Cleveland Clinic Journal of Medicine, 79*(2), 90; Misra-Hebert, A. D., & Isaccson, J. H. (2012). Overcoming health care disparities via better cross-cultural communication and health literacy. *Cleveland Clinic Journal of Medicine, 79*(2), 127–133; and Weiss, B. D. (2007). *Health literacy and patient safety: Help patients understand* (2nd ed.). American Medical Association Foundation and American Medical Association. Retrieved from http://www.ama-assn.org/ama1/pub/upload/mm/367/healthlitclinicians.pdf

nurse's ability to properly diagnose and treat patients. **Table 3–3** provides strategies to improve cross-cultural communication that the nurse can utilize.

BARRIERS TO HEALTH CARE

In order for people to receive adequate health care, a number of potential barriers need to be addressed, including the "11 A's": availability, accessibility, affordability, appropriateness, accountability, adaptability, acceptability, awareness, attitudes, approachability, and alternative practices and additional services availability. Other barriers include fragmentation of care and cultural insensitivity of healthcare providers. Quality care is not possible if the provider lacks sensitivity to the patient's culture (Giger, 2013; Purnell, 2013; Saha, Komaromy, Koepsell,

& Bindman, 1999). Effective patient care can be enhanced through awareness of one's own culture and how it may differ from other individuals' sociocultural experiences (Purnell, 2013). A healthcare provider who lacks awareness of cultural issues is culturally blind, and this type of provider requires the patient to accept the Western Biomedical Model of health, which may be in conflict with the patient's own views and beliefs. This type of narrow view, which is cultural blindness or cultural dogmatism, can lead to disaster, a tragic example of which is detailed in the book, *The Spirit Catches You and You Fall Down*, by Fadiman (1997). The healthcare provider can overcome barriers and learn a lot by watching for varying interpretations of language, nonverbal interactions, and patient and provider responsibility.

Another barrier is the lack of understanding of the impact of cultural epidemiology. Cultural epidemiology is often not emphasized in health professions training, even though the epidemiology of diseases and individual interpretation varies among populations. This means that a commitment to continuing education must be a focus of the nurse, and the nurse must seek out learning opportunities to learn more about various cultures. It is important to remember that with the vast number of ethnic and cultural groups in the United States, it is impossible for anyone to gain knowledge of all of the groups. A more reasonable approach may be to use the culture general approach. With the culture general approach, healthcare professionals develop the knowledge, skills, and approaches that may be effectively used with any group or individual who comes from a different cultural background (Taylor, 2005). This skill set would include acknowledgment of differences, advocacy for marginalized clients, and intolerance of inequity, bias, and stereotyping.

ETHNOPHARMACOLOGY

Ethnopharmacology is also an important consideration when attempting to provide culturally appropriate care. Ethnopharmacology (or ethnic pharmacology) is a field of study that investigates variant responses to drugs in ethnic and racial groups. Ethnopharmacologic research has revealed that ethnicity significantly affects response to some drugs. Genetic or cultural factors, or both, may influence a given drug's pharmacokinetics (absorption, metabolism, distribution, and elimination) and pharmacodynamics (mechanism of action and effects at the target site), as well as whether a patient will be adherent to the drug therapy and the necessary patient education that would be required for maximum benefit. As the nurse attempts to consider the impact of ethnopharmacology on a patient encounter, it leads to an important consideration—in a world of mixed heritages, how does a nurse or physician even determine a patient's race? Promoting certain drugs for race-specific markets could lead to stereotyping and discrimination. The issue is further complicated because some feel that racial categories are a societal construct and not a scientific one. In an attempt to overcome these factors, new drug research is focusing on designing drugs to target certain genes, eliminating the need to weigh race or ethnicity.

REASONS FOR HEALTH DISPARITIES

The many reasons for health disparities are complex and require further investigation. This research initiative is being spearheaded by the National Institute of Health. What has been discovered so far indicates that socioeconomic differences, differences in health-related risk factors, environmental factors, discrimination, and barriers such as access, all play a role. An important concept for the nurse to understand is that the differences in health that certain populations experience are due to factors that are beyond the individual patient's control. Not only is it not the patient's fault, but the patient is often powerless to change the situation, because the root causes of health disparities are systemic, institutionalized, and they have accumulated after many decades or even centuries. The relationships among the root causes of health disparities are multidirectional and cyclical, exacerbating one another and calling for intervention at every level. As nurses, we have a role to play in lessening the impact of health disparities through the delivery of culturally competent care. Keep in mind that Hispanics, Asian Americans, American Indians, Alaska Natives, and Black Americans are all less likely than Whites to have health insurance, have more difficulty getting health care, and have fewer choices in where to receive that care. Hispanic and Black American patients are more likely to receive care in hospital emergency rooms and are less likely than Whites to have a primary care provider.

Perhaps most disturbing is that when adjustments have been made to correct access issues, disparity still persists. Even when equivalent access to care exists, racial and ethnic minorities experience a lower quality of health services and are less likely to receive even routine medical procedures than White Americans. An example of this is that Black Americans and Hispanics are less likely than Whites to receive appropriate cardiac medication (thrombolytic therapy, aspirin, and beta-blockers) or to undergo coronary artery bypass surgery (Mickelson, Blum, & Geraci, 1997).

In summary, racial and ethnic minorities are less likely than Whites to possess health insurance, are more likely to be beneficiaries of publicly funded health insurance, and even when insured, may face additional barriers to care because of other socioeconomic factors, such as high copayments, geographic factors such as the scarcity of healthcare providers in some minority communities, and insufficient transportation. Access-related factors pose a most significant barrier to equitable care, and access must be addressed systemically in order to have any chance of eliminating healthcare disparities.

GLOBAL HEALTHCARE DISPARITIES

Public health experts have identified a significant deficit of resources to deal with the diseases that have a global impact. This deficit is referred to as the 10/90 gap. This means only 10% of the world's health research budget is spent on diseases that affect 90% of the world's population (Resnik, 2004). Global health disparities is such an apparent and pressing issue that the United Nations has set global mandates entitled the United Nations Millennium Development Goals (United Nations Development Programme, 2008). Poverty is an important component for global health disparities. The World Health Organization (WHO) estimates that diseases associated with poverty, such as tuberculosis, malaria, and HIV/AIDs, account for 45% of the disease burden in the poorest countries of the world (WHO, 2004). This does not need to be the case because many of these diseases are preventable or can be treated with medications that are already available. Vitamin A deficiency, a cause of blindness, can be eradicated through vitamin A supplementation. If there are solutions and treatments available, why does this global problem persist? It appears that lack of access is the culprit. Lack of access is an intractable political and economic problem. According to the World Health Organization (2004), an estimated 30% of the world population lacks regular access to existing drugs, with this figure rising to over 50% in the poorest parts of Africa and Asia.

Some of these patients are coming to the United States for treatment, which means nurses and other healthcare providers are being called on to care for patients from a widening and expanding range of cultural backgrounds. This explosion in diversity has resulted in an evolution in conceptualizing how nurses should function in global healthcare settings. The evolution has been from an initial awareness or sensitivity to cultural differences, to striving for competence or being able to interact effectively with people from a different culture than one's own, to cultural humility. Cultural humility does not have an end point or the objective of mastery (which some experts claim is a lofty standard that few, if any, nurses will attain). Cultural humility places the emphasis on the evolution of the nurse in a continual active process of self-reflection and self-critique (which is an activity that any nurse can participate in) and is seen as a way of engaging in the world and developing a therapeutic relationship with those who are culturally different from ourselves.

As members of the global healthcare community, all nurses must engage in an ongoing dialogue with themselves about the differences culture exerts on health outcomes, their own attitudes toward cultural differences, and their ability to objectively understand descriptions of cultural behaviors that are taken as explanatory. It is important that the descriptions they develop do not stereotype or constrain the different cultural groups that they work with and care for.

Nurses and nursing programs in the United States are expanding their focus to other healthcare systems. Nursing schools are offering cultural immersion experiences in various parts of the world, and more and more nurses and nursing faculty are having global nursing experiences. There will be more opportunities for collaboration, and learning more about our fellow nurses utilizing cultural humility may permit us to find common ground and a true appreciation for the diversity of our global partners.

GLOBAL DIVERSITY—THE ROLE OF NURSING

One would be mistaken to assume that health disparities are a problem confined to the United States. Differential treatment of minorities is not a uniquely American phenomenon. Nursing practice is a critical place to build diverse relationships for the purpose of globally providing optimal health for all. The National League for Nursing (NLN, 2011) has identified the role of nursing in global diversity as a critical priority. Our world is more open to migration than ever before. Despite our advancing technology and communication tools, there are still significant global healthcare needs and a worldwide shortage of nurses who are prepared to care for a racially and ethnically diverse patient population. The NLN is calling for nursing educational institutions to prepare an ethnically and racially diverse workforce, including faculty to mentor future nurses, and researchers to help to find solutions to the issues posed by our global diversity. What is known now is that the building of diverse relationships is key during times of a global nursing shortage. Nurses are challenged to view their patients from a variety of perspectives because of diverse global populations. Bridging the nurse/patient cultural gap can be a challenge. We must become aware of our differences to meet this challenge. Nurses are likely to feel helpless or powerless in effecting change when working with patients from another culture. Learning more about our differences may be helpful.

Disparities in health care continues to be a troubling issue for nursing, and despite attention being given to the issue, it is still a worldwide problem. Research and evidence-based nursing care are crucial to improving health care for all patients. Evidence-based nursing practice directed at how to effectively manage and treat diseases related to ethnic and racial minorities is imperative in overcoming current disparities in health care. In addition, more studies that listen to the voices of minority clients related to effective health interventions are needed to improve the quality of health care rendered to minority populations.

Cultural, ethnic, racial, language, and religious diversity exist in most nations in the world. One of the challenges to diverse democratic nation-states is to provide opportunities for different groups to maintain aspects of their community cultures while at the same time building a nation in which these groups are structurally included and to which they feel allegiance. A delicate balance of diversity and unity should be an essential goal of democratic nation-states and of teaching and learning in a democratic society. The challenge of balancing diversity and unity is intensifying as democratic nation-states such as the United States, Canada, Australia, the United Kingdom, and Japan become more diversified, and as racial and ethnic groups within these nations try to attain cultural, political, and economic rights.

These nations share the democratic ideal of inclusion of diverse groups into the mainstream society, but they are also characterized by widespread inequality through racial, ethnic, and class stratification. The discrepancy between this democratic ideal and reality can result in protest. During the 1960s and 1970s in the United States, the civil rights movement resulted in major change. A similar civil rights movement continues to spread throughout the world.

Because of technology, we are no longer just citizens of our country of origin but we are global citizens, and as such we need the knowledge, skills, and attitudes to function in this cultural community and to maintain our diversity and unity. We are becoming a multicultural global community.

CULTURE OF POVERTY

Poverty is a global phenomenon. The cycle of poverty perpetuates itself from generation to generation. Often, the motivation for immigration is the search for a better life or as a way out of poverty—to break the cycle. A child born into poverty is more likely to have poor intellectual and physical development. Often, the child lives in substandard housing in either a densely populated or remotely located rural area where water or other resources are scarce, resulting in poor nutrition and health. All of these poverty-related conditions result in high morbidity, substance abuse, and increased incidence of accidents and injury caused by violence.

UNITED STATES

According to the U.S. Census Bureau (2012) and international census data (2010), the United States is the third most populous country on Earth with a population of 312.8 million people. Despite this, the U.S. population composes only 4.5% of the total world's population. As a basis of comparison, China, with 1,339,724,852 inhabitants, makes up 58% of the world's total population. This relationship is not likely to change significantly in the future, because the world's population is continuing to grow at a rate of 1.1% annually.

The size of a country's total population tells only a small part of its demographic story. A country's population growth rate and its age–sex composition indicate the challenges it faces in providing health care for its children and elderly, providing education to its youth, providing employment opportunities for its young adults, and supporting its elderly population. According to 2010 census data, 21.2% of the U.S. population is under the age of 16 and 13% are 65 years old and over. Our country is benefitting from an increase in longevity for some populations, with 1.8% of our population now composed of people older than age 84 years. Females are now the slight majority, encompassing 50.8% of the U.S. population.

For the past 50 years, the United States (along with other more developed countries, moderately developed countries [MDCs], such as all of North America, Europe, Japan, Australia, and New Zealand) have differed from other less developed countries in fertility, mortality, and overall growth. The United States and all MDCs have typically had lower fertility, mortality, and population growth rates. This is now less true than in the past, and in the area of relative population growth is particularly alarming. From 1990 to 2000, the U.S. population increased by 13% (compared with only 2.5% for other MDCs combined). According to the most recent census data, the U.S. population continues to grow, but at a slower rate than in the previous decade (1990–2000), with a 9.8% increase (U.S. Census Bureau, 2010b). Access to these population numbers is essential for planning public policy to address many global issues. The distribution of the world's children and elderly older than age 80 indicates where the needs for children and elderly healthcare services are greatest in the world, and it is also used to predict where the needs for schooling and elderly support will be greatest in the coming years.

The country's age structure, its support ratios, and its national wealth indicate the extent to which it will be likely to address all of these age-related needs.

Alarmingly, 60% of the world's children younger than 5 years of age live in just 10 countries, of which the United States is one. Although people 24 years old or younger make up almost half of the world's population (with 1.2 billion between the ages of 10 and 19), their percentage of the population in some major developing countries is already at its peak, according to the Population Division of the United Nations Department of Economic and Social Affairs (2010a) in its *World Population Prospects: The 2010 Revision*. For example, in Mexico, reductions in fertility are already having a major impact. Mexico's population "pyramid" has been steadily shrinking at the bottom, with the birth-to-14 age group down from 38.6% of the total national count in 1990 to 34.1% in 2000, and 29.3% in 2010 (Population Division, 2010b). The country's median age has consequently risen from 19 to 26 in two decades.

The 2012 U.S. Census Bureau predicts that by 2025, the U.S. population will grow by 13%. This statistic in itself is alarming enough, but when immigration numbers are factored in, the increase swells to a 22% increase. Industrial nations as a group, including the United States, will be forced to support a growing elderly population with a smaller number of working adults. Despite this decrease in work support, the impact is expected to be less here in the United States than elsewhere worldwide because fertility and immigration tend to replenish our younger populations.

As of May 31, 2012, the population of the world was 7,016,939,519 and 313,647,805 in the United States. See **Figure 3–1** for the top 10 countries of the world ranked by population as of 2008.

Figure 3–1 Top 10 countries of the world by population.

	Country	Population
1	China	1,330,044,605
2	India	1,147,995,898
3	United States	304,228,257
4	Indonesia	237,512,355
5	Brazil	196,342,587
6	Pakistan	172,800,051
7	Bangladesh	154,037,902
8	Nigeria	146,255,306
9	Russia	140,702,094
10	Japan	127,288,419

Source: U.S. Census Bureau. (2008). International data base. Retrieved from http://www.census.gov/population/international/data/idb/sysmessage.php

UNITED KINGDOM

As of July 1, 2010, the population of the United Kingdom was ranked at 22 with a population of 62,262,000. The life expectancy at birth was 80.1 years of age (World Bank, 2009). See **Figure 3–2** for population pyramids for all countries described in this chapter from the year 2008 and estimated for the year 2025.

The transition of uniting the former countries into what today is the United Kingdom was a gradual process. Even after being recognized as one nation, there still remained hostility and cultural barriers. There had to be a new set of rules and guiding principles put into play in order to keep all satisfied. These guiding

Figure 3–2 Population pyramids showing statistics from 2008 and projections for 2025. (A) United Kingdom (B) Australia (C) Canada (D) South Africa

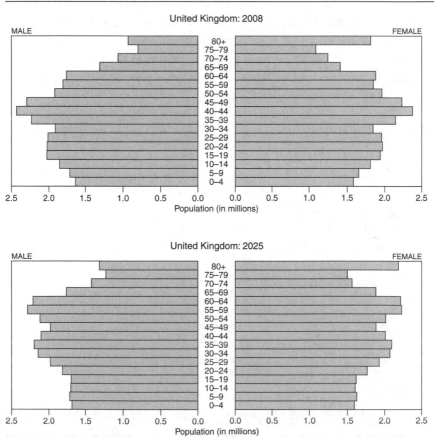

principles, such as the division of property, capitalism, and parliamentary democ-racy, along with technological advancements, are now present not only in the United Kingdom but also around the world. See **Figure 3–3** for demographic information related to the United Kingdom.

Despite a high caloric diet and minimal exercise, the average life span in the United Kingdom is 80.1 years of age. Healthcare dollars are almost entirely de-rived from taxes. The National Health Service has been criticized for long wait-ing periods and obsolete equipment and praised for its high number of qualified physicians.

Figure 3–2 *Continued*

(Continues)

Figure 3–2 *Continued*

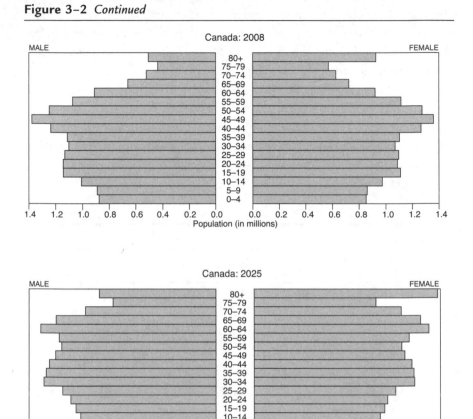

There have been published reports, since as early as 1981, which describe racism within the National Health Service in the United Kingdom. Language other than English and social class have been associated with impaired continuity of care (Hemingway, Saunders, & Parsons, 1997). Another study found that non-White patients are referred for coronary revascularization less often than White patients with similar severity of disease (Hemingway et al., 2001). According to Nazroo (2003), mortality data is not kept by ethnic group in the United Kingdom. When evaluating data on immigrant mortality rates and morbidity, heterogeneity of experience across minority groups was found. For most outcomes, Bangladeshi and Pakistani people report the poorest health, followed by Caribbean people and then Indian people, with Chinese and White people having the best health

Figure 3-2 *Continued*

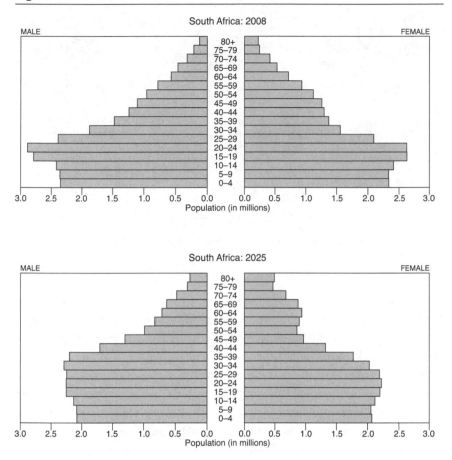

(Nazroo, 2003). Obviously, diversity is having an impact on health outcomes in the United Kingdom as well.

AUSTRALIA

The cultural competency movement is a global one and it is making itself known in Australia. Australia is an extremely diverse nation. The population of Australia as of June 2012 was 22,922,915 (Australian Bureau of Statistics, 2012). Australia's population comprises people with over 200 different ancestries. Over 200 languages are spoken and over 100 religions are observed. Almost one quarter of the population (22%) were born overseas and approximately 15% speak a

Figure 3–3 Breakdown of the demographics of the United Kingdom.

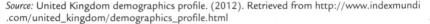

Source: United Kingdom demographics profile. (2012). Retrieved from http://www.indexmundi.com/united_kingdom/demographics_profile.html

language other than English at home (Australian Bureau of Statistics, 2012). In addition to this is the diversity within Australia's indigenous population who, at the last census, made up 2.4% of Australia's population (Australian Bureau of Statistics, 2012). Australia, like the United States, provides medical care according to the Western Biomedical Model. As has been discussed previously, for many client groups, this approach does not fit with their belief systems. When there is a mismatch between belief systems, health outcomes are likely to be poorer. The tendency of the health system (or more specifically medicine) to represent itself as a "culture of no culture" thus results in a culture-blind and ethnocentric approach. This effectively creates an exclusionary system that must be avoided.

An additional issue is the lack of health insurance among many Australians. According to the Australian Bureau of Statistics (2012), slightly over half of the population aged 15 years and over had private health insurance (53%) in 2007–2008. Of those persons with private health insurance, 77% had both hospital and ancillary coverage, 15% had hospital coverage only, and 7% had ancillary coverage only. The level and type of coverage differed across age groups, with the highest overall coverage in the 45–54-year and 55–64-year age groups (59% and 62%, respectively) and the lowest in the 25–34-year and 75-years-and-over age groups (both 45% with some form of private health insurance coverage). There is some flicker of improvement, however, for the Aboriginal Australian population. Healthcare expenditures for Aboriginal people were 3.5% of the total health expenditures for the years 2008–2009, which was an increase of 0.4% from the previous two years. The Aboriginal people make up about 2.5% of Australians. Healthcare expenditures are higher for this population ($1.39 per capita) compared to the non-Aboriginal Australian population ($1 spent per capita) (Australian Bureau of Statistic, 2012).

There is a growing body of work being produced to respond to Australasian contexts, some of it addressing the relationship between cultural respect and working with Aboriginal peoples. The health care of Aboriginal people in Australia has been criticized repeatedly during the past 20 years. It is well documented that the health status of Aboriginal and Torres Strait Islander people is substantially poorer than that of nonindigenous Australians. Disadvantages across a range of socioeconomic factors negatively impacts the health of Aboriginal and Torres Strait Islander people.

Both morbidity and mortality rates are higher, and indigenous people are more likely to experience disability and reduced quality of life because of ill health. Life expectancy of indigenous Australians is estimated to be approximately 20 years lower than for other Australians (Australian Bureau of Statistics & Australian Institute of Health and Welfare, 2003). Discrimination and stereotyping impacting the allocation of healthcare resources has also been described recently and historically (Awofeso, 2011; Lowe, Kerridge, & Mitchell, 1995). Encouragingly, Awofeso (2011) advocates for improved cultural competency skills as an effective strategy to improve healthcare outcomes for the indigenous populations of Australia.

CANADA

In Canada, the population in general, and thus the service area for health care, is becoming more diverse. As of May 2011, the total population of Canada was 33,476,688 (Statistics Canada, 2011). This is almost twice as many Canadians as there were in 1961. The average life span in Canada is 81.23 years. It has been estimated that one in eight Canadians is a member of a visible minority in a proportion that grew by 25% between 1996 and 2001, while overall population growth was just 4%. The population of First Nations peoples increased 22.2%, and there are now one million First Nations people in Canada. According to 2006 Canadian census data, 3.75% of the population is Canadian Aboriginal, which includes First Nations, Metis, and Inuit (Canadian Census Release Topics, 2006). Thus, the diversity of the country has grown rapidly, and will continue to do so in the coming 50 years. Our neighbor to the north, Canada has also been experiencing a tremendous growth in immigration, specifically of internationally trained professionals. These "new Canadians" are changing the culture of Canada. Canada has recognized the need for its nurses to become culturally competent and the Registered Nurses' Association of Ontario has established nursing best practice guidelines on this important issue (Registered Nurses' Association of Ontario, 2007). The recommendation of this best practice guideline is that as Canada becomes more diverse, so must its healthcare system. Men and women from all cultures need to be recruited and welcomed into a profession that is committed to the care of others so they can learn from these diverse groups to create an environment that capitalizes on diversity and furthers the profession and the broader healthcare system (Registered Nurses' Association of Ontario, 2007).

Although Canada has a long-standing multicultural identity and a tradition of acceptance of diversity, reinforced, for example, by the federal government's 1971 Multiculturalism Policy, government intentions have not been sufficient to achieve equity and integration. Racism and cultural oppression have been realities for many minority groups living in Canada, especially the First Nations peoples, resulting in poverty, poor health, loss of identity, and marginalization.

Numerous problems with the differential treatment of the Inuit people of Canada have also been described. These problems have resulted in a call for cultural competency in Canada to better meet the healthcare needs of the Inuit population.

SOUTH AFRICA

South Africa is characterized as a multicultural society and has great diversity in geography, language, and culture. The total population in South Africa in 2011 was 50.59 million (Statistics South Africa, 2011). The family structure in many families tends to be extended rather than nuclear and may also be multigenerational. There tends to be a fatalistic approach to disability that can result in passivity when seeking out treatment or rehabilitation. Traditional healers may form an integral part of a family's approach to health and illness. Technology and Western medical practices may be viewed as an intrusion on accepted and respected traditional activities and rituals. The community view within South Africa is that the group takes precedence over the individual, and time is only a two-dimensional phenomenon. The concept of time is one of having a long past, a present, and no future.

During the time of apartheid in South Africa, profound inequality existed in the availability and content of medical and public health services, which resulted in serious consequences for the majority non-White population (Nightingale et al., 1990). Despite the fall of apartheid, there is evidence that discrimination in treatment persists (Geiger, 2003). This painful part of South Africa's history has resulted in a push toward cultural competency within the country. The Truth and Reconciliation Commission of South Africa was established by former South African President Nelson Mandela; the commission's work has allowed the people of South Africa to openly discuss the pain and suffering caused by the intentional and enforced racial and cultural divisions within their country. The commission's activities have been credited with opening the doors to deeper cultural knowledge and positive change—key elements in the journey toward cultural competence.

RECOMMENDATIONS

It is necessary to increase recognition among all healthcare providers that racial bias persists and can be overt or covert. These biases continue to impact treatment decisions of minority patients. Quality assurance programs should be expanded to track patterns of patient care by race and ethnicity. The elephant in the room must be acknowledged, and nursing students need to be made aware that this bias is out there and that they need to advocate for their patients when treatment decisions are not evidence-based. Curriculum should be expanded, not just as has been done with cultural competency concepts, but also including the importance of the nurse developing self-awareness and understanding the culture of medicine and how it may impact on the patient experience.

For example, nurse practitioners are taught to present a case according to the medical model. This approach has traditionally included the patient's race in the clinical presentation. It has been argued that labeling a patient by race is necessary to clarify biologic risk for particular diseases, critical for differential diagnosis formation, that it provided information about socioeconomic status by proxy, and that the practice should be continued (South-Paul, 2001). Others feel that the placement of the patient's race should be moved from its traditional position in the initial patient description and placed with the other psychosocial patient data (Anderson, Moscou, Fulchon, & Neuspiel, 2001). On the surface, the placement of the patient's race in the clinical presentation may appear trivial, but small changes may ultimately result in effective change within the culture of medicine (Geiger, 2003).

SUMMARY

Diversity is a global phenomenon. As people who later become patients and as healthcare professionals immigrate into the United States, this global diversity will contribute to even greater diversity within the United States.

REVIEW QUESTIONS

1. Identify your own primary and secondary characteristics of culture.
2. How have these characteristics influenced you and your worldview?
3. Determine the racial and ethnic characteristics of the community where you practice or will practice nursing.
4. Define race and ethnicity. Differentiate the two terms.
5. Compare and contrast the healthcare delivery system of the United States and the United Kingdom, Australia, Canada, and South Africa.

REFERENCES

Anderson, M. R., Moscou, S., Fulchon, C., & Neuspiel, D. R. (2001). The role of race in the clinical presentation. *Family Medicine, 33*(6), 430–434.

Australian Bureau of Statistics. (2012). Retrieved from http://www.abs.gov.au/

Australian Bureau of Statistics & Australian Institute of Health and Welfare. (2003). *The burden of disease and injury in Australia.* Retrieved from www.aihw.gov.au/WorkArea/Download Asset.aspx?id=6442459747

Awofeso, N. (2011). Racism: A major impediment to optimal indigenous health and health care in Australia. *Australian Indigenous Health Bulletin, 11*(3). Retrieved from http://healthbulletin.org.au/articles/racism-a-major-impediment-to-optimal-indigenous-health-and-health-care-in-australia

Canadian Census Release Topics, 2006. (2011). Retrieved from http://www12.statcan.ca/census-recensement/2006/rt-td/index-eng.cfm

Collins, K. S., Hughes, D. L., Doty, M. M., Ives, B. L., Edwards, J. N., & Tenney, K. (2002). *Diverse communities, common concerns: Assessing health care quality for minority Americans.* New York, NY: The Commonwealth Fund.

Fadiman, A. (1997). *The spirit catches you and you fall down.* New York, NY: Farrar, Straus, and Giroux.

Geiger, H. J. (2003). Racial and ethnic disparities in diagnosis and treatment: A review of the evidence and a consideration of causes. In B. D. Smedley, A. Y. Stith, & A. R. Nelson (Eds.), *Unequal treatment: Confronting racial and ethnic disparities in health care* (pp. 417–454). Washington, DC: The National Academies Press.

Geronimus, A. T., Bound, J., Colen, C. G. (2011). Excess black mortality in the United States and in selected black and white high-poverty areas, 1980–2000. *American Journal of Public Health, 101*(4), 720–729.

Giger, J. N. (2013). *Transcultural nursing: Assessment and intervention* (6th ed.). Philadelphia, PA: Elsevier.

Hanson, M., Russell, L., Robb, A., & Tabak, D. (1996). *Cross-cultural interviewing: A guide for teaching and evaluation.* Toronto, Ontario: University of Toronto.

Hemingway, H., Crook, A. M., Feder, G., Banerjee, S., Dawson, J. R., Magee, P., … Timmis, A. D. (2001). Underuse of coronary revascularization procedures in patients considered appropriate candidates for revascularization. *New England Journal of Medicine, 344*(9), 645–654.

Hemingway, H., Saunders, D., & Parsons, L. (1997). Social class, spoken language and pattern of care as determinants of continuity of care in maternity services in East London. *Journal of Public Health Medicine, 19*(2), 156–161.

Institute of Medicine (IOM). (2003). *Patient safety: Achieving a new standard of care.* Washington, DC: The National Academies Press.

Institute of Medicine (IOM). (2004). *Insuring America's health: Principles and recommendations.* Washington, DC: The National Academies Press.

Institute of Medicine (IOM). (2009). *America's uninsured crisis: Consequences for health and health care.* Washington, DC: The National Academies Press.

Kaiser Family Foundation. (2004). National survey on consumers experiences with patient safety and quality information. Retrieved from http://www.kff.org/kaiserpolls/upload/National-Survey-on-Consumers-Experiences-With-Patient-Safety-and-Quality-Information-Survey-Summary-and-Chartpack.pdf

Kleinman, A. (1988). *Rethinking psychiatry: From cultural category to personal experience.* New York, NY: Free Press.

Lowe, J., & Archibald, C. (2009). Cultural diversity: The intention of nursing. *Nursing Forum, 44*(1), 11–18.

Lowe, M., Kerridge, I. H., & Mitchell, K. R. (1995). "These sorts of people don't do very well": Race and allocation of health care resources. *Journal of Medical Ethics, 21*(6), 356–360.

Mandell, B. F. (2012). Talking to patients: Barriers to overcome. *Cleveland Clinic Journal of Medicine, 79*(2), 90.

Martin, J., & Fogel, S. (2006). *Projecting the US population to 2050: Four immigration scenarios* (Federation for American Immigration Reform report). Retrieved from http://www.fairus.org/site/DocServer/pop_projections.pdf?docID5901

McGrath, B. B. (1998). Illness as a problem of meaning: Moving culture from the classroom to the clinic. *Advances in Nursing Science, 21*(2), 17–29.

Mickelson, J. K., Blum, C. M., & Geraci, J. M. (1997). Acute myocardial infarction: Clinical characteristics, outcome in metropolitan veterans. *Journal of the American College of Cardiology, 29*(5), 915–925. Retrieved from http://content.onlinejacc.org/article.aspx?articleid=1121666

Misra-Hebert, A. D., & Isaccson, J. H. (2012). Overcoming health care disparities via better cross-cultural communication and health literacy. *Cleveland Clinic Journal of Medicine, 79*(2), 127–133.

National Center on Minority Health and Health Disparities. (2002). Strategic research plan and budget to reduce and ultimately eliminate health disparities: Volume II. Retrieved from http://www.nimhd.nih.gov/our_programs/strategic/pubs/volumeii.pdf

National Library of Medicine. (2012). Health disparities. Retrieved from http://www.nlm.nih.gov/hsrinfo/disparities.html

National League for Nursing (NLN). (2011). Global diversity initatives. Retrieved from http://www.nln.org/aboutnln/globaldiversity/index.htm

National Sample Survey of Registered Nurses (NSSRN). (2008). *The registered nurse population.* Retrieved from http://bhpr.hrsa.gov/healthworkforce/rnsurveys/rnsurveyfinal.pdf

Nazroo, J. Y. (2003). The structuring of ethnic inequalities in health: Economic position, racial discrimination, and racism. *American Journal of Public Health, 93*(2), 277–284.

Nightingale, E. O., Hannibal, K., Geiger, H. J., Hartmann, L., Lawrence, R., & Spurlock, J. (1990). Apartheid medicine: Health and human rights in South Africa. *Journal of the American Medical Association, 264*(16), 2097–2102.

Passel, J., Livingston, G., & Cohn, D. (2012). *Explaining why minority births now outnumber white births*. Retrieved from Pew Research Center website: http://www.pewsocialtrends.org/2012/05/17/explaining-why-minority-births-now-outnumber-white-births/#more-12006

Passel, J., & Taylor, P. (2010). *Unauthorized immigrants and their U.S.-born children*. Retrieved from the Pew Hispanic Center website: http://www.pewhispanic.org/2010/08/11/unauthorized-immigrants-and-their-us-born-children

Population Division of the United Nations Department of Economic and Social Affairs. (2010a). *World population prospects, the 2010 revision*. Retrieved from http://esa.un.org/wpp/

Population Division of the United Nations Department of Economic and Social Affairs. (2010b). *World population prospects, the 2010 revision: Frequently asked questions*. Retrieved from http://esa.un.org/wpp/other-information/faq.htm

Purnell, L. D. (Ed.). (2013). *Transcultural health care: A culturally competent approach* (4th ed.). Philadelphia, PA: F. A. Davis.

Registered Nurses' Association of Ontario. (2007). *Embracing cultural diversity in health care: Developing cultural competence*. Toronto, Canada: Author.

Resnik, D. B. (2004). The distribution of biomedical research resources and international justice. *Developing World Bioethics, 4*(1), 42–57.

Rubio-Stipec, M., Hsiao-Rei Hicks, M., & Tsuang, M. T. (2000). Cultural factors influencing the selection, use, and interpretation of psychiatric measures. In *Handbook of psychiatric measures* (pp. 33–41). Washington, DC: American Psychiatric Association.

Saha, S., Komaromy, M., Koepsell, T. D., & Bindman, A. B. (1999). Patient–physician racial concordance and the perceived quality and use of health care. *Archives of Internal Medicine, 159*(9), 997–1004.

South-Paul, J. E. (2001). Racism in the examining room: Myths, realities, and consequences. *Family Medicine, 33*(6), 473–475.

Sowell, T. (1991). A worldview of cultural diversity. *Society, 29*(1), 37–44.

Statistics Canada. (2011). 2011 census. Retrieved from http://www12.statcan.gc.ca/census-recensement/index-eng.cfm

Statistics South Africa. (2011). Mid-year population estimates 2011. Retrieved from http://www.statssa.gov.za/publications/P0302/P03022011.pdf

Stein, H. F. (1985). The culture of the patient as a red herring in clinical decision making: A case study. *Medical Anthropology Quarterly, 17*(1), 2–5.

Taylor, R. (2005). Addressing barriers to cultural competence. *Journal for Nurses in Staff Development, 21*(4), 135–142.

United Nations Development Programme. (2008). *Annual report: Capacity development: Empowering people and institutions*. Retrieved from http://www.undp.org/content/undp/en/home/librarypage/corporate/undp_in_action_2008.html

Urban Institute & Kaiser Commission on Medicaid and the Uninsured. (2006). *Analysis of March 2006 current population survey*. Retrieved from http://www.statehealthfacts.org/profileind.jsp?cat59&sub5106&rgn51

U.S. Census Bureau. (2008). International Data Base. Retrieved from http://www.census.gov/population/international/data/idb/sysmessage.php

U.S. Census Bureau. (2010a). *2010 Census data*. Retrieved from http://2010.census.gov/2010census/data/

U.S. Census Bureau. (2010b). U.S. population clock. Retrieved from http://www.census.gov/population/www/popclockus.html

U.S. Census Bureau. (2012). Census and international census data. Retrieved from http://www.census.gov/population/international/data/idb/informationGateway.php

Weiss, B. D. (2007). *Health literacy and patient safety: Help patients understand* (2nd ed.). American Medical Association Foundation and American Medical Association. Retrieved from http://www.ama-assn.org/ama1/pub/upload/mm/367/healthlitclinicians.pdf

World Bank. (2009). U.S. Census Bureau. Retrieved from http://data.worldbank.org/indicator/SP.DYN.LE00.IN

World Health Organization. (2004). *Diseases of poverty and the 10/90 gap*. Retrieved from http://www.who.int/intellectualproperty/submissions/InternationalPolicyNetwork.pdf

For a full suite of assignments and additional learning activities, see the access code at the front of your book.

www

CHAPTER 4

Organization of Healthcare Delivery in the 21st Century

KEY TERMS www

Biopsychosocial Model

Health Belief Model

Interdisciplinary health care

Patient-centered health care

Unidisciplinary practice

Western Biomedical Model

INTRODUCTION

This chapter will describe the organization of healthcare delivery in the 21st century, such as the use of interdisciplinary or multidisciplinary teams for patient care. There is no doubt that the current U.S. healthcare system faces serious challenges on multiple fronts. Healthcare expenditures have more than doubled between 1994 and 2012, yet nearly 45 million Americans do not have healthcare insurance. The Affordable Care Act will decrease the number of Americans who presently do not have healthcare insurance. Nurses must also work within a system that has exploded with new technology, including electronic health records.

In this chapter, national standards related to quality, safety, and culturally appropriate care will be described. The shift in focus from the Western Biomedical Model (provider-focused model) to a Health Belief Model (patient-focused model) will be included. Keeping the patient central to the planning process will help to ensure that cultural beliefs will be incorporated into the plan of care. Barriers impacting the patient and the system will also be described, and some potential solutions will be offered. These barriers are communication issues, lack of access to preventive care, history of discrimination and abuse in some cultures, distrust of healthcare providers, nonadherence, and the refusal of some to enter the healthcare system for any care or treatment. The impact of the provision of primary care by NPs will be described as well. The integration of cultural competency into primary care practice has been clarified in the National Organization of Nurse Practitioner Faculties (NONPF) document on cultural competency (Green-Hernandez, Quinn, Denman-Vitale, Falkenstern, & Judge-Ellis, 2004), as well as the U.S. Department of Health and Human Services (2002) *Nurse Practitioner Primary Care Competencies in Specialty Areas* which was submitted by NONPF and the American Association of Colleges of Nursing (AACN). These competencies include the requirement that the NP provide culturally competent health care. The NP role in providing culturally competent care, delivering patient care with respect for the cultural and spiritual beliefs of all patients, and ensuring that healthcare resources are available to all patients from diverse cultures is also included.

How does the NP demonstrate cultural competence? When she or he can show respect for the inherent dignity of every human being, whatever their age, gender, religion, socioeconomic class, sexual orientation, and ethnic or cultural group; accepts the rights of individuals to choose their care provider, participate in care, and refuse care; acknowledges personal biases and prevents these from interfering with the delivery of quality care to persons of other cultures; recognizes cultural issues and interacts with clients from other cultures in culturally sensitive ways and incorporates cultural preferences, health beliefs, behaviors, and traditional practices into the management plan; develops client-appropriate educational materials that address the language and cultural beliefs of the client and accesses culturally appropriate resources to deliver care to clients from other cultures; and finally, assists clients to access quality care within a dominant culture. Opportunities for the nurse to obtain cultural competency certification will conclude the content in this chapter.

NATIONAL STANDARDS: CULTURALLY AND LINGUISTICALLY APPROPRIATE SERVICES

The Office of Minority Health of the U.S. Department of Health and Human Services (USDHHS) (Office of Minority Health, 2001) issued its final report of national standards for culturally and linguistically appropriate services (CLAS). The 2001 report describes culturally competent care as care that is effective, compatible with the patient's culture, and communicated in a language that the patient fully understands (Office of Minority Health, 2001). The CLAS standards were enhanced in 2012 by the Office of Minority Health (OMH). The enhancement was to designate the CLAS recommendations into one of three categories: mandate (a federal requirement for all entities receiving federal funds), guideline (recommended by the OMH for adoption), and recommendation (suggestion for voluntary adoption by healthcare organizations) (Office of Minority Health, 2012). CLAS was powerful in that it highlighted the need for culturally and linguistically appropriate healthcare services for diverse populations. CLAS consists of 14 national standards for providing CLAS in health care. These standards are based on a review of the law, regulation, and federal and state standards currently in place. Input was also provided by a national advisory committee made up of healthcare providers, researchers, and policy makers. The objectives for the CLAS standards were that they should be inclusive of all cultures, ensure equitable and effective treatment for all patients, and contribute to the elimination of health disparities (Office of

Minority Health, 2012). In addition to the CLAS standards, the recommendation for cultural mapping was also included. Cultural mapping requires healthcare organizations to be aware of the cultures of the patients that they may treat beyond just an appreciation for the language(s) spoken. Language may be a starting point, but a more thorough cultural understanding (such as health disparities experienced and health beliefs associated with the cultural group) is required for the healthcare institution to better plan for appropriate programs and delivery of healthcare services (Office of Minority Health, 2012).

The CLAS standards are primarily directed at healthcare organizations but are helpful to the individual healthcare professional as well. The CLAS standards (**Box 4–1**) are organized by theme: culturally competent care (standards 1–3), language access services (standards 4–7), and organizational supports for cultural competence (standards 8–14). Each of the standards has varying stringency ranging from recommendations, to guidelines, to mandates. There are four CLAS

Box 4–1 National Standards for Culturally and Linguistically Appropriate Services in Health Care

1. Healthcare organizations should ensure that patients/consumers receive from all staff members effective, understandable, and respectful care that is provided in a manner compatible with their cultural health beliefs and practices, in their preferred language. (Guideline)

2. Healthcare organizations should implement strategies to recruit, retain, and promote at all levels of the organization a diverse staff and leadership that are representative of the demographic characteristics of the service area. (Guideline)

3. Healthcare organizations should ensure that staff at all levels and across all disciplines receives ongoing education and training in culturally and linguistically appropriate service delivery. (Guideline)

4. Healthcare organizations must offer and provide language assistance services, including bilingual staff and interpreter services, at no cost to each patient with limited English proficiency at all points of contact, in a timely manner, during all hours of operation. (Mandate)

5. Healthcare organizations must provide to patients in their preferred language both verbal offers and written notices informing them of their right to receive language assistance services. (Mandate)

6. Healthcare organizations must ensure the competence of language assistance provided to patients with limited English proficiency by interpreters and bilingual staff. Family and friends should not be used to provide interpretation services (except upon request by the patient/consumer). (Mandate)

7. Healthcare organizations must make available easily understood patient-related materials and post signs in the languages of the commonly encountered groups and/or groups represented in the service area. (Mandate)

8. Healthcare organizations should develop, implement, and promote a written strategic plan that outlines clear goals, policies, operational plans, and management accountability/oversight mechanisms to provide culturally and linguistically appropriate services. (Guideline)

9. Healthcare organizations should conduct initial and ongoing organizational self-assessments of CLAS-related activities and are encouraged to integrate cultural- and linguistic-competence-related measures into their internal audits, performance improvement programs, patient satisfaction assessments, and outcomes-based evaluations. (Guideline)

10. Healthcare organizations should ensure that data on the individual patient's/consumer's race, ethnicity, and spoken and written language are collected in health records, integrated into the organization's management information systems, and periodically updated. (Guideline)

11. Healthcare organizations should maintain a current demographic, cultural, and epidemiologic profile of the community, as well as a needs assessment to accurately plan for and implement services that respond to the cultural and linguistic characteristics of the service area. (Guideline)

12. Healthcare organizations should develop participatory, collaborative partnerships with communities and utilize a variety of formal and informal mechanisms to facilitate community and patient/consumer involvement in designing and implementing CLAS-related activities. (Guideline)

13. Healthcare organizations should ensure that conflict and grievance resolution processes are culturally and linguistically sensitive and capable of identifying, preventing, and resolving cross-cultural conflicts or complaints by patients/consumers. (Guideline)

14. Healthcare organizations are encouraged to regularly make available to the public information about their progress and successful innovations in implementing the CLAS standards and to provide public notice in their communities about the availability of this information. (Recommendation)

Source: U.S. Department of Health and Human Services, Office of Minority Health. (2012). *National standards for culturally and linguistically appropriate services in health care* (Final report). Rockville, MD: Author. Retrieved from http://minorityhealth.hhs.gov/templates/browse. aspx?lvl=2&lvlID=15

mandates that are required to be followed by all recipients of federal funds. The nine guidelines are recommendations made by the Office of Minority Health to be adopted by all accrediting agencies, while one CLAS recommendation was suggested for voluntary adoption by healthcare organizations.

STANDARDS OF CARE: INSTITUTE OF MEDICINE

In 1999, the recognition of the existence and persistence of healthcare disparities resulted in Congress requesting that the Institute of Medicine (IOM) conduct a study. The study was to assess disparities in the kinds and quality of health care received by U.S. racial and ethnic minorities and nonminorities. Congress requested that the IOM assess the extent of racial and ethnic differences in health care that are not attributable to known factors (such as access to care), evaluate potential sources of disparities in health care (including bias, discrimination, and stereotyping), and perhaps most importantly, to provide recommendations regarding interventions to eliminate the disparities. The IOM committee defined health care as the continuum of services provided in traditional healthcare settings (public and private clinics, hospitals, community health centers, nursing homes, and home-based care). Disparities were defined by the IOM as racial or ethnic differences in the quality of health care that were not results of access-related factors or clinical needs, preferences, and appropriateness of intervention. Racial and ethnic groups were placed into the five categories for racial groups and two categories for ethnic groups established by the Federal Office of Management and Budget (2001) (**Box 4–2**).

The IOM study committee reviewed well over 100 studies that assessed the quality of health care for various racial and ethnic minority groups, while holding constant variations in insurance status, patient income, and other access-related factors. Many of these studies also controlled for other potential confounding factors, such as racial differences in the severity or stage of disease progression, the presence of comorbid illnesses, where care is received (e.g., public or private hospitals and health systems), and other patient demographic variables, such as age and gender. Some studies that employed more rigorous research designs followed patients prospectively, using clinical data abstracted from patients' charts, rather than administrative data used for insurance claims. The study findings indicated that minorities are less likely than Whites to receive needed services, including clinically necessary procedures. Minorities may experience a range of barriers to accessing care, even when they have health insurance comparable to Whites. These barriers include language, geography, and cultural factors. Financial, institutional, legal, regulatory, and policy factors also have a negative effect on a minority patient's ability to get quality health care. Health disparities were found to exist in a number of disease areas including cancer, cardiovascular disease, human immunodeficiency virus (HIV) and acquired immunodeficiency syndrome (AIDS),

---

Box 4–2 Revised Standards for the Classification of Federal Data on Race and Ethnicity

---

Categories for Race

- American Indian or Alaska Native: A person having origins in any of the original peoples of North or South America (including Central America) who maintains tribal affiliation or community attachment.
- Asian: A person having origins in any of the original peoples of the Far East, Southeast Asia, or the Indian subcontinent including, for example, Cambodia, China, India, Japan, Korea, Malaysia, Pakistan, the Philippine Islands, Thailand, and Vietnam.
- Black or African American: A person having origins in any of the Black racial groups of Africa. Terms such as *Haitian* or *Negro* can be used in addition to Black or African American.
- Native Hawaiian or Other Pacific Islander: A person having origins in any of the original people of Hawaii, Guam, Samoa, or other Pacific Islands.
- White: A person having origins in any of the original peoples of Europe, the Middle East, or North Africa.

Categories for Ethnicity
- Hispanic or Latino: A person of Cuban, Mexican, Puerto Rican, South or Central American, or other Spanish culture or origin, regardless of race. The term *Spanish origin* can be used in addition to *Hispanic or Latino*.
- Not Hispanic or Latino

Source: U.S. Department of Education. (2007). *Appendix A: Revisions to the standards for the classification of federal data on race and ethnicity*. Retrieved from http://nces.ed.gov/programs/handbook/data/pdf/appendices.pdf

---

diabetes, and mental illness, and were found across a range of procedures, including routine treatments for common health problems. Alarmingly, the literature review conducted by the IOM (Smedley, Stith, & Nelson, 2003) found that racial and ethnic minorities experience a lower quality of healthcare services and are less likely to receive even routine medical procedures than are White Americans.

Even more alarming is the discovery that racial and ethnic minorities receive lower quality health care than Whites, even when they are insured to the same degree and when other healthcare-access-related factors, such as the ability to pay for care, are the same. The IOM report (Smedley et al., 2003) concluded that prejudice and stereotyping on the part of healthcare providers may contribute to the differences in care. This conclusion was met with controversy within the healthcare community because the vast majority of healthcare professionals work hard under challenging circumstances to ensure that our patients receive the best possible health care. How could bias, prejudice, and stereotyping contribute to unequal treatment, particularly given that healthcare providers are sworn to beneficence and cannot, by law, discriminate against any patient on the basis of race, ethnicity, color, or national origin? Our professional organization, the American Nurses Association, states that all nurses are sworn to beneficence and cannot by law discriminate against any patient (American Nurses Association, 2004).

The IOM report (Smedley et al., 2003) found that many factors may contribute to the healthcare disparities observed in the reviewed studies. They found that some researchers suggest that there may be subtle differences in the way that members of different racial and ethnic groups respond to treatment, particularly with regard to some pharmaceutical interventions, suggesting that variations in some forms of treatment may be justified on the basis of patient race or ethnicity. In addition, patients vary in help-seeking behavior, and some racial and ethnic minorities may be more likely than Whites to avoid or delay seeking care. However, the majority of studies find disparities in clinical services that are equally effective for all racial and ethnic groups. Further, the studies that the IOM reviewed suggest that racial differences in patients' attitudes, such as their preferences for treatment, do not vary greatly and cannot fully explain racial and ethnic disparities in health care. This landmark report identified cultural competence training of health professionals as a potential strategy to improve the quality of care and to reduce health disparities between ethnic minorities and Whites (Smedley et al., 2003). The report advocates cross-cultural education from three conceptual approaches. The first focus is attitudes (cultural sensitivity/awareness), the second approach is knowledge (multicultural/categorical approach), and the third is skills (cross-cultural approach) (Smedley et al., 2003). Research does support this approach, as training is effective in improving provider knowledge of cultural and behavioral aspects of health care and building effective communication strategies. The IOM report (Smedley et al., 2003) recommended that a broad sector approach, including healthcare providers, their patients, payers, health plan purchasers, and society at large, must work to ensure that all patients receive quality health care. This type of healthcare training shows promise as a strategy for improving healthcare professionals' knowledge, attitudes, and skills, and patients' ratings of care.

The IOM study (Smedley et al., 2003) determined that despite scientific medical advances, the poor and non-White ethnic minorities ranked lower in health status on numerous measures. It states that a small number of studies find that Blacks are slightly more likely to reject medical recommendations for some treatments, but these differences in refusal rates are generally small (Blacks are only 3 to 6% more likely to reject recommended treatments, according to these studies). The IOM report recommends that more research is needed to fully understand the reason(s) for the refusal of treatment, as this may lead to the development of different strategies to help patients make informed treatment decisions. The report also highlighted the need to recruit more minorities to enter the health professions and for those already in practice to develop cultural competence. The report states that as the number of patients of diverse racial, ethnic, cultural, and linguistic backgrounds continues to increase in the United States, so will the need to produce culturally competent providers who incorporate the patients' worldview into patient management decisions (Smedley et al., 2003). Cross-cultural training should have a significant role in improving quality of care for minorities and in attempting to eliminate racial and ethnic disparities.

Since the landmark 2003 IOM report, much work has been done in the area of health disparities. Most recently, the focus has enlarged to include patient-centeredness and the pediatric population. Reflection on what has been accomplished has also occurred. In 2010 the Institute of Medicine conducted a workshop, "Ten years later: How far have we come in reducing disparities?" The workshop indicated that some progress has been made. For example, awareness of the importance of cultural competence for healthcare access and quality has significantly increased. This is supported by gains in funding, research and standards development. There is still a need for further improvement. The IOM recommended that future studies focus on identifying effective strategies for tailoring disease management to diverse patients, supporting research that charges healthcare organizations to identify strategies to eliminate or reduce health disparities, and the creation and testing of appropriate interventions that will inform medical providers to better treat and manage disease and promote health (Andrulis, 2010).

IDENTIFIED BARRIERS THAT CONTRIBUTE TO HEALTHCARE DISPARITIES

Classification by race and ethnicity is not an issue-free process. Definitions for race and ethnicity vary according to the source utilized, and they are often rife with criticism. Arguably, the most relevant criticism is that the use of the federal classifications does not permit a person to choose the label with which they self-identify. The five racial categories used are American Indian or Alaska Native, Asian, Black or African American, Native Hawaiian or other Pacific Islander, and White. The two ethnic categories are Hispanic or Latino and not Hispanic or Latino. This criticism was addressed when a newer classification system was adopted that permits a more individualized process of self-identification. It also allows for a separation of race from ethnicity. Now everyone has to be identified as either Hispanic or Latino or Not Hispanic or Latino, regardless of race. Individuals may self-select from more than one racial category as well (U.S. Department of Education [USED], 2007).

It is difficult to attempt to determine the reasons why healthcare disparities exist in this country; it is a daunting process. To separate or attempt to quantify or qualify the relative contribution of any one factor, or the interrelationship between factors, increases the risk of not seeing the whole picture. For example, when trying to determine the reasons why segregation of housing persists, one must recognize that it is a by-product of discrimination in the past and present, past and contemporary racism, socioeconomic differences, and the legacy of less or poorer opportunities being available to minority groups in this country. Recognizing that the problems are a result of both historic and contemporary forces reinforces the importance of considering the impact of these forces that contribute to differences in access to quality health care when searching for solutions. Despite the inherent difficulty in the task, many connections and relationships were identified by the IOM study (Smedley et al., 2003).

Individual risk factors for poor health are pronounced among many racial and ethnic minorities. These risks are increased by the disproportionate representation of minorities in the lower socioeconomic levels. Socioeconomic status seems to be the most important predictor of health status. Socioeconomic position, in and of itself, is correlated with a health status independent of individual risk factors. This is a powerful discovery. As people move up the socioeconomic ladder, they tend to have better health.

Cultural factors also play an important part. Korenbrot and Moss (2000) found that among some immigrant Hispanic populations, birth outcomes were better than among those of their U.S.-born peers. This may suggest that the risk of poor health status increases with each subsequent generation living in the United States. Negative environmental factors, such as air and water pollution, are more likely to exist in poorer communities. House and Williams (2000) conclude that these and other risk factors that are associated with health and poor health illustrate that racial and ethnic disparities in health status largely reflect differences in social, socioeconomic, and behavioral risk factors and environmental living conditions. If one accepts this conclusion to be true, then it becomes apparent that the solution to the problem of healthcare disparities cannot be solved by addressing the issue of healthcare delivery alone.

There were two other factors that may be associated with healthcare disparities, assuming that all populations have equal access to health care. The first set of factors is related to the operation of healthcare systems and the legal and regulatory climate in which they operate. These include factors such as cultural or linguistic barriers (e.g., the lack of interpreter services for patients with limited English proficiency), fragmentation of healthcare systems (as noted earlier, these include the possibility that minorities are disproportionately enrolled in lower-cost health plans that place greater per-patient limits on healthcare expenditures and available services), the types of incentives in place to contain costs (e.g., incentives to physicians to limit services), and where minorities tend to receive care (e.g., minorities are less likely to access care in a private physician's office, even when insured at the same level as Whites).

The second set of factors emerges from the clinical encounter. Three mechanisms might be operative in healthcare disparities from the provider's side of the exchange: bias (or prejudice) against minorities, greater clinical uncertainty when interacting with minority patients, and beliefs (or stereotypes) held by the provider about the behavior or health of minorities. Patients might also react to providers' behaviors associated with these practices in a way that also contributes to disparities. The IOM report (Smedley et al., 2003) states that research on how patient race or ethnicity may influence physician decision making and the quality of care for minorities is still emerging, and as yet there is no direct evidence to illustrate how prejudice, stereotypes, or bias may influence care. In the absence of conclusive evidence, the study committee decided to draw upon a mix of theory and relevant research in an attempt to understand how these processes might operate in the clinical encounter.

CLINICAL UNCERTAINTY

A powerful concept that emerged from the IOM report was that of clinical uncertainty. Clinical uncertainty is the uncertainty a healthcare professional has relative to the condition of the patient. Clinical uncertainty can contribute to disparities in treatment. The diagnosis that is formulated by the NP or physician must depend on inferences made about the severity of the illness. These inferences are made based on what is seen during the clinical encounter (this also includes the patient's race or ethnicity), often within a very short time frame.

Clinical uncertainty has been described as the single most important influence on provider behavior (Balsa, Seiler, McGuire, & Bloche, 2003). In the process of care, health professionals must come to judgments about patients' conditions and make decisions about treatment, often without complete and accurate information. In most cases, they must do so under severe time pressure and resource constraints. The responses of racial and ethnic minority patients to healthcare providers during the clinical encounter are also a potential source of disparities. Little research has been conducted as to how patients may influence the clinical encounter, but in the IOM report (Smedley et al., 2003), it was speculated that if patients convey mistrust, refuse treatment, or comply poorly with treatment, the provider may become less engaged in the treatment process, which can result in the patient being less likely to be provided with vigorous treatment and services. This type of patient response or reaction is understandable as a response to prior negative racial experiences, whether they include real or perceived mistreatment by other providers in the past. Research indicates that minority patients perceive higher levels of racial discrimination in health care than nonminorities do. Patients' and providers' behaviors and attitudes may therefore influence each other concurrently.

BIASES

Biases may exist subconsciously even among people who are strongly opposed to bigotry and discrimination and in people who strongly believe that they are not prejudiced. The rate of prejudice among White Americans is very high; estimates range from one-half to three-quarters of White Americans believe that relative to Whites, minorities—and particularly African Americans—are less intelligent, more prone to violence, and prefer to live off welfare (Smedley et al., 2003). With such a high prevalence rate, it would be unrealistic to assume that all healthcare professionals are without at least some of these prejudicial beliefs or the manifestation of these prejudicial beliefs in their own behaviors.

The IOM report (Smedley et al., 2003) states that there is significant evidence that well-intentioned Whites who are not overtly biased and who do not believe that they are prejudiced typically demonstrate unconscious implicit negative racial attitudes and stereotypes. Both implicit and explicit stereotypes significantly shape interpersonal interactions, influencing how information is recalled and guiding expectations and inferences in systematic ways. They can also produce self-fulfilling prophecies when the perceived stereotype influences the interaction in ways that conform to the stereotypical expectations.

Some of the identified areas requiring intervention from the IOM study (Smedley et al., 2003) are improving minority socioeconomic status, desegregating housing and making housing more equitable, improving educational opportunities, modifying individual behavioral risk factors, and improving access to and use of healthcare services. Healthcare delivery must strive to be egalitarian. Health care is a resource that should be tied to social justice. Society expects our healthcare providers to adhere to the highest ethical standards to ensure fairness to all. Opposing this is the need for providers to be managers of the available healthcare resources. Poor decisions can result in the allocation of more resources for one person or group than for others. An unequal distribution of healthcare resources can have serious consequences. First, some will receive inadequate care. Second, the trust of the public (already tenuous within some minority populations) will be further weakened. Finally, a lack of access or lack of trust will negatively impact a patient's willingness to seek care and adhere to treatment recommendations.

ROLE OF EDUCATION

Because of the identified factors/barriers that can impact treatment decisions, it appears that education is the key tool to attempt to overcome healthcare disparities. Education needs to focus on all healthcare professionals as well as the patients. Healthcare providers should be made aware of racial and ethnic disparities in health care and the fact that these disparities exist, often despite providers' best intentions. In addition, all current and future healthcare providers can benefit from cross-cultural education. Cross-cultural education programs have been developed to enhance health professionals' awareness of how cultural and social factors influence health care, while providing methods to obtain, negotiate, and manage this information clinically once it is obtained. Cross-cultural education can be divided into three conceptual approaches focusing on attitudes (cultural sensitivity/awareness approach), knowledge (multicultural/categorical approach), and skills (cross-cultural approach), and has been taught using a variety of interactive and experiential methodologies. Based on the strength of current research data, the Agency for Healthcare Research and Quality and the Department of Health and Human Services both support the use of cross-cultural training as an effective way to improve provider knowledge of cultural and behavioral aspects of health care and for establishing effective communication strategies.

Focus needs to be on patient education as well. Health literacy is an important issue and is an important component of Healthy People 2020, a federal healthcare initiative. The Department of Health and Human Services has developed the National Action Plan to Improve Health Literacy, which has two main principles: (1) every patient has the right to health information that helps them make informed decisions, and (2) health services should be delivered in ways that are understandable and beneficial to health, longevity, and quality of life (USDHHS, 2010a). Limited health literacy affects people of all ages, races, incomes, and education levels, but it impacts patients from lower socioeconomic and minority groups at a significantly disproportionate level. Lack of health literacy impacts the ability of the patient to seek out accurate health information, which limits their ability to adopt health-promoting behaviors or to be aware of important public health alerts. A patient with limited health literacy has worse health outcomes and higher medical costs (Berkman et al., 2004). The nurse must be aware of health literacy issues, so that he or she can develop patient educational strategies that ensure effective learning for all patients.

IMPACT ON PUBLIC HEALTH

The productivity of the workforce is inextricably linked to the health of the workforce. If some members of the workforce receive substandard medical care, there will be both an individual and societal consequence. The individual impact on those workers is that they will become further disadvantaged and unable to advance both economically and professionally. The costs to society are loss of productivity and increased healthcare costs. The higher burden of disease and mortality among minorities has profound financial implications (higher costs for health care and rehabilitative care) and public health implications. All members of a community are affected by the health of other community members. This is the tenet of public health. All members of a community are affected by the poor health status of its least healthy members. An infectious disease outbreak can and will have devastating consequences to the entire community. Infectious diseases do not discriminate and do not recognize any racial or ethnic boundaries. This principle is so well recognized by public health advocates and the federal government that it guides policy for our country. For example, Healthy People 2020 has an overarching goal to achieve health equity, eliminate disparities, and improve health for all groups. Healthy People 2020 calls for a shared responsibility for health equity, which is defined as the "principle underlying a commitment to reducing disparities in health and its determinants." (Braveman et al., 2011).

From an economic standpoint, failure to treat properly has repercussions. In the long run, it will cost more to treat the complications associated with a chronic disease process than the cost of doing the job right in the first place. For example, a patient with diabetes who is brought to control (hemoglobin A1C of less than 6) is less likely to develop serious complications of diabetes. A patient that is not well controlled is vulnerable to many serious and potentially life-threatening complications including dialysis, kidney transplantation, or amputation. This fact should be of importance to every taxpayer in the United States. Minority patients who are the beneficiaries of publicly funded health insurance are less likely to receive high-quality health care, which will result in higher future healthcare costs not only for the beneficiary but also for the taxpayers. It is cheaper to do it right in the first place but it is also, according to distributive justice theory, the correct thing to do.

DISCRIMINATION AND EQUITABLE-QUALITY HEALTHCARE DELIVERY

Americans have widely held beliefs that abhor racial discrimination and believe that all Americans should (and do) enjoy equal opportunities in accessing health care (Morin, 2001). Despite the debate regarding universal healthcare coverage, many Americans are unaware that this ideal falls short in many areas of this country, most predominantly within our lower socioeconomic communities. The impact on longevity is especially startling. In a study conducted by Murray et al. (2006) the life expectancy and mortality rates for the "eight Americas" was determined. The designation of the eight America subgroups was based on race, location of the county of residence, population density, race-specific county-level per capita income, and cumulative homicide rate. Data sources for population and mortality figures were obtained from the U.S. Census Bureau and the National Center for Health Statistics. The gap between the highest and lowest life expectancies for race–county combinations in the United States was, astoundingly, greater than 35 years difference. Additionally, disparities exist in health insurance coverage as well. Murray et al. (2006) found that the self-reported health plan coverage revealed by the data showed the lowest level of coverage rates were for Native Americans and low-income southern rural Blacks.

Evidence of unequal or substandard care for some segments of the population, particularly on the basis of group membership, should raise the concern that the provision of care may be inconsistently and subjectively administered. Inequities in care expose a threat to quality care for all Americans. It also exposes the need for the public health system to improve the way it deals with managing risk factors for chronic disease and injuries that are prevalent in minority groups, so that the groups' members do not continue to be disproportionately impacted. This will require that the groups with the highest death rates (or lowest life expectancy) receive the greater benefits and attention (Murray et al., 2006).

ETHICS

Normative ethics is the primary standard utilized for ethical decision making in nursing and medicine. Normative ethics include questions about what ethical principles and values should be adopted, what reasons count as ethical reasons, what actions should be performed in a certain situation, and why some principles or values should be chosen over others (Kuhse, 1997). Our values provide the framework for decision making. Our values give meaning to our lives and are derived from our family and societal norms, and may include a religious influence. Our morals are our personal standards for determining right from wrong. Behaviors that are in accordance with group norms, customs, and traditions are considered moral. Culture can play a role in group norms; moral behaviors can be individual and associated with certain cultural groups. This is different from ethics. Ethics are societal standards of right or wrong and what ought to be and, as such, they guide conduct to ensure the protection of the rights of individuals or groups. Normative ethics have traditionally been considered impartial and possessing universal applicability.

There are several ethical frameworks under the normative umbrella. Each person utilizes the framework that is most acceptable to them. For some, one framework will be relied on exclusively, whereas others may change frameworks depending on the situation. The four main frameworks are utilitarianism, liberalism, contextualism, and deontology. See **Box 4–3** for a description of each of these frameworks. The principles of biomedical ethics are autonomy (independence), nonmaleficence (avoidance of harm), beneficence (produce benefit), and justice (fairness). Many nurse scholars, such as Hall (1996), Nash (1999), and Schwarz (2000), have attempted to set a hierarchy for these principles, but according to Leddy (2006), none have provided adequate justification for their rankings.

Informed consent arises from the ethical principle of autonomy. How much or little autonomy a patient wishes to possess is culturally mediated. In practice, obtaining consent is often done to meet an administrative requirement and as such does meet its true intent of ensuring that a patient understands and makes a rational, voluntary decision after adequate deliberation. The language on the consent form connotes compliance with the treatment plan and not collaboration— it does not permit involvement or engage the patient, and as such is not patient

Box 4–3 Categories of Ethical Frameworks

Utilitarianism	Moral behavior is behavior that results in the greatest good; the individual has the responsibility for behavior that is for the good of the community.
Liberalism	Focuses on individual rights and freedom from coercion.
Contextualism	Ethics are bound to time and place and possess cultural relativism: "There is a moral, bounded or cultural relativism where ethical standards are dictated by the society and those in power, judged by the customs, rules and norms of the society, and grounded in the history of the community" (Rothschild, 2000, p. 31).
Deontology	Proposes that ethical standards are held absolutely and categorically.

Source: Leddy, S. K. (2006). *Integrative health promotion* (2nd ed.). Sudbury, MA: Jones and Bartlett; and Rothschild, M. L. (2000). Ethical considerations in support of the marketing of public health issues. *American Journal of Health Behavior, 24*(1), 26–35.

centered. A way to become more culturally competent in one's nursing practice is to rethink the informed consent process. Engage in a meaningful discussion with your patients about healing methods and the expected or desired outcome, instead of merely providing one-way communications that spell out the patients' alternatives and the associated risks and benefits. This approach truly permits informed decision making on the patient's and family's part.

Empirical research (with an emphasis on describing, not prescribing) in bioethics attempts to describe particular states of affairs that have some moral or ethical relevance with an emphasis on the social, cultural, and cross-cultural aspects of morality. This classification is an attempt to differentiate bioethics from normative ethics by some scholars (Goldenberg, 2005). More recently, attention has been given to a type of bioethics—evidence-based ethics—in medicine and health care. This type of research was designed to provide evidence for healthcare professionals to utilize when providing patient care (evidence-based medicine). When ethical decision making is required, utilizing evidence-based ethics would involve the conscientious and judicious use of the best evidence available (relevant to the care and prognosis of the patient), to ensure that the best informed and justified medical decision is made. The purpose of evidence-based ethics is to guide clinical decision making and to help the nurse or physician move away from an intuitive-focused practice, which relies on the provider's clinical experience instead of a scientifically rigorous approach. For example, awareness of the cultural beliefs of a particular group (informed by the results of empirical studies) regarding the appropriateness of informing a patient who has been diagnosed with a life-threatening illness would guide the NP or provider on how best to proceed, and it would determine what is morally important for clinicians to include when providing information and care to patients from that particular cultural group (Goldenberg, 2005).

CROSSING THE QUALITY CHASM

The purpose of the IOM report (2001), *Crossing the Quality Chasm: A New Health System for the 21st Century*, was to identify strategies that could substantially improve the quality of health care delivered to Americans with the focus on how to redesign the healthcare system to innovate and improve care. The report provided a vision for how the healthcare system and health policy must be radically transformed to narrow the gap between theoretical quality medical care and what actually exists in practice (and hopefully close the chasm entirely). This redesign or transformation refers to a new perspective on the purpose and aims of the healthcare system, how patients and their clinicians should relate, and how care processes can be designed to optimize responsiveness to patient needs. The principles and guidance for redesign that are offered in this report represent fundamental changes in the way the system meets the needs of the people it serves. This redesign is not aimed only at the healthcare organizations and professionals that compose the delivery system. Change is also required in the structures and processes of the environment in which those organizations and professionals function. Such change includes setting national priorities for improvement, creating better methods for disseminating and applying knowledge to practice, fostering the use of information technology in clinical care, creating payment policies that encourage innovation and reward improvement in performance, and enhancing educational programs to strengthen the healthcare workforce.

Some quality gaps identified in this report include the overuse, underuse, and misuse of healthcare delivery. The challenge is to bring the full potential benefit of effective health care to all Americans while avoiding unneeded and harmful interventions and eliminating preventable complications of care. This report was the result of an 8-year literature review of more than 70 publications that revealed abundant evidence that serious and extensive quality problems exist throughout American medicine, resulting in harm to many Americans. Four key aspects were identified: the growing complexity of science and technology, the increase in chronic conditions, a poorly organized healthcare delivery system, and constraints in fully embracing the information technology revolution. Each of these four factors plays a role individually and each exacerbates the impact or effect of the other factors. The goal is quality health care, which the IOM (1990) defines as "the degree to which healthcare services for individuals and populations increase the likelihood of desired outcomes and are consistent with current professional knowledge."

The commitment to quality health care for all is evidenced by the inclusion of the following goal as one of the six overarching goals of the IOM's report (2001). The goal is to provide equitable health care that does not vary by patient race, ethnicity, gender, or age. The *Crossing the Quality Chasm* report and the desire to meet the goal of equitable health care was one of the motivating factors for Congress to request that the IOM determine if unequal or substandard health care exists.

As part of the data collection process for the IOM report, *Unequal Treatment: Confronting Racial and Ethnic Disparities in Health Care*, conducted by Smedley et al. (2003), certain themes were identified. The strongest and most consistent evidence was found in support of the existence of significant cardiovascular health disparities among minorities. This finding remained consistent even when potential confounding factors were controlled (e.g., race, ethnicity, access to care, disease severity, comorbidities, disease prevalence, tendency of Whites to overuse services), indicating that racial and ethnic disparities in cardiovascular care remain. Studies of racial disparities in cancer diagnosis and treatment are less clear and consistent than the cardiovascular studies. In any event, several studies indicate that racial and ethnic minorities are diagnosed at later stages of cancer progression, and several studies demonstrated significant racial differences in the receipt of appropriate cancer treatment and analgesics.

The preponderance of studies reviewed by the IOM committee found significant disparities among Blacks, including generally lower rates of diagnostic and therapeutic procedures for those with cerebrovascular disease. In addition, Black Americans are at greater risk for end-stage renal disease (ESRD) than Whites. Although Blacks only make up 12.3% of the U.S. population, they represent almost one-third of those with ESRD. Despite these numbers, Black American patients with ESRD are less likely than similar White patients to receive a kidney transplant (Epstein, Baldwin, & Bishop, 2000). Shockingly, this has not improved in the past 12 years: of the 92,000 Americans currently awaiting a kidney donor, one-third are Black (Hall et al., 2012). Although the rate of kidney failure is 3.5 times greater than that of White Americans, Black Americans are still less likely to receive a kidney transplant and are also less likely to have a living donor than a White patient (Hall et al., 2012). Receiving a kidney from a living donor is preferable as outcome data reveals that these patients do much better post operatively (Hall et al., 2012). It is important to keep in mind that in general, fewer Blacks than

Whites desire or are appropriate for transplantation, and immunologic matching criteria result in fewer donor matches for Blacks than Whites. The bottom line is that several studies are consistent in finding that Black American patients (and in some instances, other ethnic minority patients) are less likely to be judged as appropriate for transplantation, are less likely to appear on transplantation waiting lists, and are less likely to undergo transplantation procedures, even after patients' insurance status and other factors are considered.

HIV infection continues to spread more rapidly among Black and Hispanic populations than any other racial/ethnic group in the United States. Black Americans with HIV infection are less likely to receive antiretroviral therapy, less likely to receive prophylaxis for pneumocystis pneumonia, and less likely to receive protease inhibitors than nonminorities with HIV. These disparities remain, even after adjusting for age, gender, education, and insurance coverage.

Black Americans, particularly those living in urban areas characterized by concentrated poverty, are at greater risk for morbidity and mortality caused by asthma. Management and control of the disease is affected by socioeconomic and cultural considerations. Black Americans are more likely to receive treatment for asthma in the emergency department and are more likely to use inhaled bronchodilator medications than inhaled corticosteroids, suggesting the management of the disease in this population has been focused more on acute symptom control as opposed to suppression of chronic airway inflammation. Black Americans, Hispanics, and Native Americans experience a 50 to 100% higher burden of illness and mortality caused by diabetes than White Americans, yet the disease appears to be more poorly managed among minority patients.

Given the role of cultural and linguistic factors in both patients' perception of pain and in physicians' ability to accurately assess patients' pain, it is reasonable to suspect that healthcare disparities might be greater in pain treatment and other aspects of symptom management than in treatment of objectively verifiable disease.

Although large increases in Internet access have occurred among most groups of Americans regardless of income, education, race or ethnicity, location, age, or gender (U.S. Department of Commerce, 2002), the IOM quality report (2001) identifies a "digital divide" in the use of technology within the disabled Black and Hispanic communities. Access to the Internet and other information technology gives the patient access to healthcare information unavailable before. The quality and completeness of this Internet information has a high degree of variability that may result in more problems than answers for patients.

Placing a focus on patient-centered care is another recommendation from the quality report (IOM, 2001). Obviously, culture plays an important role here. As with communication styles, patients differ in their views about how active they wish to be in decision making. In some cases, patients demand a large role, in others, they may wish a large role but are passive in making this known. In still other cases, the patient may delegate decision making to another person—this could be a family member of the patient. The goal of patient centeredness is to customize care to the specific needs and circumstances of each individual patient. The care must be modified to respond to the person and their culture, not force the patient to modify to the care. Health care is not just any service industry, as its fundamental nature is the delivery of care to people and their families in a time of illness. Because the outcome is uncertain, the stress and strain are considerable. The establishment of a trusting relationship between patient and nurse is essential and critical, and its absence contributes to a poor outcome. Change is a difficult concept for many. This appears to be especially true of healthcare professionals, who traditionally are a conservative group who stress precedent and the avoidance

---

Box 4–4 Barriers to Healthcare Delivery: The 12 A's

- **Availability**—Is the service available at times when it will be needed?
- **Accessibility**—Is transportation available? Are there geographic boundaries that are impenetrable?
- **Affordability**—Does the patient have the financial resources to cover the cost?
- **Appropriateness**—Are the offered services appropriate to the community?
- **Accountability**—Do members of the healthcare team demonstrate accountability for their own education regarding the cultures being served?
- **Adaptability**—Is the system designed for maximum flexibility or is it rigid?
- **Acceptability**—Are the services culturally and linguistically acceptable to the patient population?
- **Awareness**—Are potential patients and community members aware of all available services?
- **Attitudes**—Are the attitudes of healthcare providers open to the inclusion of neutral or nonharmful traditional interventions?
- **Approachability**—Do patients feel welcome when accessing care?
- **Alternative Practices**—Are the patient's alternative/complementary practices incorporated into the plan of care?
- **Additional Services**—Is care delivery designed so that multiple services are available during the same hours?

Source: Lattanzi, J. B., & Purnell, L. D. (2006). *Developing cultural competence in physical therapy practice*. Philadelphia, PA: F. A. Davis.

Box 4–5 Pertinent Research Studies

1. A retrospective study conducted by Enriquez et al. (2008) examined the impact of a bicultural/bilingual healthcare team on health-related outcomes among Hispanic/Latino adults who received care at an academic HIV specialty center (N = 43 subjects). The HIV center program manager brought together three Hispanic/Latino bilingual/bicultural care providers made up of an NP, a case manager, and a peer educator. All of the patient education and case management materials were revised and evaluated to ensure that they were culturally and linguistically appropriate. This was done by clinic staff and the director of interpreter services for the institution, who was also bicultural/bilingual. Demographic and health data extracted from medical records were compared over two time periods: 1 year before and 1 year after the implementation of the care team. Results indicated that there were more clinic visits per patient and that a higher percentage of individuals had suppressed HIV viral loads to less than 50 copies/mL during the year after the team was implemented, compared with the previous year. Results from this study suggest that provision of care by healthcare workers who are bilingual/bicultural, together with the use of linguistically and culturally appropriate materials, may enhance health outcomes among Hispanic/Latino adults living with HIV infection. The team believed that the ability to interact with patients within the patient's cultural context improved communication, enhanced patient understanding of the treatment plan, and increased patient trust in the healthcare system.

2. An observational cohort study conducted by Hall and colleagues (2012) evaluated the 247,707 adults who were registered for first-time kidney transplants from 1995 to 2007 to determine center-specific estimates of living donor kidney transplant (LDKT) attainment in Black Americans versus non-Black patients. Racial parity was not seen at any of the 275 kidney centers. Individual kidney center racial disparities ranged from 35 to 76% lower odds of receiving LDKT for Black Americans, compared to non-Black American patients. In addition, higher rates of LDKT (interaction term, 1.25; $P < 0.001$) were associated in patients with less racial disparity. Thus, the study concluded that every transplant center in the United States had racial disparity in the attainment of LDKT, and that the centers with the highest rates of LDKT attainment for all races had the lowest level of disparity. The study authors recommend that these higher-performing kidney centers be further evaluated to see if any insights regarding their policies may be helpful to reduce this particular health disparity.

Source: Enriquez, M., Farnan, R., Cheng, A. L., Almeida, A., Del Valle, D., Pulido-Parra, M., & Flores, G. (2008). Impact of a bilingual/bicultural care team on HIV-related outcomes. *Journal of the Association of Nurses in AIDS Care, 19*(4), 295–301; and Hall, E. C., James, N. T., Garonzik Wang, J. M., Berger, J. C., Montgomery, R. A., Dagher, N. N., . . . Segev, D. L. (2012). Center-level factors and racial disparities in living donor kidney transplantation. *American Journal of Kidney Diseases, 59*(6), 849–857.

of risk in practice (IOM, 2001). The result is that change is slow and difficult to achieve, especially when the perceived benefit is unclear or not valued.

Another important issue raised in this report is equity. The aim of equity is to ensure that all Americans receive the same benefit from our healthcare system. The goal of health care is to improve health status and to reduce health disparities by providing universal access—a promise that has not yet been kept. The report states unequivocally that with regard to equity in caregiving, all individuals rightly expect to be treated fairly by social institutions, including healthcare organizations. The availability of care and quality of services should be based on individuals' particular needs and not on personal characteristics unrelated to the patient's condition or to the reason for seeking care. In particular, the quality of care should not differ because of such characteristics as gender, race, age, ethnicity, income, education, disability, sexual orientation, or location of residence.

MULTIDISCIPLINARY AND INTERDISCIPLINARY TEAMS

One approach advocated to provide for greater equity is the use of teams so that professionals from various disciplines contribute to patient care. Because some of the skills of NPs overlap with those of physicians, tension can often develop. Despite a difference in the training and education provided to all advance practice nurses who practice clinically (NPs, nurse–midwives, certified RN assistants), there are subsets of skills that overlap with physicians. This complexity of rules across settings and across state lines makes it difficult for true multidisciplinary or interdisciplinary teams to be developed and fully implemented. Because licensure and scope of practice is determined at the state level, there is a great deal of variability in advance practice nursing roles. State licensure permits regulations that are tailored to meet local needs, resources, and patient expectations. The resulting state-by-state variation is not always logical given the growth of the Internet and the formation of large, multistate provider groups that cut across geographic boundaries. The National Council of State Boards of Nursing has endorsed a mutual recognition model for interstate nursing practice that retains state licensure authority, but provides a mechanism for practice across state lines (similar to a driver's license that is granted by one state and recognized in other states). Still others have argued the relative merits of state-based versus national licensing systems. In any event, the care that is delivered must meet the individual needs of each patient to ensure quality health care for all Americans.

Clinical encounters are an interaction between the patient's culture and the culture of nursing/medicine. The patient's culture and the medical culture both possess unique perspectives, knowledge, attitudes, skills, and behaviors. The patient and the nurse will each approach a clinical encounter from a different viewpoint. The ability to find common ground is key to working together effectively to meet patient goals. To help find this common ground, it is important for the nurse to recognize that the patient will have an illness perspective (the subjective feeling of being unhealthy) while the nurse will plan care around the diagnosis of the patient (a medical label). The patient's beliefs provide the guidelines for how the patient will perceive, interpret, understand, and respond to the illness.

The practice of nursing, with its emphasis on patient response to illness, is compatible with a patient-centered approach. Medicine has a disease-focus interpretation, which is not the same as the experience of illness related to individual perception. When a patient's beliefs about health and illness are closely aligned to the Western Biomedical Model, there is a high degree of likelihood of compatibility between patient and provider. On the other hand, when there is incompatibility between the patient's illness beliefs and the provider's approach, there is the likelihood of resistance to biomedical treatment recommendations. The advance practice nurse, by virtue of education and philosophical focus, is in the best position to bridge such a gap if it is present. Taking the emphasis off achieving medical goals and placing the emphasis on the concerns of the patient is the preferred approach. The nurse must attempt to understand the patient's health, illness, and health beliefs and not impose his or her own cultural beliefs on them. Doing this is necessary in order to provide patient-centered care.

NEED TO IMPROVE DIVERSITY OF NURSING AND HEALTHCARE WORKFORCE

The National Advisory Council on Nursing Education and Practice (NACNEP) advises the Secretary of the U.S. Department of Health and Human Services and the U.S. Congress on policy issues related to programs authorized by Title VIII of the U.S. Public Health Service Act and administered by the Health Resources and Services Administration, Bureau of Health Professions, Division of Nursing, including nurse workforce supply, education, and practice improvement. NACNEP in its sixth report (2008), entitled *Meeting the Challenges of the New Millennium: Challenges Facing the Nurse Workforce in a Changing Health Care Environment*, stated that although more nurses are needed in the workforce, this is not the complete answer. The end goal of our healthcare workforce needs to be inclusion, not just increased diversity. This means involvement by underrepresented minorities in all aspects of the healthcare institution, including decision making. Inclusion will result in less workplace tension and increased productivity. Ultimately, a diverse workforce can attract a more diverse patient population. Our increasingly diverse population requires increased cultural competence and sensitivity to receive the most effective care (NACNEP, 2008). Nurses play a critical role in making this a reality because nurses are the single largest component of the workforce in health care. Nurses not only provide the majority of direct care to patients, but also are major partners in healthcare management and policy. NACNEP predicts a nursing shortage that could expand to potentially insurmountable levels over the next 10 to 15 years because of an aging workforce and a faculty shortage that limits student enrollment, among other factors. Practicing nurses will also need to establish and further develop skills in critical thinking and provide innovations in patient care delivery and increased cultural competence that corresponds to the patient population for which the nurse provides care (NACNEP, 2008).

The organization and delivery of health care in the United States is continually changing in order to meet new economic challenges and to adopt improvements and innovations in patient care. Delivery of healthcare services in the United States is becoming more demanding as the healthcare system is becoming more complex and the expectation for services is growing. At the same time, financial pressures are driving organizations to reduce costs and increase efficiency, and funders and consumers are demanding greater focus on the quality of health care and its impact on patient outcomes. The healthcare system in the United States is becoming ever more complex at a time when an expanding, aging, and diverse population is demanding increasing amounts of healthcare services.

NACNEP (2008) has identified the capabilities, skills, and nursing resources required for today's modern nursing practice. The rapidly changing healthcare environment requires nurses with strong critical thinking and analytical skills as well as the ability to provide professional and compassionate care. These critical thinking and analytical skills are required to acquire and assimilate data in order to make appropriate patient care decisions. Nurses need interdisciplinary competencies supported by backgrounds in the sciences as well as the humanities. In order to ensure patient safety, provide quality care, and deliver patient care efficiently, nurses must be able to gather and synthesize new information and identify and address needs as soon as they emerge. This is critical not only for nursing and the healthcare delivery system to provide for routine medical situations, but it is also complicated by the need for the healthcare workforce to be prepared to provide the necessary emergency response in the event of either natural or man-made disasters.

With the prospect of the nursing shortage worsening, nurse–patient staffing ratios also need to be considered when planning for nursing workforce design. There is a growing body of research that associates inadequate nurse staffing with adverse patient outcomes. A study by Aiken, Clarke, Sloane, Sochalski, and Silber (2002) found that each additional patient per nurse results in a 7% increase in the likelihood of dying within 30 days of hospital admission. Other studies have found associations between low nurse staffing levels and hospital-acquired pneumonia, urinary tract infection, sepsis, nosocomial infections, pressure ulcers, upper gastrointestinal bleeding, shock and cardiac arrest, medication errors, falls, and longer than expected length of stay (Needleman & Buerhaus, 2003). Evidence shows that having more nurses in the workforce is associated with better hospital outcomes (Needleman & Buerhaus, 2003).

Consideration must be given to the fact that inadequate or poor staffing not only increases the chance of a poor patient outcome, but its impact is felt by the nurse as well. Aiken et al. (2002) found RN job dissatisfaction levels were more elevated in hospitals with high patient-to-nurse ratios than in hospitals with lower patient-to-nurse ratios. The health of the nurse is also negatively impacted. Aiken et al. (2010) found that only 29% of California RNs (CA has mandated nursing staffing ratios) experienced high burnout compared with 34% in New Jersey and 36% of nurses in Pennsylvania (both states do not have minimum staffing ratios). Increased levels of nurse staffing means improved nurse-to-patient ratios. This leads to better patient safety (including more opportunities for patient monitoring and interaction) and reduces risks for unsafe conditions, thereby yielding better patient outcomes. Another study found that the increase of one RN per patient was associated with a 24% reduction in the time spent in the intensive care unit and a 31% reduction in time spent in a surgical unit (Kane, Shamliyan, Mueller, Duval, & Wilt, 2007). Improved nurse-to-patient ratios also mean more opportunities for patient monitoring and interaction, which includes attending to patients' psychosocial needs. Having more nurses available at a patient care site also improves the availability of cross coverage when one patient's care demands a greater proportion of an individual nurse's time.

The National Sample Survey of Registered Nurses (USDHHS, 2010b), a survey of only RNs that is conducted every four years (conducted in 2008 and published in 2010), found the RN workforce hit an all-time high of 3.1 million; a growth of more than 5% between 2004 and 2008. The United States has one-fifth of all of the world's nurses. The latest survey data showed a growth in the number of RNs under the age of 30—the first increase seen in 30 years. There is also improvement noted in the number of men entering the RN profession as well as other minority groups. While the 2008 survey found that 16.8% of the nurses were ethnic minorities, an increase from 12.2% in 2004, there is still much more recruitment that needs to be done to make the nursing workforce better reflect the population of the patients that are being served. Despite this growth in total numbers, the demographic characteristics of RNs remain relatively unchanged from its majority of White females. The percentage of male RNs only increased very slightly from 5.4% in 2000 to 5.8% in 2009. Although there has been some increase in male student enrollment numbers, the representation of men in nursing education programs remains low. Men accounted for 8.8% of all baccalaureate graduates, 10.6% of master's graduates, and only 4.0% of doctoral program graduates in the year 2004 (Berlin, Wilsey, & Bednash, 2005). The numbers for minority student enrollments are also low. Racial and ethnic minorities accounted for 23.8% of undergraduate enrollees and 21.5% of graduate-level enrollees (Berlin et al., 2005). The average age of RNs increased by 6.5 years since 1980, to an average of 46.8 years in 2004, and 73.4% of all RNs were age 40 years or older. (USDHHS, 2010b).

Between 1977 and 1997, the number of RNs from minority backgrounds grew from 6.3% to 9.7% of the total population of RNs (Buerhaus & Auerbach, 1999). The 2008 National Sample Survey of Registered Nurses found 16.8% of RNs identified as non-White. Comparisons of racial/ethnic composition of the RN population across time are complicated because of changes in definitions of race/ethnicity initiated with the U.S. census. Regardless of the difficulty of closely tracking changes over time, the U.S. RN population in 2008 remained significantly less racially and ethnically diverse than the overall population of the United States: 83.2% of RNs identified as White and non-Hispanic, compared with 65.6% for the overall U.S. population (USDHHS, 2010b). Approximately 3.5% of RNs are foreign born and educated. The bottom line is that the nursing population in the United States does not reflect the population for whom we are asked to deliver care. The majority of RNs today are female, White, and aging.

IMPACT ON PROVISION OF PRIMARY CARE BY NURSE PRACTITIONERS

According to the National Survey of Registered Nurses 2008 data (USDHHS, 2010b), there are 138,600 nurse practitioners in the United States, an increase of 4.2% from 122,800 in 2004. Advance practice nurses (which include NPs, nurse anesthetists, nurse–midwives, and clinical nurse specialists) now make up 8.2% of the total RN population. Even more growth is needed in the NP numbers to meet the primary care needs of many underserved Americans. Some healthcare advocates are calling for even more advanced practice nurses to provide primary care to patients, because there is a shortage of primary care physicians. The Institute of Medicine has recommended permitting advance practice nurses a larger and more independent role in patient care. It is clear that a further expanded role for nurses is urgent as the potential for more people seeking health care with the implementation of healthcare reform legislation. In addition, NPs need to continue the advocacy role of nursing and apply it to minority populations to help make a difference in the incidence of healthcare disparities over time. The movement to improve the quality of patient care and to minimize healthcare disparities places the focus on improving access to patient-centered and linguistically appropriate services (Nailon, 2007). NPs have traditionally gone to underserved areas to improve patient access throughout the years. Because NPs come from the nursing workforce, they are representative of the demographic characteristics of the global U.S. nursing workforce in general. Because only about 11% of NPs are minorities, it is likely the NP may not share the same cultural, racial, or ethnic background of the patients they care for. This underscores the need for all NPs to be educated in the area of cultural competence and to provide appropriate patient education to help decrease health disparities (Edmunds, 2008). NPs, just like other nurses, must acknowledge their beliefs and biases about specific groups of people because these biases and beliefs may be inadvertently communicated to the patient and his or her family through both verbal and nonverbal communication. This can result in potentially offensive situations for both the patient and his or her family. NPs must find adaptive and creative ways to cross the cultural divide and to negotiate any language barriers so that all patients receive the quality health care they deserve and require.

The integration of cultural competency into primary care practice has been clarified in the NONPF document on cultural competency (Green-Hernandez et al., 2004). It states that the NP demonstrates cultural competence when she or he shows respect for the inherent dignity of every human being, whatever their age, gender, religion, socioeconomic class, sexual orientation, and ethnic or cultural group; accepts the rights of individuals to choose their care provider, participate in care, and refuse care; acknowledges personal biases and prevents these from interfering with the delivery of quality care to persons of other cultures; recognizes cultural issues and interacts with clients from other cultures in culturally sensitive ways and incorporates cultural preferences, health beliefs, behaviors, and traditional practices into the management plan; develops client-appropriate educational materials that address the language and cultural beliefs of the client and accesses culturally appropriate resources to deliver care to clients from other cultures; and finally, assists clients in accessing quality care within a dominant culture.

The American Association of Colleges of Nursing standards that are outlined in the Essentials of Masters Education for Advanced Practice Nurses states that NPs be exposed and complete diverse learning experiences in order to develop understanding of the impact of cultural diversity on human behavior (Van Zandt, Sloand, & Wilkins, 2008). Presently, NP educational guidelines do not specifically identify all of the unique skills that are required to provide advance practice nursing care to vulnerable groups.

An attempt to meet this challenge is the development and utilization of nurse-managed academic health centers, which are community-based health practices that provide care to vulnerable populations. Because these institutions are often staffed by NPs, RNs, health educators, community health workers, social workers, dietitians/nutritional support, and collaborating or supervising physicians, among other healthcare professionals, they provide the opportunity for student NPs to have a clinical placement to meet their educational requirements as well as the opportunity to watch a multidisciplinary, and perhaps even an interdisciplinary, team in action.

OPPORTUNITIES FOR NURSES TO ATTAIN CULTURAL COMPETENCY CERTIFICATION

There are several opportunities already in existence for nurses to attain cultural competency certification. One such program is Cultural Competence Certification for Clinicians, which is offered by the Center for Professional Development at the School of Nursing at the University of Pennsylvania. Topics covered for the certification include appraisal of personal attitudes, values, and beliefs; impact of racial and ethnic disparities on quality of care; conceptual framework for discussions on ethnic diversity; and concerns of special populations. Other areas covered are assessments of diverse cultural health values and beliefs, strategies to facilitate cross-cultural communication, and working effectively with interpreters. The program also addresses issues surrounding ethnic pharmacology, dietary concerns, the use of complementary and alternative therapies, and religious issues with emphasis on healthcare decision making and treatment.

The City University of New York College of Staten Island (CSI) offers an advanced certificate in cultural competence that can be taken for college credit or continuing education units. The program is accredited by the New York State Department of Education. The program consists of three courses and can be completed in two semesters (one year).

The Leadership Fellowship is a program designed to educate healthcare leaders in promoting culturally appropriate care to all patients. It was developed by the American Hospital Association in collaboration with the National Healthcare Leadership Cultural Competence and is offered by the Health Resource Educational Trust.

Nurses are also encouraged to consider joining the Transcultural Nursing Society or at a minimum to read its journal to become more informed and to enhance nursing care delivery. The Transcultural Nursing Society was founded in 1974 and it offers the nation's first certification program, which began in 1987. Since then there have been modifications and changes in the certification process. According to the Transcultural Nursing Society website (http://tcns.org) the nurse who possesses or attains either a basic or advanced certification in transcultural nursing "demonstrates to nurse colleagues, patients, employers, and others, the knowledge, experience, and commitment to transcultural nursing" (Transcultural Nursing Society, 2012).

FUTURE RESEARCH

Future research should be designed to rely on standardized data collection. This IOM recommendation (Smedley et al., 2003) would result in improved identification of factors that are associated with healthcare disparities and avoid discriminatory practices. It is a difficult recommendation to implement, however, because of privacy concerns, cost, and resistance within the healthcare system. Research should also focus on the development of clinical practice guidelines that are culturally competent as well. In summary, a broad and comprehensive approach is required, with full participation from all stakeholders, to keep the promise to all Americans of receiving high-quality health care.

SUMMARY

Making the commitment to provide culturally competent nursing care within the changing healthcare environment takes time and dedication. The organization's mission statement, policies and procedures, and stated goals must reflect this commitment as well. Areas of diversity that exist within the practice area must be identified, analyzed, and respected so that more can be learned about cultural beliefs and factors and the community's true healthcare needs. Finally, the organization, often at the nurses' urging, needs to provide training and education for all interdisciplinary and multidisciplinary team members on how to provide culturally appropriate care in the 21st century healthcare environment. The provision of culturally competent care will result in greater patient satisfaction, and if current research studies are correct, improved patient outcomes. This is an area that is ripe for further research opportunities as there are questions that still require answers and studies that need replication that are available for nurse researchers to tackle.

REVIEW QUESTIONS

1. Which potential areas of diversity exist in your practice community?
2. How might you learn more about your local community and its unique needs?
3. What reasons have you identified for you to make the commitment to strive toward cultural competence? What barriers are in your way? Can they be overcome?

REFERENCES

Aiken, L. H., Clarke, S. P., Sloane, D. M., Sochalski, J., & Silber, J. H. (2002). Hospital nurse staffing and patient mortality, nurse burnout, and job dissatisfaction. *Journal of the American Medical Association, 288*(16), 1987–1993.

Aiken, L. H., Sloane, D. M., Cimiotti, J. P., Clarke, S. P., Flynn, L., Seago, J. A., . . . Smith, H. L. (2010). Implications of the California nurse staffing mandate for other states. *Health Services Research, 45*(4), 904–921.

American Nurses Association. (2004). *ANA position statements*. Retrieved from http://www.nursingworld.org

Andrulis, D. P. (2010). *Disparities knowledge gaps, cultural competence status and progress, and potential future directions*. Retrieved from http://iom.edu/~/media/Files/Activity%20Files/SelectPops/HealthDisparities/2010-APR-08/Dennis%20Andrulis2_1.pdf

Balsa, A. I., Seiler, N., McGuire, T. G., & Bloche, M. G. (2003). Clinical uncertainty and healthcare disparities. *American Journal of Law and Medicine, 29*(2–3), 203–219.

Berkman, N. D., DeWalt, D. A., Pignone, M. P., Sherican, S. L., Lohr, K. N., Lux, L., . . . Bonito, A. J. (2004). *Literacy and health outcomes*. Retrieved from http://archive.ahrq.gov/downloads/pub/evidence/pdf/literacy/literacy.pdf

Berlin, L. E., Wilsey, S. J., & Bednash, G. D. (2005). *2004–2005 Enrollment and graduations in baccalaureate and graduate programs in nursing*. Washington, DC: American Association of Colleges of Nursing.

Braveman, P. A., Kumanyika, S., Fielding, J., Laveist, T., Borrell, L. N., Manderscheid, R., & Troutman, A. (2011). Health disparities and health equity: The issue is justice. *American Journal of Public Health, 101*(Suppl. 1), S149–S155.

Buerhaus, P. I., & Auerbach, D. (1999). Slow growth in the United States of the number of minorities in the RN workforce. *Image—The Journal of Nursing Scholarship, 31*(2), 179–183.

Edmunds, M. W. (2008). Join us in resolving health disparities [Editorial]. *The Journal for Nurse Practitioners, 4*(1), 7.

Enriquez, M., Farnan, R., Cheng, A. L., Almeida, A., Del Valle, D., Pulido-Parra, M., & Flores, G. (2008). Impact of a bilingual/bicultural care team on HIV-related outcomes. *Journal of the Association of Nurses in AIDS Care, 19*(4), 295–301.

Epstein, N. B., Baldwin, L. M., & Bishop, D. S. (2000). Family assessment device. In K. Corcoran & J. Fischer (Eds.), *Measures for clinical practice: A sourcebook*. New York, NY: Free Press.

Federal Office of Management and Budget. (2001). *Reports and bulletins*. Retrieved from http://www.whitehouse.gov/omb

Goldenberg, M. J. (2005). Evidence-based ethics? On evidence-based practice and the "empirical turn" from normative bioethics. *BMC Medical Ethics, 6*, E11. doi:10.1186/1472-6939-6-11

Green-Hernandez, C., Quinn, A. A., Denman-Vitale, S., Falkenstern, S. K., & Judge-Ellis, T. (2004). Making primary care culturally competent. *The Nurse Practitioner, 29*(6), 49–55.

Hall, E. C., James, N. T., Garonzik Wang, J. M., Berger, J. C., Montgomery, R. A., Dagher, N. N., . . . Segev, D. L. (2012). Center-level factors and racial disparities in living donor kidney transplantation. *American Journal of Kidney Diseases, 59*(6), 849–857.

Hall, J. K. (1996). *Nursing ethics and law*. Philadelphia, PA: Saunders.

House, J. S., & Williams, D. R. (2000). Understanding and reducing socioeconomic and racial/ethnic disparities in health. In B. D. Smedley & S. L. Syme (Eds.), *Promoting health: Intervention strategies from social and behavioral research* (pp. 81–124). Washington, DC: National Academy Press.

Institute of Medicine. (1990). *Medicare: A strategy for quality assurance: Executive summary*. Washington, DC: National Academy Press.

Institute of Medicine. (2001). *Crossing the quality chasm: A new health system for the 21st century*. Washington, DC: National Academy Press.

Kane, R. L., Shamliyan, T. A., Mueller, C., Duval, S., & Wilt, T. J. (2007). The association of registered nurse staffing levels and patient outcomes: Systematic review and meta-analysis. *Medical Care, 45*(12), 1195–1204.

Korenbrot, C. C., & Moss, N. E. (2000). Preconception, prenatal, perinatal, and postnatal influences on health. In B. D. Smedley & S. L. Syme (Eds.), *Promoting health: Intervention strategies from social and behavioral research* (pp. 125–169). Washington, DC: National Academy Press.

Kuhse, H. (1997). *Caring: Nurses, women and ethics*. Oxford, UK: Wiley.

Lattanzi, J. B., & Purnell, L. D. (2006). *Developing cultural competence in physical therapy practice*. Philadelphia, PA: F. A. Davis.

Leddy, S. K. (2006). *Integrative health promotion: Conceptual bases for nursing practice* (2nd ed.). Sudbury, MA: Jones and Bartlett.

Morin, R. (2001, July 11). Misperceptions cloud whites' views of blacks. *The Washington Post*, p. A1.

Murray, C. J., Kulkarni, S. C., Michaud, C., Tomijima, N., Bulzachelli, M. T., Iandiorio, T. J., & Ezzati, M. (2006). Eight Americas: Investigating mortality disparities across races, counties and race-counties in the United States. *PLoS Medicine, 3*(9), e260. doi:10.1371/journal.pmed.0030260

Nailon, R. E. (2007). The assessment and documentation of language and communication needs in healthcare systems: Current practices and future directions for coordinating safe, patient-centered care. *Nursing Outlook, 55*(6), 311–317.

Nash, R. A. (1999). The biomedical ethics of alternative, complementary, and integrative medicine. *Alternative Therapies in Health and Medicine, 5*(5), 92–95.

National Advisory Council on Nursing Education and Practice. (2008). *Meeting the challenges of the new millennium: Challenges facing the nurse workforce in a changing health care environment*

(6th annual report). Retrieved from http://www.hrsa.gov/advisorycommittees/bhpradvisory/nacnep/Reports/sixthreport.pdf

Needleman, J., & Buerhaus, P. (2003). Nurse staffing and patient safety: Current knowledge and implications for action. *International Journal for Quality in Health Care, 15*(4), 275–277.

Office of Minority Health. (2001). *National standards for culturally and linguistically appropriate services in health care.* (Final report). Rockville, MD: Author. Retrieved from http://www.omhrc.gov/assets/pdf/checked/finalreport.pdf

Office of Minority Health. (2012). *National standards for culturally and linguistically appropriate services in health care* (Final report). Rockville, MD: Author. Retrieved from http://www.mhsoac.ca.gov/meetings/docs/Meetings/2012/Mar/CLCC_030712_Tab5_DrCarneiro-sCLASPresentation.pdf

Rothschild, M. L. (2000). Ethical considerations in support of the marketing of public health issues. *American Journal of Health Behavior, 24*(1), 26–35.

Schwarz, J. K. (2000). Have we forgotten the patient? *American Journal of Nursing, 100*(2), 61, 64.

Smedley, B. D., Stith, A. Y., & Nelson, A. R. (Eds.). (2003). *Unequal treatment: Confronting racial and ethnic disparities in health care.* Washington, DC: National Academies Press.

Transcultural Nursing Society. (2012). Transcultural nursing certification. Retrieved from http://www.tcns.org/Certification.html

U.S. Department of Commerce. (2002). How and where America goes online. In *A nation online: How Americans are expanding their use of the Internet* (pp. 35–41). Retrieved from http://www.ntia.doc.gov/files/ntia/publications/anationonline2.pdf

U.S. Department of Education. (2007). *Appendix A: Revisions to the standards for the classification of federal data on race and ethnicity.* Retrieved from http://nces.ed.gov/programs/handbook/data/pdf/appendices.pdf

U.S. Department of Health and Human Services (USDHHS). (2002). *Nurse practitioner primary care competencies in specialty areas.* Retrieved from http://www.aacn.nche.edu/education-resources/npcompetencies.pdf

U.S. Department of Health and Human Services (USDHHS). (2010a). *Healthy People 2020.* Retrieved from http://www.healthypeople.gov/2020/about/DOHAbout.aspx

U.S. Department of Health and Human Services (USDHHS). (2010b). *The Registered Nurse Population: Initial findings from the 2008 National Sample of Registered Nurses.* Retrieved from http://bhpr.hrsa.gov/healthworkforce/rnsurveys/rnsurveyinitial2008.pdf

Van Zandt, S. E., Sloand, E., & Wilkins, A. (2008). Caring for vulnerable populations: Role of academic nurse–managed health centers in educating nurse practitioners. *The Journal for Nurse Practitioners, 4*(2), 126–131.

For a full suite of assignments and additional learning activities, see the access code at the front of your book.

Impact of Culture on Health and Illness for Selected Cultural Groups

OVERVIEW

Unit 2 consists of five chapters; each chapter describes a different racial and/or ethnic group, with an emphasis on what the nurse needs to know regarding the potential impact health and illness has on each group. The cultures selected for inclusion represent those most likely, based on the most recent census population numbers, to require nursing and advanced practice nursing from the nursing workforce currently practicing in the United States.

When reviewing the information contained in Unit 2, the reader is asked to keep in mind that although the information is current and evidence based, it will not be applicable to all patients or to all members of a particular racial or ethnic group. There are vast differences among all people and within group affiliations. This means that certain cultural characteristics will be presented in the chapters within Unit 2, that may or may not be associated with the individual patients to whom you may need to deliver nursing care. The intent of the book is not to be stereotypical but to provide a starting point for knowledge acquisition regarding the selected racial or ethnic groups. The ultimate goal is for patients to receive individualized nursing care that meets their unique needs. The difference between a stereotype and a generalization is determined by timing. A stereotype is an ending point, because no further effort will be made to ascertain whether the information is appropriate for application to the individual patient. A generalization, on the other hand, serves as a starting point. The nurse who possesses knowledge of these generalizations regarding cultural customs and beliefs can use the information to avoid misunderstandings and to enable nurses and nurse practitioners to ultimately provide evidence-based, culturally appropriate, individualized care.

Chapter 5—Black Americans

Background/statistics, definition of health and illness, traditional healing methods, alternative and complementary folk medicine, current healthcare problems including mortality and morbidity data, barriers impacting care (communication, time, space, environment, biologic variations, and social organization), faith and spirituality, case studies, and pertinent research studies.

Chapter 6—Hispanics/Latinos

Background/statistics, distinction between Hispanics and Latinos, various types of Hispanics/Latinos, definition of health and illness, traditional healing methods, alternative and complementary folk medicine, current healthcare problems including mortality and morbidity data, barriers impacting care (communication, time, space, environment, biologic variations, and social organization), faith and spirituality, case studies, and pertinent research studies.

Chapter 7—Asians/Pacific Islanders

Background/statistics, distinctions between Asians and Pacific Islanders, various types of Asians, definition of health and illness, traditional healing methods, alternative and complementary folk medicine, current healthcare problems including mortality and morbidity data, barriers impacting care (communication, time, space, environment, biologic variations, and social organization), faith and spirituality, case studies, and pertinent research studies.

Chapter 8—Native Americans/Alaska Natives

Background/statistics, distinction between Native Americans and Alaska Natives, various types of Native Americans, definition of health and illness, traditional healing methods, alternative and complementary folk medicine, current healthcare problems including mortality and morbidity data, barriers impacting care (communication, time, space, environment, biologic variations, and social organization), faith and spirituality, case studies, and pertinent research studies.

Chapter 9—Whites (Non-Hispanic)

Background/statistics, various types of White Americans of European descent, definition of health and illness, traditional healing methods, alternative and complementary folk medicine, current healthcare problems including mortality and morbidity data, barriers impacting care (communication, time, space, environment, biologic variations, and social organization), faith and spirituality, case studies, and pertinent research studies.

DISCLAIMER

Every consideration will be given to be as accurate and comprehensive as possible. With that said, any attempt to provide cultural information has the potential to be viewed as discriminatory, an oversimplification, offensive, or at worst, all three. It is important that the reader recognizes that individual interpretation of the book's content by the reader will vary, but the intent of the writer will not. The intent is to provide evidence-based information that is associated with the cultural groups being described in the book. The nurse has a responsibility to strive to learn as much as possible about each individual patient under his or her care and to find what, if any, of the included cultural information the individual patient actually ascribes to. Every attempt was made to avoid stereotyping and to focus on generalizations as a starting point to providing culturally competent nursing care. Although the book strives to be a one-stop resource for the busy practicing nurse, the author does not in any way wish to imply that the culturally specific information that is included in the book is all-inclusive or that it will be applicable to each and every patient under your care. Ultimately, experience is the best teacher; the nurse should attempt to broaden his or her practice—the best way to truly learn a culture is to work with patients and staff from that culture. Select the cultures that are most commonly seen in your practice's geographical area to learn about first. Learning about cultural diversity will not only increase your understanding of the world in which we live but multicultural education is an important aspect of our personal and professional development.

CHAPTER 5

Black Americans

www

CHAPTER OBJECTIVES

Upon completion of this chapter, the nurse will be able to:

- Identify ways the Black American culture may impact healthcare beliefs and behavior.
- Recognize biologic variations associated with the Black American patient.
- Plan for the delivery of culturally aware nursing care for the Black American patient.

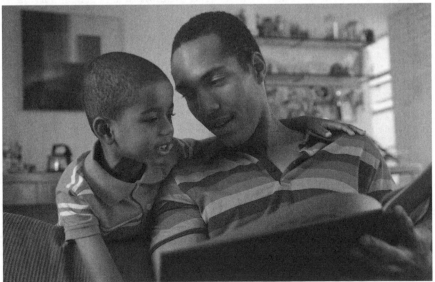

© Jupiterimages/Polka Dot/Thinkstock

INTRODUCTION

All members of a cultural group are not the same. After reading this text, the assumption may be to generalize and stereotype members of various cultures as one. Striving to understand cultural trends should never overshadow the importance and uniqueness of the individual. Other factors can impact the situation as well, such as length of time in the United States, education, social status, whether people live in groups with other members of their cultural group or in isolation, or if they have assimilated into the mainstream culture.

It is neither possible nor necessary for every nurse to learn everything about every culture. What is important is for all nurses to recognize that there are major cultural differences not only in the beliefs and practices of the patients they care for, but also in their needs and expectations regarding care. Nurses should make an effort to learn more about the health beliefs of the particular cultural groups they are most likely to serve. This knowledge and awareness will boost nurses' competence even when they approach patients who belong to cultures with which they are unfamiliar. The key to cultural competence is an awareness and ability to identify differences in beliefs and practices about health maintenance and care and to evaluate their impact on patient satisfaction and adherence to care. Nurses need to view the practices of other cultures without judging them according to their own.

The nurse must always strive to understand the individual patient and to establish a therapeutic relationship. Recognizing that culture may have an impact on the patient's health beliefs and response to treatment is essential as a starting point to avoid a cultural mismatch or cultural gaffe, and the nurse must strive to learn as much as she or he can about the patient and be responsive to this information in planning nursing care. When nurses have developed these sensitivities, they will be better equipped to encourage the patients they care for to disclose any beliefs and practices that may have an impact on care and respond to them in an appropriate manner. The Giger and Davidhizar (Giger, 2013) Transcultural Assessment Model is used as a framing guide for this textbook. Because not all Black Americans are from Africa, the term *Black Americans* will be used in place of *African Americans*. When caring for patients, the nurse should ask the patient how he or she wishes to be identified, as some prefer African American, some prefer Black, some prefer person of color, and so on. Dark-skinned patients from the Caribbean may identify with the African culture but may prefer to be identified by their countries of origin such as West Indian, Dominican Republican, Jamaican, or Haitian. Newer immigrants from the continent of Africa may prefer to be called by their country of origin, such as Nigerian, and may feel disenfranchised from the Black American community in the United States that has its roots in slavery.

HISTORICAL BACKGROUND

The only racial group with ancestors who were forced immigrants to our country is Black Americans. Most Black Americans have their roots in Africa and the majority are descended from people who were brought here from the west coast of Africa, against their will, to be enslaved.

According to some sources, the first Black people to enter the United States arrived in 1618, a year earlier than the Pilgrims, whereas other sources claim that Blacks arrived with Columbus in the 15th century (Bullough & Bullough, 1982). This means that the very first Blacks who came to the North American continent did not come as slaves.

Between 1619 and 1860, more than 4 million people were transported to America as slaves. In 1619, the first African slaves arrived in Virginia. In 1808, Congress banned the importation of slaves from Africa. In 1820, the Missouri Compromise banned slavery north of the southern boundary of Missouri. A setback to the antislavery movement occurred when Congress passed the Kansas-Nebraska Act in 1854, establishing those two territories but repealing the Missouri Compromise. This inflamed tensions between proslavery and antislavery factions. In 1857, the Dred Scott case held that Congress does not have the right to ban slavery in states and, further, that slaves are not citizens. In 1861, the Confederacy was founded when the South seceded from the nation and the Civil War began. In 1863, President Abraham Lincoln signed the Emancipation Proclamation stating that all slaves "are and henceforward shall be free." In 1865, the Civil War ended, President Lincoln was assassinated, and the Thirteenth Amendment to the U.S. Constitution abolished slavery throughout the United States. On June 19, 1865, slavery effectively ended when the last remaining slaves in Texas finally received word that the Civil War had ended 2 months earlier.

Despite the tremendous hardships and inhumane treatment endured by the slaves, the Black culture survived and continued to grow (Eiser & Ellis, 2007). Despite forced separations, Black people managed to maintain community awareness and family structure. The rich variety of traditional beliefs and practices that came with them from West Africa were maintained, continued, and passed down throughout the years. These religious traditions respected the spiritual power of ancestors. Many gods were initially worshipped, including gods who oversaw daily life (change of seasons, fertility, health, healing practices, etc.). Many aspects of current Christian religious practice are believed to have originated in these early practices. It has been estimated that between 10 and 30% of the slaves brought to America between 1711 and 1808 were Muslim, and some of these early religious customs have persisted until today (Eiser & Ellis, 2007).

Today, immigrants come voluntarily from African countries, the Dominican Republic, and other island countries such as Haiti, Jamaica, and the West Indian Islands.

Census data reveals that immigrants from Africa and the Caribbean are a growing component of the U.S. population. They are part of the racial and ethnic transformation of the United States in the 21st century. According to U.S. census data, in 1800, about 20% of the 5 million people in the United States were Black compared to 13.6% of the nearly 313.7 million people in the country as of 2010. Although far outnumbered by non-Black Hispanic and Asian immigrants, the number of Black immigrants is growing at a remarkable rate. More than one-fourth of the Black population in New York, Boston, and Miami is foreign-born. Immigration contributed at least one-fifth of the growth in the U.S. Black population between 2001 and 2006. From 1980 to 2009, the African-born population in United States grew from just under 200,000 to almost 1.5 million. As of 2010, immigrants from Africa make up a small (3.9%) but growing share of the country's 38.5 million immigrants (Terrazas, 2009).

According to Batalova and Terrazas (2010), the foreign-born Black population from all sources increased nearly sevenfold between 1960 and 1980, and more than tripled between 1980 and 2005. The number of Haitians—the second largest Caribbean group—nearly quadrupled between 1980 and 2005 (Terrazas, 2010), and the number of Jamaicans—the largest Caribbean group—more than doubled (McCabe, 2011). The increases were even more dramatic among African groups. The number of Ethiopians in 2005 was 13 times the 1960 number (Terrazas, 2009).

Overall, the number of foreign-born U.S. Blacks rose from 125,000 in 1980 to 2,815,000 in 2005, with a majority arriving since 1990. About two-thirds of Black foreign-born persons in the United States are from the Caribbean and Latin America, and one-third are from Africa. Only a small fraction of the new Black immigrants were born in Europe, Canada, or elsewhere. But the African share is growing. More African-born Blacks arrived between 2000 and 2005 than in the previous decade. Nearly two-thirds of Caribbean-born Blacks live in the New York or Miami metropolitan areas. African-born Blacks are more dispersed throughout the United States. Among the top cities of residence for African-born Blacks are New York; Washington, DC; Minneapolis; and Atlanta; three-fifths live in other metropolitan areas, such as Philadelphia, Los Angeles, or Dallas. These immigrants have high educational attainment—38% of African-born and 20% of Caribbean or Latin American–born Blacks have a college degree. They tend to have low rates of unemployment and poverty compared with the general population, but they often are underpaid and underemployed given their educational achievements and experience. This new 21st-century Black immigration will have a tremendous impact on the American Black population as well as the whole population in general. According to the *New York Times* (Library Index, n.d.), these immigrants from Africa have been "redefining what it means to be African American." Immigrants from Africa lack the perspective of American history that drove affirmative action and diversity programs. Many speak English, have been raised in large cities with capitalist economies, live in families headed by married couples, and are generally more highly educated than American-born Blacks. They also tend to have higher paying jobs.

For purposes of this text, Black or African American terminology is based on the definition used in the 2010 U.S. census. Most members of the present Black American community have their roots in Africa and the majority descended from people who were brought here as slaves from the west coast of Africa. Today, a number of Blacks have immigrated to the United States voluntarily from some African countries, the West Indian Islands, the Dominican Republic, Haiti, and Jamaica. It is for the reason of inclusion that the term *Black Americans* or *Blacks* is used in this textbook. There is no general agreement as to a preferred name for this racial group, so it is recommended to ask the patient how they prefer to be identified. According to Office of Management and Budget for the 2010 census, "Black or African American" refers to a person having origins in any of the Black racial groups of Africa. The Black racial category includes people who marked the "Black, African American, or Negro" checkbox. It also includes respondents who reported entries such as African American; sub-Saharan African entries, such as Kenyan and Nigerian; and Afro-Caribbean entries, such as Haitian and Jamaican.

There is a long history of blatant discrimination and racism that the Black population of the United States has had to endure. In the early 20th century, separate healthcare facilities were developed for Black Americans. Churches were one of the most common sites used. Blacks who wished to become doctors were unable to attend White medical colleges. Black medical schools opened, but were not as well funded as their White counterparts. When Blacks were forced to have interactions with the White healthcare system, inequalities in care often resulted. This history, coupled with the ethical violations that occurred at Tuskegee, has contributed to a legacy of mistrust of the healthcare system that persists today. In the past, Blacks and other minorities were sent to either "all Black" hospitals, charity wards, or the basements of White hospitals for medical care (Myrdal, 1944). The scars from this segregation persist. Now the differential treatment that exists is much more subtle than in years past. Progress perhaps has been achieved but much more is required. The healthcare system has been slow to follow the governmental shift from policy that supported discrimination toward one that supports the establishment of policies to dismantle healthcare discrimination, and one of the consequences of this is healthcare disparities within the Black population.

STATISTICS

According to the most recent U.S. census data from September 2011, 42,020,743 people responded as Black or African American, alone or in combination (13.6% of the total U.S. population). This was up from 12.3% of the total U.S. population in the year 2000. Of those 42,020,743 people, 38.9 million (13%) responded as Black or African American alone. Although Blacks live in all parts of the United States, the vast majority live in the South (55%), while 18% live in the Midwest, 17% in the Northeast, and 10% in the West (U.S. Census Bureau, 2010). It is predicted that by the year 2050, this group may make up 19% of the total population (U.S. Census Bureau, 2008).

According to the 2010 census data, the median age for Blacks of both genders is 32.5 years old. The languages spoken by U.S. Blacks include English, French, Spanish, and African dialects. Overall, Blacks are considered an economically deprived group, which impacts access to and quality of health care received: 12.7% of Blacks of all ages are in fair or poor health, and 12.3% of Black persons of all ages have a limitation in usual activities caused by one or more chronic health conditions.

The state of health for Black Americans is especially precarious. Chronic disease has an excessive impact on this minority population.

- The prevalence of diabetes among Blacks is dramatically higher than among White Americans. The Office of Minority Health reported in 2012 that Black Americans were twice as likely to be diagnosed with diabetes as non-Hispanic Whites. In addition, they were more likely to suffer complications from diabetes, such as end-stage renal disease and lower extremity amputations (Office of Minority Health, 2012b). Although Black Americans had the same or lower rate of high cholesterol as their non-Hispanic White counterparts, they were more likely to have high blood pressure.

Figure 5–1 U.S. minority population by race/ethnicity.

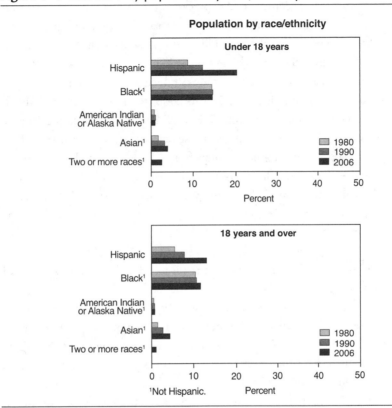

Population by race/ethnicity

Source: National Center for Health Statistics. (2007). *Health, United States, 2007 with chartbook on trends in the health of Americans.* Hyattsville, MD: Author.

- Black Americans have 2.4 times the infant mortality rate as non-Hispanic Whites. Blacks are four times as likely to die as infants due to complications related to low birth weight as compared to non-Hispanic White infants (Office of Minority Health, 2011).
- The 5-year survival rate for cancer among Blacks diagnosed in 1986 to 1992 was about 44%, compared with 59% for White Americans. Today the situation has only worsened. According to the Office of Minority Health (2012a), Black Americans have the highest mortality rate of any racial and ethnic group for all cancers combined and for most major cancers.
- Overall death rates for all major causes of death are higher for Black Americans than for Whites, contributing in part to a lower life expectancy for both Black American men and Black American women.

The incidence of pregnancy is higher in this population. There has been some improvement in life expectancy in the Black population. Between 1990 and 2004, life expectancy at birth increased more for the Black than for the White population, thereby narrowing the gap in life expectancy between these two racial groups. In 1990, life expectancy at birth for the White population was 7.0 years longer than for the Black population. A study conducted by Harper, Rushani, and Kaufman (2012) reported that from 2003 to 2008, the life expectancy at birth for non-Hispanic Black men rose from 68.8 to 70.8 years and for non-Hispanic White men rose from 75.3 to 76.2 years. These new statistics lowered the differences in the average life spans for both groups from 6.5 to 5.4 years. Improvements in racial disparities of women's life spans were also reported. Non-Hispanic White women's life expectancy from 2003 to 2008 went up from 80.3 to 81.2 years, and for non-Hispanic Black women, increased from 75.7 to 77.5 years, cutting the difference from 4.6 to 3.7 years (Harper et al., 2012).

According to Harper et al. (2012), the good news ends there, however. Between 2003 and 2008, the leading cause of death in all men was heart disease (22% of deaths) and homicide (19%). Women were more likely to die from heart disease (29%) or diabetes (11%). Overall mortality was 31% higher for Black Americans than for White Americans in 2004, compared with 37% higher in 1990. In 2004, age-adjusted death rates for the Black population exceeded those for the White population by 46% for stroke (cerebrovascular disease), 32% for heart disease, 23% for cancer (malignant neoplasm), and increased 787% for HIV disease. Large disparities in infant mortality rates among racial and ethnic groups continue to exist. In 2004, infant mortality rates were highest for infants of non-Hispanic Black mothers (13.6 deaths per 1,000 live births). The homicide rate for Black males 15 to 24 years of age decreased sharply from the early to the late 1990s and has remained relatively stable since then. Homicide continues to be the leading cause of death for young Black males 15 to 24 years of age (Centers for Disease Control and Prevention [CDC], 2009).

BLACKS AND THE U.S. HEALTHCARE SYSTEM

Black Americans understand and subscribe to the U.S. Biomedical Model and, with little variation, hold mainstream cultural views about health and management of illness. It is important to keep in mind that caring for patients with English as their primary language does not eliminate the possibility of language impacting the delivery of health care. Some Black Americans believe they are treated unfairly and with disrespect in the healthcare system based on the way they speak English. This finding lends support to the belief that cultural differences between Black Americans and their predominantly White physicians may exist despite language concordance (Johnson, Roter, Powe, & Cooper, 2004). Research shows that the quality of communication between patient and provider is impacted by race/ethnicity. When there is concordance in patient–provider race/ethnicity (the patient identifies as having the same race and/or ethnicity as the provider) better communication and an enhanced understanding by the patient results, because the patient has more trust in the provider and they therefore are more comfortable (Traylor, Schmittdiel, Uratsu, Mangione, & Subramanian, 2010).

Consequences are still reverberating from historical events as they apply to race. Research findings suggest that the Tuskegee study has negatively impacted medical decision making by and for Blacks. For example, in a survey of physicians, 88% of U.S.-born Black American physicians, compared to 35% of White physicians, believed that the Tuskegee study has negatively impacted medical decision making among Black Americans (Wallace et al., 2007). In addition, government and societal policies, however well-intentioned on paper, have limited minority access (including for Blacks) and have resulted in a continuing mistrust and perception of racism in the healthcare system (Fowler-Brown, Ashkin, Corbie-Smith, Thaker, & Pathman, 2006).

Blacks exhibit resilience and adaptive coping mechanisms when dealing with racism and poverty. They tend to have a strong religious affiliation. Nearly one out of every three Black households (29%) are headed by a single woman, the highest percentage of female-headed households in the United States (U.S. Census Bureau, 2010). There is an extended network of caregivers from the family and the community. There is a high level of respect for elders, and small children are highly valued within this culture.

DEFINITIONS OF HEALTH AND ILLNESS

The Black American definitions for health and illness have their roots in African beliefs. Blacks have a long tradition of health and healing practices that contribute to how they care for themselves today. Traditional medicine used by Blacks has its roots in immigrants from Africa, Native Americans, and the European colonists who came to the United States. Magical and herbal cures from Africa were enhanced with practices from Native Americans. Later, European approaches such as blood letting or use of purgatives were added to further enhance and expand the original traditional treatments. Throughout history there has been an emphasis on a higher power and the importance of the spiritual power in action (Becker, Gates, & Newsom, 2004).

The major assumption here is that all things, either living or dead, influence each other. It is felt that all people have control over their destiny and they can also have control over others, either through behavior or knowledge. The possession of health means you are in harmony with nature, whereas illness is defined as disharmony with nature. Illness can result when a person is possessed by demons or evil spirits, which causes illness or disharmony. The goal of treatment is to remove the demon or evil spirit through voodoo or intervention by traditional healers. Folk medicine is characterized by a belief in supernatural forces. From this perspective, health and illness are viewed as natural and unnatural, respectively. Some Blacks who were born and raised in the rural South may have grown up being treated by folk practitioners and/or herbal products and may not have encountered a medical physician until adulthood, if at all (Groover & Baumann, 1996). It is for this reason that it is essential for the nurse to question a patient about their geographic history. Careful questioning of Black American women regarding menstruation is important. People steeped in Black American folk tradition view menstrual blood as a pollutant. They believe that menstruation is the body's way of ridding itself of "bad blood." Some Blacks may consider medications that alter or reduce this flow to be harmful, fearing that this bad blood may back up and thicken, causing possible hemorrhage and death (Salimbene, 2000).

The traditional healers have extensive knowledge regarding the use of herbs and roots (Groover & Baumann, 1996). Because the elderly have knowledge that resulted in their living a long and healthy life, they are held in high esteem in African society. Death is described as the passing from one realm to another (Mokaila, 2001). Funerals are often joyous events with a party following the burial.

Today, many of the preventive treatments used by Blacks have their roots in Africa, combined with approaches from Native Americans, and tempered by the attitudes of the Whites with whom they interacted. Folk medicine still persists in the Black community for many reasons: lack of trust or respect in the system and its workers; fear; lack of money; lack of access, especially in rural areas; and a history of bad experiences and humiliation encountered in the healthcare system. Because of these reasons, seeking out healthcare services is often delayed. Blacks tend to seek prenatal care later, usually after the first trimester is completed. Haitian women are less likely than other groups to seek prenatal care.

Health is maintained by eating three meals a day, including a hot breakfast. Proper rest and a clean environment are also valued. Laxatives are used to prevent constipation and to keep the system open, and cod liver oil is taken to prevent colds. Physicians are not consulted routinely and they are not generally viewed as important or necessary for disease prevention and health promotion.

The most common method today of treating illness in Blacks is prayer, which, for many, includes the laying on of hands.

TRADITIONAL HEALING METHODS

Providing health care to this group may be complicated by folk practices, including the belief that all animate and inanimate objects have good or evil spirits. Educational level and socioeconomic status do not appear to impact how some Blacks perceive folk practitioners. There are distinct types of folk practitioners. The healers may include family, a "granny," or a spiritualist. The granny or old lady acts as a local consultant. She is knowledgeable about home remedies made from spices, herbs, and roots that can be used to treat common illnesses. She may also give advice or make referrals to other folk practitioners with different expertise.

The spiritualist, another type of practitioner, is very prevalent. The spiritualist combines rituals, spiritual beliefs, and herbal medicines to effect a cure. Another type of practitioner is the voodoo priest or priestess. Voodoo is still practiced in some areas of the country. It is not just confined to the rural south and New Orleans, but can also be found in some northern urban areas as well. It is a belief in magic, both white magic, which is harmless, and black magic, which is considered quite harmful. The nurse should be alert for terms such as "fix," "hex," or "spell." Many Black people continue to fear voodoo and become fearful when they fall ill. This view of unnatural illness is based on the belief that illness results from evil influences that are negatively impacting God's plan. These beliefs are more commonly found in Black American members of the lower socioeconomic groups (Welch, 2003).

Voodoo came to the United States around 1724 and was brought by slaves who had initially been sold in the West Indies (Tallant, 1994). They were called "snake worshippers" and worshipped the god Vodu. Over time, the term changed to the more inclusive term *voodoo* (which also includes not only the god but the sect, the members, the priests and priestesses, the rites of passage, and all of the teachings). There are a large number of rituals associated with voodoo. The ceremonies are held with large groups, usually at night in the open air, and include blood drinking (animal blood, such as from a young goat or cat, or from children) and animal sacrifice.

In some urban settings, the voodoo practitioner can be a man, but in some rural areas of the United States, the practitioner must be a woman who has inherited the title by birthright or by a perceived special gift. In New Orleans, the priestess must possess certain physical characteristics as well: She must be Black American and, more specifically, she must be of mixed ancestry, either of one-eighth (octoroon) or one-fourth (quadroon) Black ancestry for her powers to be superior. In contrast to this type of voodoo priestess, the type of voodoo priest or priestess found in some larger urban areas such as Chicago, Queens, New York, or Los Angeles can be male or female and does not have to have inherited the right to practice by special powers or birth. The voodoo ceremonies that exist today have evolved from primitive African rites to include Christian rituals.

Folk practices may include the use of pica (ingestion of nonfood items such as starch and clay) and the wearing of garlic, amulets, and copper or silver bracelets.

The practice of witchcraft is also widespread throughout the world. The practice of witchcraft is not limited to any one particular cultural group. Persons who believe in witchcraft feel that it can be used to cure illness or disease—but also to cause it. The fundamental belief of witchcraft is that some people possess the ability to use the forces of good and evil utilizing the principles of sympathetic magic. The principle of sympathetic magic is an important concept to all folk medicine practice, and its basic premise is that everything in the universe is connected. Any action taken against any part of the body or person causes an action against the whole of the person. A recurring theme is that dead animals that have been pulverized and ingested in one's food or drink can cause illness. Therefore, it is not uncommon for those who believe in witchcraft to refuse food or drink from someone they believe may have put a hex on them. The nurse should be aware that many patients who believe they have been hexed present at health fairs or healthcare settings with symptoms that refer to reptiles, snakes, lizards, toads, and spiders. Convincing these patients to see a physician can be very difficult if not impossible, as they do not believe the hex can be fixed by Western medicine.

Folk medicine in the Black community is viewed as effective—tried and tested. The terminology that may be used to describe folk medicine practitioners in the Black community are unique from titles used by other cultural groups. Some of the titles used by Blacks include "conjure doctor," "underworld man," "father divine," the "root doctor," or "root worker" (Jacques, 1976). One of the reasons the use of folk medicine practices has persisted is because of the fundamental practice of equality, fairness, and honesty. This tradition of equality of care contributes to the faith of the people in its effectiveness. Another reason folk medicine has persisted is access. In rural areas where access to health care is difficult, folk medicine may be the difference between living and dying.

CURRENT HEALTH PROBLEMS

Despite steady improvement in the overall health of Americans, racial and ethnic minorities, with few exceptions, linger behind. This is especially true of Black Americans, as numerous research studies point out that Black Americans experience the highest rates of mortality from heart disease, cancer, cerebrovascular disease, and HIV/AIDS than any other U.S. racial or ethnic group. As a group, they are also less likely to utilize hospice or palliative care measures at the end of life, or to have planned for end-of-life care through the use of advance directives or living wills (Laguna, Enguídanos, Siciliano, & Coulourides-Kogan, 2012).

The prevalence of hypertension in Black Americans is among the highest in the world (Welch, 2003). Compared with Whites, hypertension develops earlier in life and average blood pressures are much higher in Black Americans. Black Americans have higher rates of stage 3 hypertension than Whites, causing a greater burden of hypertension complications. This earlier onset, higher prevalence, and greater rate of stage 3 hypertension in Black Americans is accompanied by an 80% higher stroke mortality rate, a 50% higher heart disease mortality rate, and a 320% greater rate of hypertension-related end-stage renal disease (ESRD) than seen in the general population (Martins & Norris, 2004).

Available evidence indicates that, compared with Whites, Black Americans receiving adequate treatment will achieve similar overall declines in blood pressure and may experience a lower incidence of cardiovascular disease. However, Black Americans often do not receive treatment until blood pressure has been elevated a long time and target organ damage is present (Martins & Norris, 2004). This may also account for the higher incidence of hypertension-related morbidity and mortality in the Black American population, including ESRD. Because of the high prevalence of cardiovascular risk factors in Black Americans, such as obesity, cigarette smoking, and type 2 diabetes, as well as increased responsiveness to reduced salt intake, lifestyle modifications are particularly important.

In Black Americans, as well as in Whites, diuretics have been proven in controlled trials to reduce hypertensive morbidity and mortality; thus, diuretics should be the agent of first choice in the absence of conditions that prohibit their use. Calcium antagonists and alpha-beta blockers are also effective in lowering blood pressure. Monotherapy with beta-blockers or angiotensin-converting enzyme (ACE) inhibitors is less effective, but the addition of diuretics markedly improves response. However, these agents are indicated regardless of ethnicity when patients have other specific indications (e.g., beta-blockers for angina or postmyocardial infarction, ACE inhibitors for diabetic nephropathy, or left ventricular systolic dysfunction). Large, long-term clinical trials of antihypertensive treatment have included both men and women and have not demonstrated clinically significant sex differences in blood pressure response and outcomes. Recent trials of older persons support a similar approach to hypertension management in men and women. Because of their greater prevalence of stage 3 hypertension, many Black American patients require multidrug therapy. Every effort should be made to achieve a goal blood pressure of below 130/80 mm Hg; tight control is especially important in hypertensive patients with renal insufficiency.

Despite the high prevalence of heart disease in the Black American population, this group is less likely than White patients to receive the appropriate medication therapy (thrombolytics, aspirin, and beta-blockers) or to receive coronary artery bypass surgery (Ayanian, Udvarhelyi, Gatsonis, Pashos, & Epstein, 1993; Canto et al., 2000; Hannan, Kilburn, O'Donnell, Lukacik, & Shields, 1991; Johnson, Lee, Cook, Rouan, & Goldman, 1993). As just one example of healthcare disparities between Black Americans and Whites, recent studies indicate that differences persist between these two racial groups in terms of coronary reperfusion therapy

---

Box 5–1 Pertinent Research Studies

1. Jacobs, Rolle, Ferrans, Whitaker, and Warnecke (2006) attempted to determine what trust and distrust in physicians means to Black Americans. They found in their study that the establishment of trust is determined by a perception of interpersonal and technical competence. Trust appears to facilitate care-seeking behavior and promotes patient honesty and adherence. Conversely, distrust inhibits care-seeking behavior; it can result in the patient changing physicians and also result in nonadherence. Perhaps even more alarming was the finding in this study that the subjects had an expectation that discrimination would occur during interactions with physicians. Many of the study subjects reported experiences with racial and financial discrimination by physicians in the past; in fact, it was reported as having occurred in all of the focus groups. This finding corresponds with the Institute of Medicine (IOM) report (Smedley, Stith, & Nelson, 2003) report that discrimination (and perceived discrimination) by physicians and healthcare organizations is a cause of health disparities. The IOM report (Smedley et al., 2003) was congressionally mandated. Its publication contributed greatly to the cultural competency movement. The report concluded that minority patients receive a lower quality of health care than Whites—even after taking into account differences in health insurance and other economic and health factors. It was authored by a blue-ribbon panel assembled by the nation's foremost health and science advisory body

(the IOM). The report went on to say that such inequalities in health care carry a significant human and economic toll and therefore are "unacceptable" (Smedley et al., 2003), concluding that minority patients receive a lower quality of health care than Whites. The report was critically important because it highlights that unequal opportunity exists in terms of accessing and receiving quality health care, which runs contrary to our national value that everyone should be treated equally. Smedley and Jenkins (2007) stated that while inequality continues to persist today in many ethnic groups, it is especially true in the Black American population. Insured Black patients are less likely than insured Whites to receive many potentially life-saving or life-extending procedures—particularly high-tech care such as cardiac catheterization, bypass graft surgery, or kidney transplantation. Black cancer patients fail to get the same combinations of surgical and chemotherapy treatments that White patients with the same disease presentation receive. Even routine care suffers. Black (as well as Latino) patients are less likely than Whites to receive aspirin upon discharge following a heart attack, to receive appropriate care for pneumonia, and to have their pain—such as the kind resulting from broken bones—appropriately treated (Smedley & Jenkins, 2007).

2. In a research study conducted in 2005, the first national study of its kind, a University of California, Irvine, sociologist found that Black immigrants who arrive in America from Black majority regions of the world are healthier than those from White majority regions; still, regardless of how healthy Black immigrants are when they come to the United States, the longer they stay, the more their health erodes. The findings suggest racial discrimination is a major cause of poor health for American Blacks—native and foreign born alike (Read & Emerson, 2005).

   University of California, Irvine, professor Jen'nan Ghazal Read and Rice University professor Michael O. Emerson examined the health of more than 2,900 Black immigrants coming from the top regions of emigration: the West Indies, Africa, South America, and Europe. Compared to U.S.-born Blacks, those born in Europe—a majority-White region that most closely resembles the U.S. racial structure—are the least healthy, faring no better than American-born Blacks. Blacks born in Africa and South America, where Whites are the minority, are much healthier than U.S.-born Blacks. Those born in the West Indies, a racially mixed region, are healthier than U.S.-born Blacks, but less healthy than those from Black-majority regions. According to Read and Emerson (2005), racial minorities are exposed to more stressful life events caused by discrimination. Stress, a key risk factor for many ailments, accumulates over the life course to harm health. "These findings do not bode well for the persistent Black/White health gap in America. . . . Any health advantage that Black immigrants have when they arrive is lost as they, and then their children, blend into America's racial landscape and suffer the consequences of being Black in the United States." The authors explain that although this study does not provide the definitive explanation for the Black/White health gap in America, it encourages researchers and policy makers to take a much harder look at how racial discrimination harms health (Read & Emerson, 2005).

(Continues)

Box 5–1 *Continued*

The researchers looked at three measures to assess peoples' health: self-rated health, disability, and hypertension. Their primary data came from the 2000 to 2002 National Health Interview Surveys, which were conducted by the National Center for Health Statistics and Centers for Disease Control and Prevention, and included a question on region of birth for the first time in 2000. Additional data for the study came from the U.S. Census Bureau, the Office of Immigration Statistics, and the CIA's *World Factbook*. The study was published in the September 2005 issue of *Social Forces* (Read & Emerson, 2005).

Highlight on Nurse Practitioner Cultural Competence Research on the Black Population

3. A study published by Matteliano and Street (2012) in the *Journal of the American Academy of Nurse Practitioners* highlights the positive contributions that nurse practitioners (and all nurses) can have on patient care and the provision of culturally competent care. The authors attempted to document the unique ways nurse practitioners (NPs) contribute to the delivery of culturally competent health care to diverse and underserved patient populations in urban primary care practices. They collected and evaluated data from a multiyear, multisite study and included 50 intensive interviews with healthcare professionals and repeated observations at three urban primary health clinics in a northeastern U.S. city. The results indicated that different healthcare professionals reported common perspectives on cultural competence dealing with distinctive patient communities, including altruistic motivations, advocacy, and addressing root causes while treating diverse patients. What was unique to NPs compared to other healthcare workers studied was the comprehensive nature of the culturally competent approaches that were utilized during patient interactions and while working as a member of the interdisciplinary healthcare team. The NPs established a partnership with the patient that encouraged patient self-advocacy, and practices were adjusted (when needed) to better meet the patient's needs. Holistic approaches were emphasized to establish trust and to help cross any cultural boundaries when providing independent or team-based nursing care (Matteliano & Street, 2012).

4. A quasi-experimental pretest–posttest research design was used to evaluate the impact of a culturally competent educational intervention on pain scale, functional status, and quality-of-life indicators in Black American chronic pain patients in a study conducted by Linda Dayer-Berenson (2011). The educational intervention consisted of two components: a health beliefs questionnaire and a 15-minute narrative teaching session from a pain management NP that described cultural beliefs associated with Black American chronic pain patients. The study results were encouraging, although the sample size was small ($N = 26$). Statistical significance was found on two of the three outcome measures: functional status was improved at a highly statistical level of $p = 0.005$ as was quality of life in the spiritual domain ($p = 0.05$). Although statistical significance was not achieved for pain scale, a level of clinical significance was achieved on reduction in pain on post testing for the experimental group. Replication of this study is needed, as well as further content validity testing of the culturally competent educational intervention, which, will be done in the near future.

and coronary angiography (Canto et al., 2000; Cromwell, McCall, Burton, & Urato, 2005). White patients were more likely than Black American patients to undergo the potentially lifesaving procedures such as coronary revascularization or reperfusion (Canto et al., 2000; Cromwell et al., 2005). Black Americans with ESRD are less likely to receive peritoneal dialysis and to receive a kidney transplant (Barker-Cummings, McClellan, Soucie, & Krisher, 1995; Gaylin et al., 1993; Kasiske, London, & Ellison, 1998). Black Americans (along with Hispanics) are less likely to receive analgesia than Whites for a bone fracture (Todd, Deaton, D'Adamo, & Goe, 2000; Todd, Samaroo, & Hoffman, 1993). This is especially distressing in light of the studies that show that the Black American pain experience is unique. One study found, after subjecting 108 women of different ethnicities to the same pain stimulus by immersing an extremity in cold water, that White non-Hispanics showed greater pain tolerance than Black Americans (Reid, 1992). A study of Black American Medicare patients revealed that patients with congestive heart failure or pneumonia received care that was inferior to that of White patients and that this receipt of substandard care was associated with increased mortality for the Black patients (Ayanian, Weissman, Chasan-Taber, & Epstein, 1999; Peterson et al., 1997).

As has been demonstrated, many Black Americans tend to be suspicious of healthcare professionals, which means they may see a physician or nurse only when absolutely necessary. Also, many Black Americans take medications differently from how they were prescribed. This is especially problematic when medications are used to treat hypertension. Many Black American patients take their antihypertensive medicine on an "as needed" basis (Lewis, 2012). Lewis (2012) found some of the reasons for nonadherence to medication regimes were self-efficacy, depression, and lack of patient–provider communication.

Research studies conducted with Black subjects that investigated disparities of disease management and interventions are startling and indicate that the patient's Black race influenced physician perceptions and attitudes toward that patient's treatment, prognosis, and outcome. One study found that the physicians studied were less likely to believe that renal transplantation improves survival, when compared to White patients (Ayanian et al., 2004). Another study found that physicians were more likely to find their Black patients uncooperative or less cooperative than White patients (Green et al., 2007). Black patient perceptions of the healthcare system are also revealing and sobering. Blacks are more likely to report negative experiences, especially regarding the speed of services, the helpfulness of the healthcare office staff, the timeliness of receipt of care, and the overall rating of healthcare delivery provided by specialists (Fongwa, Cunningham, Weech-Maldonado, Gutierrez, & Hays, 2008).

Clearly, despite the major medical advances of the 20th century, Black Americans are still lagging behind. This population suffers disproportionately with health disparities, which must be addressed and eliminated.

DISPARITIES

Psychiatric Care

Numerous studies have documented overrepresentation of the Black population in psychiatric inpatient settings. Black Americans are more likely than Whites to be diagnosed as psychotic but are less likely to be given antipsychotic medications. They are also more likely to be hospitalized involuntarily, to be regarded as potentially violent, and to be placed in restraints or isolation—differences that are found at every age level and in both outpatient and inpatient services (Benson, 1983; DelBello, Lopez-Larson, Soutullo, & Strakowski, 2001; Kales, Blow, Bingham, Copeland, & Mellow, 2000; Mukherjee, Shukla, Woodle, Rosen, & Olarte, 1983; Rosenfield, 1984; Sleath, Svarstad, & Roter, 1998; Snowden, Hastings, & Alvidrez, 2009; Whaley, 1998). Snowden et al. (2009) found that, after controlling for demographic and clinical factors, Black Americans and Caribbean Blacks had higher odds than Whites of having a psychiatric hospitalization in their lifetime, while U.S.-born Caribbean Blacks had much higher odds of hospitalization than Whites did.

Asthma

The Office of Minority Health reports that in 2007, Black Americans were three times more likely to die from asthma-related causes than the White population. In addition, data from 2003 to 2005 reveals that the death rate for Black American children from asthma was seven times that of non-Hispanic White children (Office of Minority Health, 2011). From 2003 to 2005, Black American children had a death rate seven times that of non-Hispanic White children.

A study of Black and White Medicaid-insured children in Detroit found that Black American children were much more likely than their White counterparts to receive inadequate therapy, obsolete fixed-combination medications rather than the recommended single-entity prescriptions, and were less likely to receive steroid or an adrenergic inhaler (Bosco, Gerstman, & Tomita, 1993; Joseph, Havstad,

Ownby, Johnson, & Tilley, 1998), despite higher rates of healthcare visits and higher rates of hospitalization.

Diabetes

Diabetes strikes 1 out of every 14 Blacks. Blacks are twice as likely to be diagnosed with diabetes mellitus as Whites, and are more likely to suffer from diabetes-related complications (Office of Minority Health, 2012b). Once diagnosed, Black Americans are less likely than Whites to undergo hemoglobin A1C testing, have lipids tested, have an ophthalmology visit, have a physician visit, and have vaccinations. Black Americans with diabetes are also more likely to visit an emergency room or have a hospitalization than other groups.

Twenty-six percent of Black American women and 16% of Black American men qualify to have metabolic syndrome (Clark & El-Atat, 2007). The Black American population is at a very high cardiovascular risk. Blacks have the highest rate of strokes among different populations in the United States. They have very high rates of hypertension, which certainly increases the risk for cardiovascular disease. Seven out of 10 (70%) of all Black Americans between the ages of 18 to 64 are obese or overweight. Sixty-five percent of Black American women are overweight (compared to the general population which has a rate of 50 to 60%). Fifty-seven percent of Black American men are overweight (Grand Rapids African American Health Institute, 2011). Overall, lipid levels are good (triglycerides and high-density lipoprotein), yet stroke level remains very high for these reasons, as well as the prevalence of hypertension in this population as was previously described.

Preventive Care

Medicare-insured Black Americans were less likely than Whites to receive preventive services (Gornick et al., 1996). In a study conducted by Greiner, Born, Nollen, and Ahluwalia (2005) to determine knowledge and perceptions of colorectal cancer screening among urban Black Americans, it was found that a lack of colorectal cancer knowledge and fear are major barriers to screening, as is patient mistrust and fatalism. A report conducted by the Robert Wood Johnson Foundation (2007) found that Blacks (as well as Hispanics and Asians) lag behind Whites in the use and access to preventive care services. It was felt that this was a complex issue that resulted from a lack of continuity in health care and a lack of a primary care provider who could ensure proper utilization of the required preventive services. Most alarmingly, it was reported that screening rates for both breast and cervical cancer was lower in 2005 than they had been in 2000 for Blacks (as well as all of the major racial minority categories).

MISTRUST OF THE HEALTHCARE SYSTEM

There are many studies, some very recent, that reveal that Blacks generally mistrust the healthcare system (Armstrong et al., 2008; Boulware, Cooper, Ratner, LaVeist, & Powe, 2003; Voils et al., 2005), receive lower quality of care (Saha, Arbelaez, & Cooper, 2003; Smedley et al., 2003), and use fewer medical services in general than Whites (Chandler, 2010; Mayberry, Mili, & Ofili, 2000; Wallace, Levy-Storms, Kington, & Andersen, 1998).

BARRIERS TO CARE

Due to the lack of healthcare workforce diversity, Blacks often receive culturally discordant care. Unfortunately, these medical interactions between Black patients and non-Black physicians or providers are usually less positive and productive than racially concordant interactions (Penner et al., 2010). In addition to the lack of Black physicians/providers, Black Americans are less likely to have access to and to use all types of healthcare services, including preventive care. Studies show colorectal cancer screening disparities between Whites and Black Americans, especially for sigmoidoscopy. Black Americans have exhibited higher rates of late-stage colorectal cancer diagnosis and less overall decline in colorectal deaths than Whites over the past decade. There is significant fear of the healthcare system in general and fatalism associated with cancer in the Black population.

Black Americans are less likely than Whites to receive arthritis-related joint replacement, even when controlling for other demographic factors and access to care. Black Americans are also more likely to be dissatisfied with the interpersonal aspects of the medical encounter than Whites (Barr, 2004).

Needed healthcare services may not be affordable for those in lower socioeconomic groups, or if they are available, they may not be culturally relevant. There are several identified barriers to health care that Black Americans perceive. One major barrier, according to Jacobs et al. (2006) and Underwood (1999), is that the history of discrimination and abuse against Black Americans causes some to believe that their lives are not valued by most healthcare professionals, who may provide differential care according to race. Another perception of some Black Americans is that some providers take risks with their lives when rendering care (Underwood, 1999) as well as a prevalent view of fatalism, which impacts compliance with all aspects of health care including receipt of preventive services such as mammography (Spurlock & Cullins, 2006). There is a general distrust of healthcare professionals, practitioners, and the healthcare system within the Black American community (Jacobs et al., 2006; Kennedy, Mathis, & Woods, 2007; Underwood, 1999; among many others). For example, Saha, Komaromy, Koepsell, and Bindman (1999) found in their study that Black American respondents who had Black physicians were more likely than those with non-Black physicians to rate their physicians as excellent (adjusted odds ratio 2.40; 95% confidence interval) and reported receiving preventive care (adjusted odds ratio 1.74; 95% confidence interval), and all required medical care (adjusted odds ratio 2.94; 95% confidence interval). This study emphasizes the importance of providing racially concordant care whenever possible to Black Americans, and in the alternative, at a minimum, the provision of culturally competent care.

Physicians are somewhat less likely to have positive perceptions of Black than White patients on a number of dimensions. Blacks are often perceived as having a higher risk of substance abuse, more likely to be noncompliant than Whites, less likely to desire an active lifestyle compared to Whites, and less likely to participate in cardiac rehabilitation if it is prescribed (van Ryn, Burgess, Malat, & Griffin, 2006; van Ryn & Burke, 2000). In addition, Black patients are rated as less intelligent and educated than Whites (even when controlling for socioeconomic status and other standard covariates), and it is felt that they will have less social support (van Ryn & Burke, 2000). Van Ryn and Burke concluded that this study found that physicians are applying general race characteristics to their impressions of individual patients and failing to incorporate disconfirming individual information.

Other studies have focused on distrust of the motives of the medical profession in withdrawal of life-sustaining technology, pursuit of organ donation, research, and health care overall (Gamble, 1997; Mechanic & Meyer, 2000; Thom & Campbell, 1997). A finding of importance in the Jacobs et al. (2006) study that has major implications for the cultural competence movement is that sharing the same race as the patient is not what was deemed important; what was deemed important by the majority of respondents was the ability of the provider to communicate across language and cultural barriers.

Many Black Americans are still dealing with the impact of slavery. The legacy of slavery causes a serious mistrust of the medical establishment by the Black American population. According to Smith (1999), the Black American community's response to the AIDS epidemic has been in response to and has reflected the profound mistrust of the medical establishment that many Black Americans feel. Among Blacks, the belief that the epidemic originated in a genocidal plot is widespread (Smith, 1999). It is thought that organized medicine has been significantly involved in this plot. If we look at Black Americans' historical relationship to the medical establishment from the era of slavery to the recent past, the suspicious attitudes that make such beliefs possible may be seen as an intelligible response to a new disease that disproportionately affects Black Americans. Successful medical and public health responses have depended and will continue to depend on overcoming the historical legacy of suspicion of the medical establishment and gaining the trust of the Black community. This view was stated even earlier by Charatz-Litt (1992), with an indictment of medical care to Black Americans. According to Charatz-Litt, at no time in history has the health of Black Americans equaled that of White Americans. This is particularly evident in the South, where Blacks have been subjected to governmental policies promoting discrimination and segregation (Charatz-Litt, 1992). The rationale presented in the Charatz-Litt article to explain this unequal health status is that the health of Blacks in the United States has been greatly affected by the attitudes and perceptions of White physicians. This belief is supported in later studies conducted by Malat, van Ryn, and Purcell (2006) and van Ryn and Burke (2000).

IMPACT OF COMMUNICATION

Differences in dialect are based on geography and social stratification (ethnic orientation, economic level, and class status). African American Vernacular English (AAVE), also referred to as African American English (AAE) or "Black English," refers to the dialect that is spoken by many Black Americans (Thomas, 2007). AAVE relates specifically to a vernacular form, spoken principally by working-class Black Americans. AAE refers to the speech of all Black Americans, including that of middle-class Black Americans. It is significantly different from standard English in pronunciation, grammar, and syntax. The use of Black English by most Black Americans is systematic and predictable, making it possible for others to understand it. This ability for understanding is key. It was estimated that approximately 80% of Black Americans use Black English at least some of the time (Dillard, 1972). The use of Black English is not consistent among all Black Americans, nor is it consistently used all of the time. It is felt that this variability is related to educational level and socioeconomic status. Black English has been described as a way for Black Americans to maintain their cultural and ethnic identity. It is not uncommon for some Black Americans to speak standard English while interacting with general society and to use Black English when interacting with peers. A lack of comfort with standard English can serve as a barrier to the delivery of health care, as the caregiver may perceive a quiet Black American as hostile or submissive when in reality, they may be uncomfortable because of language. It is also important for the caregiver not to impart any judgment regarding the speaker's speech being substandard or ungrammatical because it is possible for Black English to be readily understood.

Some characteristic traits of Black English are to pronounce certain syllables differently. For example *th* can be pronounced as *d*, so *the* becomes *de*, *these* becomes *dees*, and *them* becomes *dem* (Dillard, 1972; Wolfram & Clark, 1971). There can also be the tendency to drop the final *r* or *g* from words. According to Thomas (2007), examples of AAVE include "the invariant *be* (*we be cold all the time*), copula deletion (*we cold right now*), third person singular *s* absence (*He think he look cool*) and *ain't* in place of *didn't*" (p. 450).

Slang may be a part of the language, and these slang words may not convey the same meaning and may be different from the slang words used in other dialects (Center for Applied Linguistics, 2010). For example, the word "bad" in Black English can mean good—the opposite of its definition in standard English. For this reason, it is essential that the nurse seek clarification if the Black patient states a medical experience was "bad." It is always essential to seek clarity of definition when slang words are used. It is also important to consider nonverbal communication. While the speech of some Black Americans is very colorful and dynamic, they also tend to use a wide range of body movements (facial gestures, hand/arm movements, hand signals and unique handshakes, expressive dance). The nurse must recognize when working with the Black American population that frequent head nodding, good eye contact, or frequent smiling do not necessarily indicate that the patient is paying attention or is fully accepting of the message being sent (Giger, 2013). With that said, the nurse still needs to focus on all communication (verbal and nonverbal) in an attempt to fully grasp the context of the message. This is especially important when the language of the patient and the caregiver are technically the same (in this case, English) to ensure that the perception of the message is matches the intent of the message being sent (Ashton et al., 2003).

Giger (2013) states that it is essential that the nurse fully comprehends what is happening to the patient psychologically and physiologically, and to help with this process, they advocate substituting terms commonly understood by Black Americans for complicated medical terminology. It is felt that this substitution will improve care delivery and patient satisfaction. **Box 5–2** shows some examples from Stokes (1977) of commonly used medical terms with equivalent Black English words that can be substituted.

IMPACT OF TIME AND SPACE

The time orientation of the Black American is dependent on how they have assimilated into the mainstream (Utsey, Hook, Fischer, & Belvet, 2008). The mainstream dominant American culture is time conscious and future oriented. This means being effective and on time is valued and punctuality is strived for. Some Blacks have a present time orientation. It is felt that this is a legacy from slavery (Utsey et al., 2008). Planning for the future is viewed as hopeless, because the future will be unchanged from the person's present and past. Blacks who are present time-oriented are unlikely to value time. This can result in being tardy for or missing medical appointments. The nurse should be aware that some Blacks believe that lateness of 30 minutes, or even up to 60 minutes, is acceptable.

Other Blacks are future oriented because of a strong religious belief (Utsey et al., 2008). Future-oriented people are so future focused that they plan for their funerals, even purchasing burial plots, long before illness even sets in. Nurses should consider that Black Americans view time as elastic and flexible. The nurse should help the patient identify activities where time can be flexible, such as grooming or exercising as opposed to activities where time is inflexible such as medication

---

Box 5–2 Commonly Used Medical Terms with Equivalent Black English Substitution Words

Medical Condition	Equivalent Black English Term
Diabetes	Sugar
Pain	Miseries
Syphilis	Bad blood, pox
Anemia	Low blood, tired blood
Vomiting	Throw up

Medical Function	Equivalent Black English Term
Constipation	Locked bowels
Diarrhea	Running off, grip
Menstruation	Red flag, the curse
Urinate	Urine/pass water, pee pee, tinkle

Source: Stokes, L. G. (1977). Delivering health services in a Black community. In A. M. Reinhardt & M. B. Quinn (Eds.), *Current practice in family centered community nursing.* St. Louis, MO: Mosby.

administration. When dealing with the present-oriented patient, remember that they may be more likely to be flexible with keeping appointments and will feel that their immediate concerns are more important than any possible future ones.

Black Americans tend to prefer closeness in personal space. Personal space refers to the amount of actual physical closeness a person is comfortable with during interactions with others. Whites prefer a personal space distance of 18 to 36 inches, whereas Black Americans are comfortable with a much shorter personal distance span of only 5 to 10 inches (Hegner, Acello, & Caldwell, 2004). The nurse should consider this personal space difference when planning for and delivering nursing care. A violation in the personal space provided by the nurse may lead to patient discomfort during nursing interactions, especially if this need for closeness is violated or not respected.

IMPACT OF ENVIRONMENT

It is important for the nurse to recognize whether a patient's personal health practices are helpful (efficacious), neutral, or harmful (dysfunctional). Practices that are helpful should be actively encouraged by the nurse because a treatment plan that includes the patient's own health beliefs is more likely to be followed and successful. If the practice is deemed neutral, it should still be considered for incorporation in the plan of care because there may be psychological benefits to its inclusion for the patient. Difficulty is encountered when the patient wishes to have dysfunctional health practices included in the plan of care.

The nurse must also determine whether the patient perceives his or her illness as natural or unnatural. Natural illnesses occur because the patient is affected by natural forces without adequate protection.

Patient education by the nurse may help the patient avoid these types of illnesses (e.g., cold or flu) in the future. As was previously described, some Black American patients believe in unnatural illnesses that are the result of evil influences (such as voodoo and witchcraft). In this case, it is often very difficult for the nurse to get the patient to accept that the treatment plan can be effective. Although the nurse may not believe in these cultural beliefs, it is essential that the nurse recognize that the patient does, and that these beliefs must be identified and incorporated, whenever possible, into the plan of care for treatment to be effective.

Lastly, the nurse should recognize the importance of the church to Black Americans and their recovery from illness. The Black American minister can be a bridge between the client and the healthcare team because the Black American minister fully understands the culture and beliefs of the patient.

IMPACT OF BIOLOGIC VARIATIONS

Most healthcare providers, unless very recently educated, were taught the bio-psychosocial characteristics of the dominant White culture in the United States. This resulted in members of the nondominant culture, such as Black Americans, receiving care that was less than optimal. An essential component of providing culturally competent care is the recognition of differences and then incorporation of these differences from the dominant White culture into our plans of care. Understanding biologic variations is essential. This understanding needs to be more than just skin deep, which means recognizing that racial differences involve more than just skin color and the texture of hair. Black Americans have unique and distinctive genotypes and phenotypes that characterize them as a racial group and as different from other racial groups. In addition, there are ethnic and cultural differences from other ethnic and cultural groups. Understanding biologic variations is essential in avoiding racial and ethnic disparities in health care. Important biologic variations include body size, birth weight, and body proportion. Black American children younger than the age of 2 tend to weigh less and be shorter than White children. Black American children tend to have less subcutaneous fat than White children but are taller and heavier by 2 years of age. The average weight for a Black American woman is consistently higher than that for her White counterpart. There has been found a direct relationship between skin pigmentation and hypertension, which supports the need for hypertension screening in the Black American population. According to Gravelee & Dressler (2005) the relationship between skin color and blood pressure is mediated by sociocultural processes. There is also a higher incidence of lactose intolerance in this population that should be considered when providing nutritional education. Because about 11% of the male Black American population has glucose-6-phosphate dehydrogenase (G6PD) deficiency (an X-linked recessive condition that causes a hematologic problem), it is essential that nurses advocate for screening for this deficiency through the use of the fluorescent spot test.

The seven major chronic illnesses that impact Black Americans are HIV/AIDS, asthma, coronary heart disease (CHD), diabetes, hypertension, sickle-cell anemia, and cerebral vascular accident/stroke.

Human Immunodeficiency Virus Infection/Acquired Immunodeficiency Syndrome

According to the U.S. Centers for Disease Control and Prevention (CDC), the prevalence of AIDS is six times higher in Black Americans and three times higher among Hispanics than among Whites (CDC, 2009).

Asthma

Asthma affects more than 5% of the U.S. population. Black Americans are three to four times more likely than Whites to be hospitalized for asthma, and are four to six times more likely to die from asthma than Whites (Asthma and Allergy Foundation of America, 2005).

Coronary Heart Disease

Research on CHD has contributed to the decline in cardiovascular disease morbidity and mortality that has occurred during the past three decades in the United States. However, life expectancy and rates of illness and death from CHD have not improved as much for Blacks as they have for Whites. Blacks have not experienced the full benefit of research advancements for a variety of reasons, including insufficient scientific data, lack of research focused on minority populations, and limited access to healthcare resources and technology. Consistent and universally accepted racial and ethnic categories have not been established, and definitions may vary according to the social and scientific context. The limited database currently available leaves a number of paradoxes unresolved. Controversy remains, in particular, regarding both chest pain and sudden death. The probability of dying from CHD is greater in Black Americans than in White Americans. According to the CDC (2011) the age-adjusted death rates for cardiovascular disease are 37% higher among African Americans than among Whites and there is a higher prevalence of smoking, hypertension, diabetes, obesity, and left ventricular hypertrophy (LVH) in Blacks. Blacks are also less likely to receive coronary angiography or coronary revascularization.

Although major advances in therapy for CHD have occurred in recent years, few data are available on the clinical value, effectiveness, and efficacy of newer therapeutic modalities in Blacks. Innovative therapeutic approaches to CHD have been based on data obtained primarily in White male populations. Blacks, especially women, are at greater CHD risk. Therapeutic algorithms focused primarily on the relief of chest pain have been refined in majority populations, but other algorithms may be more efficacious in populations with higher prevalence of hypertension, diabetes, and differing clinical presentations. Although information regarding the interactions of LVH, hypertension, and CHD has increased, there are few data in Blacks.

Diabetes

Approximately 14.4% of all Black Americans aged 20 years or older have diabetes (CDC, 2011a). However, one-third of them do not know it. The following additional statistics (National Institute of Diabetes and Digestive and Kidney Diseases, 2007) illustrate the magnitude of diabetes among Black Americans.

- For every Black American diagnosed with diabetes, there is at least one undiagnosed case.
- For every White American who gets diabetes, 1.6 Black Americans get diabetes.
- One in four Black women, 55 years of age or older, has diabetes. (Among Black Americans, women are more likely than men to have diabetes.)
- Twenty-five percent of Blacks between the ages of 65 and 74 have diabetes.
- Black Americans with diabetes are more likely to develop diabetes complications and experience greater disability from the complications than White Americans with diabetes.

There are genetic risk factors impacting Black Americans. Research suggests that Black Americans and recent African immigrants to America have inherited a "thrifty gene" from their African ancestors (Neel, 1962). Years ago, this gene enabled Africans, during "feast and famine" cycles, to use food energy more efficiently when food was scarce. Today, with fewer feast and famine cycles, the thrifty gene that developed for survival may instead make weight control more difficult. This genetic predisposition, along with impaired glucose tolerance, often occurs together with the genetic tendency toward high blood pressure.

Black American ancestry is also an important predictor of the development of diabetes. To understand how rates of diabetes vary among Black Americans, it is important to look at the historical origins of Black populations in America. Genetic predisposition to diabetes is based, in part, on a person's lineage. The Black American population formed from a genetic admixture across African ethnic groups and with other racial groups, primarily European and North American White.

Another concern is the incidence of impaired glucose tolerance (IGT). People with IGT have higher-than-normal blood glucose levels but not high enough to be diagnosed as diabetes. Some argue that IGT is actually an early stage of diabetes. Some recent evidence shows that the degree to which obesity is a risk factor for diabetes may depend on the location of the excess weight. The presence of truncal, or upper body, obesity is a greater risk factor for type 2 diabetes, compared to excess weight carried below the waist. Blacks have a greater tendency to develop upper-body obesity, which increases their risk of type 2 diabetes. Although Blacks have higher rates of obesity, researchers do not believe that obesity alone accounts for their higher prevalence of diabetes. Even when compared to White Americans with the same levels of obesity, age, and socioeconomic status, Black Americans still have higher rates of diabetes. Other factors, yet to be understood, appear to be at work.

Compared to White Americans, Black Americans experience higher rates of three diabetes complications: blindness, kidney failure, and amputations (CDC, 2012). They also experience greater disability from these complications. Some factors that influence the frequency of these complications, such as delay in diagnosis and treatment of diabetes, denial of diabetes, abnormal blood lipids, high blood pressure, and cigarette smoking, can be influenced by proper diabetes management.

Kidney Failure

Black Americans experience kidney failure, also called ESRD, from 2.5 to 5.5 times more often than White Americans. Interestingly though, hypertension, not diabetes, is the leading cause of kidney failure in Black Americans. Hypertension accounts for almost 38% of ESRD cases in Blacks, whereas diabetes causes 32.5%. In spite of their high rates of the disease, Black Americans have better survival rates from kidney failure than White Americans (Cooper, Brinkman, Petersen, & Guyton, 2003).

Visual Impairment

The frequency of severe visual impairment is 40% higher in Black Americans with diabetes than in White Americans. Blindness caused by diabetic retinopathy is twice as common in Blacks than in Whites. Compared to White women, Black women are three times more likely to become blind from diabetes. Black American men have a 30% higher rate of blindness from diabetes than White American men. Diabetic retinopathy may occur more frequently in Black Americans than Whites because of their higher rate of hypertension (Roy & Affouf, 2006).

Amputations

Black Americans undergo more diabetes-related lower-extremity amputations than White or Hispanic Americans (CDC, 2012).

Hypertension

Black Americans are at higher risk for this serious disease than any other race or ethnic group. High blood pressure tends to be more common, happens at an earlier age, and is more severe for many Black Americans (Hertz, 2005).

Sickle-Cell Anemia

The sickle-cell disorders are found in people of African, Mediterranean, Indian, and Middle Eastern heritage (Human Genome Project, 2005). In the United States, these disorders are most commonly observed in Black Americans and Hispanics from the Caribbean, Central America, and parts of South America (Human Genome Project, 2005). An additional and less recognized problem is that sickle-cell patients live under considerable psychosocial stress. Not only do they experience stresses common to other painful chronic illnesses, but they must also cope with the unpredictable nature of their illness. The recurrent and unpredictable nature of the disease can adversely affect both school and work attendance and has the potential of reducing the patient's sense of self-esteem.

Cerebral Vascular Accident/Stroke

Age-adjusted stroke deaths are higher in Black Americans and men (CDC, 2011b). High blood pressure has long been established as the major risk factor for stroke. More recently, cigarette smoking and obesity also have been found to be significant risk factors for stroke.

The bottom line is that the nurse who denies or who does not believe that race is a factor denies a significant part of the patient's being. All aspects of care must be adapted to the patient's culture, socioeconomic status, and educational background.

IMPACT OF SOCIAL ORGANIZATION

The majority of Black homes have a female-headed family structure. Black American female-headed families with children under the age of 5 account for the majority of American families living in poverty today. Most Blacks are demonstrative and comfortable with physical contact and emotional sharing. The legacy of slavery is that Black Americans are the only cultural group in the United States that has not been fully assimilated into mainstream society. Historically, as a result of slavery, Black Americans were kept isolated or segregated from other cultural groups. Even today, Black Americans maintain separate and, in most cases, a lower socioeconomic lifestyle compared to mainstream society. Slavery also resulted in negatively impacting the role of the man in the family. Because the Black American male was someone else's property, it kept him from being the head of the household or the protector of the family. This resulted in the female becoming the dominant force in the family, which to this day is still true in the majority of Black households in the United States. It is important for the nurse to recognize that the Black American family is matrifocal, which means the woman is responsible for the health of the family. The woman is responsible for sharing information and assisting the patient with all decision making, including treatment decisions. The recognition of the importance of the female role to the family should not permit the nurse to ignore or minimize the role of the Black man in the decision-making process.

IMPACT OF FAITH AND SPIRITUALITY

Black people have a strong religious foundation and commitment. Religion appears to be especially salient for Black women and has been shown to play an important role in health and disease management (Chatters, 2000; Holt & McClure, 2006). The most popular religions are Southern Baptist, fundamentalist, and Muslim. Many Black Americans believe in the power of some people to heal and help others. Many have a belief in the healing powers of religion. A reliance on healers reflects the deep religious faith within this group.

An understanding of religion is also important because of its impact on nutrition and the patient's diet. This is especially true of the Muslim religion (for more on this religion see Appendix 1). Islamic dietary restrictions consist of eating a strictly halal diet (no pork, pork products, or "soul foods," such as black-eyed peas, kidney beans, ham hocks, bacon, or pork chops) and the philosophy that "a person is what he eats" (ElGindy, 2005). These foods are considered to be filthy. It is felt that food affects the way a person thinks and acts. Alcohol is avoided because it dulls the senses and it is felt that it causes illness. Muslims fast for a 30-day period during the year (fast of Ramadan), which means no consumption of meat from land animals and only one meal per day in the evening. Nothing is taken by mouth from 5:00 A.M. until sundown. Ill Muslims, small children, and pregnant women are exempt from this rule. Muslims believe in self-help and assisting in uplifting each other, and the lifestyle is not so rigid that people are not permitted to have a good time. To Muslims, life is precious. They will accept blood transfusions but no treatments that have a pork base (e.g., some gelatin has a pork base) because of the belief that it is unclean and the avoidance of pork and pork products in a halal diet (University of New Castle, 2012). It is important to realize that many Muslims differ in their practice and philosophy of Islam. Some Muslims dress in distinctive clothing (e.g., long skirts and head coverings for women); other sects are less strict regarding dress (ElGindy, 2004). Some do not follow the halal diet and are allowed to smoke and drink alcoholic beverages in moderation. Although polygamy is illegal in the United States and most mosques discourage plural marriages, in some sects, it is considered acceptable for men to practice polygamy and for men to have many sexual partners. Therefore, it is important for the nurse to determine which sect the Muslim Black American patient belongs to in order to provide culturally competent care.

SUMMARY

When caring for Black patients, the nurse must not only recognize the impact that culture has on the Black patient's experience, but also incorporate this knowledge of culture into the plan of nursing care. Adjustments in care may be necessary when the culture of the patient does not match the culture of the nurse. Even when the cultures match, there still is the potential for cross-cultural clashes because the nurse has been assimilated into the philosophy of Western medicine. Failing to recognize the impact of culture makes it impossible for the nurse to fully know the patient because race and culture contribute so much to the patient's entire being.

Black people, as a group, have disproportionate morbidity and mortality rates compared to the White majority group. Research to date, including the IOM report (Smedley et al., 2003), concludes that this is caused by discriminatory practices as well as inequalities in educational preparation, social status, and economics. This is considered to be of much more significance than racial or genetic/biologic factors. According to census data, Blacks are more likely to live in poverty and have less education than other racial and ethnic groups, and these two factors underlie many of the health disparities in this country. A public health focus that only considers the factors of socioeconomic status, access to care, and poverty would not be adequate. Even when these variables are controlled, health disparities remain constant along racial lines, and this was especially true among Blacks (Braithwaite & Taylor, 2001). Healthcare providers must be aware that unequal treatment and cultural incompetence is prevalent and that changing health outcomes requires all team members to recognize and acknowledge the patient's racial, cultural, and ethnic background, because it is in these areas that the patient experience becomes unique. Nurses must consider and plan for any required changes in care to ensure that nursing care has been individualized. This requires the care to be adapted to consider the patient's cultural experiences, educational level, and socioeconomic background. As patient advocates, it falls to the nurse to ensure that a cultural assessment is performed, documented, and communicated clearly among all healthcare team members in order to narrow the gap in health-care disparities in the United States.

CASE STUDY 5–1 www

The "Hexed" Patient

C. I., a 56-year-old migrant Black construction and farm worker, had consider-able difficulty explaining and describing his symptoms of back pain, right upper quadrant pain, and jaw pain. When nothing was found to explain his symptoms by radiograph or laboratory studies, he began to feel that they were secondary to a hex. He felt that a man was working "roots" on him and he wanted to see a root doctor. Suddenly, he developed paraplegia and a granulomatous lesion was found in his vertebral column with cord compression. He has not had a return of function since surgery but still tends to think that the hex might have caused his problems.

REVIEW QUESTIONS www

1. What does the nurse need to know to provide culturally competent patient care to a patient who feels he (or she) has been hexed?
2. Design a plan of culturally competent plan of care for a "hexed" patient.

Rationale: The perception of the nurse versus the patient in this situation will be very different. The potential for a cultural gaffe is great. While the patient be-lieves he has been hexed, the nurse may believe the patient is delusional. Hex and voodoo are cultural beliefs that an illness is caused by hexing or an evil influence brought about by another person. These traditional beliefs have persisted and vary in prevalence in different parts of the United States and the world. These beliefs can even be found in some developed areas. A distinction is made between natural conditions that are perceived as God's will or unnatural conditions that are a result of disharmony or conflict with God's will or the result of evil influence. Symptoms can be quite varied but frequently include those associated with a generalized anxi-ety disorder: nausea, vomiting, dizziness, weakness, diarrhea, and fears ranging from being poisoned to being killed (Voodoo death). A culture-bound treatment for this is rootwork, which is the use of dried roots from plants in charms and spells and is quite common in the South among the Black American population.

CASE STUDY 5–2

www

Female Genital Mutilation

Female genital mutilation (FGM) was not known about widely in the United States until the case of Fauziya Kassindja, a then 17-year-old from Togo, who was requesting political asylum in the United States in 1994 (Center for Gender and Refugee Studies). She had run away on the eve of her arranged wedding to avoid FGM. At that time, our government thought she was attempting to immigrate to our country and held her for 1.5 years in prison, often in solitary confinement. Despite human rights advocates speaking out on her behalf, the court did not deem her case to be credible. It was only when the story gained widespread notice in the media that she was freed and the spotlight began to shine on the issue of FGM. It has taken many years for the public to become aware of this practice and still more awareness needs to occur, as it is still practiced in many countries. The practice began 2000 years ago either in Egypt or the Horn of Africa (what is now Eritrea, Djibouti, Ethiopia, and Somalia). The World Health Organization in 2008 called for the elimination of FGM. The WHO emphasized the need for a global concerted effort because it is such a firmly entrenched ritual that is valued by several cultures. Because it is a practice that will likely continue for some time, nurses need to be aware of it and how best to proceed with caring for these women and their families.

REVIEW QUESTIONS

www

1. What does the nurse need to know to provide culturally competent patient care to a patient who has experienced female genital mutilation?
2. Design a culturally competent plan of care for the FGM patient.

Rationale: An increasing number of the countries with a long tradition of performing circumcision rites, widely referred to as FGM, are beginning to reexamine and legislate against this practice. However, the custom of circumcising young girls may take several generations to change. The World Health Organization (2012), which promotes the elimination of FGM, has estimated that about 140 million women worldwide have undergone FGM. The U.S. Centers for Disease Control and Prevention has estimated that 168,000 women (48,000 under the age of 18) who have had FGM are living in the United States today (World Health Organization, 2012).

FGM is typically performed when a girl is between 4 and 8 years old. It is practiced in about 28 African countries, Asia, the Middle East, and increasingly in Europe, Australia, Canada, and the United States. The World Health Organization (2012) has identified four types of FGM. Type 1, which is the only type that can accurately be referred to as female circumcision, is a clitoridectomy. The prepuce and all or parts of the clitoris are removed. This does not usually result in long-term complications. Type 2 involves an excision by which the clitoris and inner labia are removed. Women who have undergone this procedure may suffer from pain during intercourse and experience other long-term problems. Type 3 is infibulation, or an extreme form of circumcision. The clitoris is removed, and at least two-thirds of the labia majora are cut off, as well as the entire labia minora. Incisions are made in the majora to create raw surfaces, which are then stitched or held together (sometimes by tying the woman's legs together), until a hood of skin grows to cover the urethra and vagina. A small hole, about the diameter of a matchstick, is made to allow menstrual blood and urine to escape. Type 4 is pricking, piercing, or incising the clitoris and/or labia or cauterization by burning of the clitoris and surrounding tissue. Adverse effects include formation of cysts, abscesses, and scar tissue; sexual dysfunction; dysmenorrhea and chronic pelvic infections; damage to the urethra; incontinence; chronic pelvic and back pain; chronic urinary tract infections; and difficulties with childbirth (World Health Organization, 2012).

FGM refers to a range of practices involving the cutting, removal, and sometimes sewing up of the female genitalia for cultural or other nontherapeutic reasons. Women who have undergone FGM have been taught to believe that this rite of passage is normal. Reasons for having FGM include identification with cultural heritage and the initiation of girls into womanhood. The possible consequences of FGM are numerous including psychological trauma, difficulty with childbirth, gynecological problems, infection, and even death.

Nursing implications: Nurses working with women are likely to encounter women who have had FGM in their clinical practice. It is important not to assume that all these women want this condition reversed. In their culture, reversal of circumcision would make them unsuitable for marriage, liable for divorce, and virtually an outcast in their communities. Make sure that your assessment questions are culturally appropriate, asking how the circumcision is impacting their life, urination, and menstruation. If the patient seems open to the possibility of surgical correction, it is recommended to refer the patient to healthcare providers and counselors that share her same cultural background.

REFERENCES

Armstrong, K., McMurphy, S., Dean, L. T., Micco, E., Putt, M., Halbert, C. H., ... Shea, J. A. (2008). Differences in the patterns of health care system distrust between Blacks and Whites. *Journal of General Internal Medicine, 23*(6), 827–833.

Ashton, C. M., Haidet, P., Paterniti, D. A., Collins, T. C., Gordon, H. S., O'Malley, K.,... Street, Jr., R. L. (2003). Racial and ethnic disparities in the use of health services. *Journal of General Internal Medicine, 18*(2), 146–152.

Asthma and Allergy Foundation of America. (2005). *Ethnic disparities in the burden and treatment of asthma.* Retrieved from https://www.aafa.org/pdfs/Disparities.pdf

Ayanian, J. Z., Cleary, P. D., Keogh, J. H., Noonan, S. J., David-Kasdan, J. A., & Epstein, A. M. (2004). Physicians' beliefs about racial differences in referral for renal transplantation. *American Journal of Kidney Diseases, 43*(2), 350–357.

Ayanian, J. Z., Udvarhelyi, I. S., Gatsonis, C. A., Pashos, C. L., & Epstein, A. M. (1993). Racial differences in the use of revascularization procedures after coronary angiography. *Journal of the American Medical Association, 269*(20), 2642–2646.

Ayanian, J. Z., Weissman, J. S., Chasan-Taber, S., & Epstein, A. M. (1999). Quality care by race and gender for congestive heart failure and pneumonia. *Medical Care, 37*(12), 1260–1269.

Barker-Cummings, C., McClellan, W., Soucie, J. M., & Krisher, J. (1995). Ethnic differences in the use of peritoneal dialysis as initial treatment for end-stage renal disease. *Journal of the American Medical Association, 274*(23), 1858–1862.

Barr, D. A. (2004). Race/ethnicity and patient satisfaction: Using the appropriate method to test perceived differences in care. *Journal of General Internal Medicine, 19*(9), 937–943.

Batalova, J., & Terrazas, A. (2010). *Frequently requested statistics on immigrants and immigration in the United States.* Retrieved from http://www.migrationinformation.org/feature/display.cfm?ID=818

Becker, G., Gates, R. J., & Newsom, E. (2004). Self-care among chronically ill African Americans: Culture, health disparities, and health insurance status. *American Journal of Public Health, 94*(12), 2066–2073.

Benson, P. R. (1983). Factors associated with antipsychotic drug prescribing by southern psychiatrists. *Medical Care, 21*(6), 639–654.

Bosco, L. A., Gerstman, B. B., & Tomita, D. K. (1993). Variations in the use of medication for the treatment of childhood asthma in the Michigan Medicaid population, 1980–1986. *Chest, 104*(6), 1727–1732.

Boulware, L. E., Cooper, L. A., Ratner, L. E., LaVeist, T. A., & Powe, N. R. (2003). Race and trust in the health care system. *Public Health Reports, 118*(4), 358–365.

Braithwaite, R. L., & Taylor, S. E. (2001). *Health issues in the Black community* (2nd ed.). San Francisco, CA: Jossey-Bass.

Bullough, V. L., & Bullough, B. (1982). *Health care for the other Americans.* East Norwalk, CT: Appleton-Century-Crofts.

Canto, J. G., Allison, J. J., Kiefe, C. I., Fincher, C., Farmer, R., Sekar, P., ... Weissman, N. W. (2000). Relation of race and sex to the use of reperfusion therapy in Medicare beneficiaries with acute myocardial infarction. *New England Journal of Medicine, 342*(15), 1094–1100.

Center for Applied Linguistics. (2010). *Dialects: African American English.* Retrieved from http://www.cal.org/topics/dialects/aae.html

Centers for Disease Control and Prevention (CDC). (2009). Retrieved from http://www.cdc.gov/mmwr/preview/mmwrhtml/00001849.htmv

Centers for Disease Control and Prevention (CDC). (2011a). Table 50: Diabetes among adults 20 years of age and over, by sex, age, and race and Hispanic origin: United States, selected years 1988–1994 through 2005–2008. *Health, United States, 2010*. Retrieved from http://www.cdc.gov/nchs/data/hus/hus10.pdf

Centers for Disease Control and Prevention (CDC). (2011b). *Heart disease and stroke prevention: Addressing the nation's leading killers at a glance*. Retrieved from http://www.cdc.gov/chronicdisease/resources/publications/AAG/dhdsp.htm

Centers for Disease Control and Prevention (CDC). (2012). National Diabetes Surveillance System. Retrieved from http://minorityhealth.hhs.gov/templates/content.aspx?ID=3017

Chandler, D. (2010). The underutilization of health services in the Black community: An examination of causes and effects. *Journal of Black Studies, 40*(5), 915–931.

Charatz-Litt, C. (1992). A chronicle of racism: The effects of the White medical community on Black health. *Journal National Medical Association, 84*(8), 717–725.

Chatters, L. M. (2000). Religion and health: Public health research and practice. *Annual Review of Public Health, 21*, 335–367.

Clark, L. T., & El-Atat, F. (2007). Metabolic syndrome in African Americans: Implications for preventing coronary heart disease. *Clinical Cardiology, 30*(4), 161–164.

Cooper, W. A., Brinkman, W., Petersen, R. J., & Guyton, R. A. (2003). Impact of renal disease in cardiovascular surgery: Emphasis on the African-American patient. *Annals of Thoracic Surgery, 76*(4), S1370–S1376.

Cromwell, J., McCall, N. T., Burton, J., & Urato, C. (2005). Race/ethnic disparities in utilization of lifesaving technologies by Medicare ischemic heart disease beneficiaries. *Medical Care, 43*(4), 330–337.

Dayer-Berenson, L. (2011). The effect of a culturally competent educational intervention with African American chronic low-back pain patients. Doctoral dissertation. (UMI Number 3515745).

DelBello, M. P., Lopez-Larson, M. P., Soutullo, C. A., & Strakowski, S. M. (2001). Effects of race on psychiatric diagnosis of hospitalized adolescents: A retrospective chart review. *Journal of Child and Adolescent Psychopharmacology, 11*(1), 95–103.

Dillard, J. L. (1972). *Black English: Its history and usage in the United States*. New York, NY: Vintage Books.

Eiser, A. R., & Ellis, G. (2007). Cultural competence and the African American experience with healthcare: The case for specific content in cross-cultural education. *Academic Medicine, 82*, 176–183.

ElGindy, G. (2004). Treating Muslims with cultural sensitivity in a post-9/11 world. *Minority Nurse*. Retrieved from http://www.minoritynurse.com/cultural-competency/treating-muslims-cultural-sensitivity-post-911-world

ElGindy, G. (2005). Meeting Jewish and Muslim patients' dietary needs. *Minority Nurse*. Retrieved from http://www.minoritynurse.com/cultural-competency/meeting-jewish-and-muslim-patients%E2%80%99-dietary-needs

Fongwa, M. N., Cunningham, W., Weech-Maldonado, R., Gutierrez, P. R., & Hays, R. D. (2008). Reports and ratings of care: Black and White Medicare enrollees. *Journal of Health Care for the Poor and Underserved, 19*(4), 1136–1147.

Fowler-Brown, A., Ashkin, E., Corbie-Smith, G., Thaker, S., & Pathman, D. E. (2006). Perception of racial barriers to health care in the rural South. *Journal of Health Care for the Poor & Underserved, 17*(1), 86–100.

Gamble, V. N. (1997). Under the shadow of Tuskegee: African Americans and health care. *American Journal of Public Health, 87*(11), 1773–1778.

Gaylin, D. S., Held, P. J., Port, F. K., Hunsicker, L. G., Wolfe, R. A., Kahan, B. D., . . . Agodoa, L. Y. (1993). The impact of comorbid and sociodemographic factors on access to renal transplantation. *Journal of the American Medical Association, 269*(5), 603–608.

Giger, J. N. (2013). *Transcultural nursing: Assessment and intervention* (6th ed.). St Louis, MO: Mosby.

Gornick, M. E., Eggers, P. W., Reilly, T. W., Mentnech, R. M., Fitterman, L. K., Kucken L. E., & Vladeck, B. C. (1996). Effects of race and income on mortality and use of services among Medicare beneficiaries. *New England Journal of Medicine, 335*(11), 791–799.

Grand Rapids African American Health Institute. (2011). *Minority health report.* Retrieved from http://www.graahi.org/Portals/0/Documents/2011MinorityHealthReport.pdf

Gravlee, C. C., & Dressler, W. W. (2005). Skin pigmentation, self-perceived color, and arterial blood pressure in Puerto Rico. *American Journal of Human Biology, 17*(2), 195–206.

Green, A. R., Carney, D. R., Pallin, D. J., Ngo, L. H., Raymond, K. L., Iezzoni, L. I., & Banaji, M. R. (2007). Implicit bias among physicians and its prediction of thrombolysis decisions for Black and White patients. *Journal of General Internal Medicine, 22*(9), 1231–1238.

Greiner, K. A., Born, W., Nollen, N., & Ahluwalia, J. S. (2005). Knowledge and perceptions of colorectal cancer screening among urban African Americans. *Journal of General Internal Medicine, 20*(11), 977–983.

Groover, M. D., & Baumann, T. E. (1996). They worked their own remedy: African American herbal medicine and archaeological record. *South Carolina Antiquities, 28*(1 & 2), 21–32.

Hannan, E. L., Kilburn, H., Jr., O'Donnell, J. F., Lukacik, G., & Shields, E. P. (1991). Interracial access to selected cardiac procedures for patients hospitalized with coronary artery disease in New York State. *Medical Care, 29*(5), 430–441.

Harper, S., Rushani, D., & Kaufman, J. S. (2012). Trends in Black-White life expectancy gap, 2003–2008. *Journal of the American Medical Association, 307*(21), 2257–2259.

Hegner, B. R., Acello, B., & Caldwell, E. (2004). *Nursing assistant: A nursing process approach* (p. 190). Clifton Park, NY: Delmar Learning.

Hertz, R. P. (2005). Racial disparities in hypertension prevalence, awareness and management. *Archives of Internal Medicine, 165*(18), 2098–2104.

Holt, C. L., & McClure, S. M. (2006). Perceptions of the religion–health connection among African American church members. *Qualitative Health Research, 16*(2), 268–281.

Human Genome Project. (2005). *Genetic disease profile: Sickle cell anemia.* Retrieved from http://www.ornl.gov/sci/techresources/Human_Genome/posters/chromosome/sca.shtml

Jacobs, E. A., Rolle, I., Ferrans, C. E., Whitaker, E. E., & Warnecke, R. B. (2006). Understanding African Americans' views of the trustworthiness of physicians. *Journal of General Internal Medicine, 21*(6), 642–647.

Jacques, G. (1976). Cultural health traditions: A Black perspective. In M. F. Branch & P. P. Paxton (Eds.), *Providing safe nursing care for ethnic people of color* (pp. 115–124). East Norwalk, CT: Appleton-Century-Crofts.

Johnson, P. A., Lee, T. H., Cook, E. F., Rouan, G. W., & Goldman, L. (1993). Effect of race on the presentation and management of patients with acute chest pain. *Annals of Internal Medicine, 118*(8), 593–601.

Johnson, R. L., Roter, D., Powe, N. R., & Cooper, L. A. (2004). Patient race/ethnicity and quality of patient–physician communication during medical visits. *American Journal of Public Health, 94*(12), 2084–2090.

Joseph, C. L., Havstad, S. L., Ownby, D. R., Johnson, C. C., & Tilley, B. C. (1998). Racial differences in emergency department use persist despite allergist visits and prescriptions filled for anti-inflammatory medications. *Journal of Allergy and Clinical Immunology, 101* (4 Pt. 1), 484–490.

Kales, H. C., Blow, P. C., Bingham, C. R., Roberts, J. S., Copeland, L. A., & Mellow, M. A. (2000). Race, psychiatric diagnosis, and mental health care utilization in older patients. *American Journal of Geriatric Psychiatry, 8*(4), 301–309.

Kasiske, B. L., London, W., & Ellison, M. D. (1998). Race and socioeconomic factors influencing early placement on the kidney transplant waiting list. *Journal of the American Society of Nephrology, 9*(11), 2142–2147.

Kennedy, B. R., Mathis, C. C., & Woods, A. K. (2007). African Americans and their distrust of the health care system: Healthcare for diverse populations. *Journal of Cultural Diversity, 14*(2), 56–60.

Laguna, J., Enguídanos, S., Siciliano, M., & Coulourides-Kogan, A. (2012). Racial/ethnic minority access to end-of-life care: A conceptual framework. *Home Health Care Services Quarterly, 31*(1), 60–83.

Lewis, L. M. (2012). Factors associated with medication adherence in hypertensive Blacks: A review of the literature. *Journal of Cardiovascular Nursing, 27*(3), 208–219.

Library Index. (n.d.). *The impact of immigration on twenty-first century America—Black immigrants from Africa differ from American Black population*. Retrieved from http://www.libraryindex.com/pages/2463/Impact-Immigration-on-Twenty-First-Century-America-BLACK-IMMIGRANTS-FROM-AFRICA-DIFFERFROM-AMERICAN-BLACK-POPULATION.html

Malat, J. R., van Ryn, M., & Purcell, D. (2006). Race, socioeconomic status, and the perceived importance of positive self-presentation in health care. *Social Science & Medicine, 62*(10), 2479–2488.

Martins, D., & Norris, K. (2004). Hypertension treatment in African Americans: Physiology is less important than sociology. *Cleveland Clinical Journal of Medicine, 71*(9), 735–743.

Matteliano, M. A., & Street, D. (2012). Nurse practitioners' contributions to cultural competence in primary care settings. *Journal of the American Academy of Nurse Practioners, 24*(7), 425–35. doi: 10.1111/j.1745-7599.2012.00701.x

Mayberry, R. M., Mili, F., & Ofili, E. (2000). Racial and ethnic differences in access to medical care. *Medical Care Research and Review, 57*(Suppl. 1), 108–145.

McCabe, J. (2011). *Caribbean immigrants in the United States*. Retrieved from http://www.migrationinformation.org/usfocus/display.cfm?ID=834

Mechanic, D., & Meyer, S. (2000). Concepts of trust among patients with serious illness. *Social Science & Medicine, 51*(5), 657–668.

Mokaila, A. (2001). *Traditional Vs. Western Medicine-African Context*. Springfield, MO: Drury University.

Mukherjee, S., Shukla, S., Woodle, J., Rosen, A. M., & Olarte, S. (1983). Misdiagnosis of schizophrenia in bipolar patients: A multiethnic comparison. *American Journal of Psychiatry, 140*(12), 1571–1574.

Myrdal, G. (1944). *An American dilemma: the Negro problem and modern democracy* (Vol. 1). New York, NY: Harper & Brothers.

National Center for Health Statistics. (2007). *Health, United States, 2007 with chartbook on trends in the health of Americans*. Hyattsville, MD: Author.

National Institute of Diabetes and Digestive and Kidney Diseases. (2007). *National diabetes fact sheet*. Retrieved from http://www.cdc.gov/diabetes/pubs/pdf/ndfs_2007.pdf

Neel, J. V. (1962). Diabetes mellitus: a "thrifty genotype rendered detrimental by "progress." *American Journal of Human Genetics, 14*, 353–362.

Office of Minority Health. (2011). *Infant mortality and African Americans*. Retrieved from http://minorityhealth.hhs.gov/templates/content.aspx?ID=3021

Office of Minority Health. (2012a). *Cancer and African Americans*. Retrieved from http://minorityhealth.hhs.gov/templates/content.aspx?ID=2826

Office of Minority Health. (2012b). *Diabetes and African Americans*. Retrieved from http://minorityhealth.hhs.gov/templates/content.aspx?ID=3017

Penner, L. A., Dovidio, J. F., West, T. V., Gaertner, S. L., Albrecht, T. L., Dailey, R. K., & Markova, T. (2010). Aversive racism and medical interactions with Black patients: A field study. *Journal of Experimental Social Psychology, 46*(2), 436–440.

Peterson, E. D., Shaw, L. K., DeLong, E. R., Pryor, D. B., Califf, R. M., & Mark, D. B. (1997). Racial variation in the use of coronary-revascularization procedures: Are the differences real? Do they matter? *New England Journal of Medicine, 336*(7), 480–486.

Read, J. G., & Emerson, M. O. (2005). Racial context, Black immigration and the US Black/White health disparity. *Social Forces, 84*(1), 181–199.

Reid, V. J. (1992). Ethnicity, interpersonal factors and pain expressions: Implications for physician patient interaction (53:DA922505). In *Dissertation abstracts international*. Ann Arbor: University of Michigan.

Robert Wood Johnson Foundation. (2007). *Preventive care: A national profile on use, disparities and health benefits*. Retrieved from http://www.rwjf.org/pr/product.jsp?id=19896

Rosenfield, S. (1984). Race differences in involuntary hospitalization. Psychiatric vs. labeling perspectives. *Journal of Health and Social Behavior, 25*(1), 14–23.

Roy, M. S., & Affouf, M. (2006). Six-year progression of retinopathy and associated risk factors in African Americans with type 1 diabetes mellitus: The New Jersey 725. *Archives of Ophthalmology, 124*(9), 1297–1306.

Saha, S., Arbelaez, J. J., & Cooper, L. A. (2003). Patient–physician relationships and racial disparities in the quality of health care. *American Journal of Public Health, 93*(10), 1713–1719.

Saha, S., Komaromy, M., Koepsell, T. D., & Bindman, A. B. (1999). Patient–physician racial concordance and the perceived quality and use of health care. *Archives of Internal Medicine, 159*(9), 997–1004.

Salimbene, S. (2000). Providing culture-sensitive care to African Americans. In *What language does your patient hurt in? A practical guide to culturally competent patient care*. Amherst, MA: Diversity Resources.

Sleath, B., Svarstad, B., & Roter, D. (1998). Patient race and psychotropic prescribing during medical encounters. *Patient Education and Counseling, 34*(3), 227–238.

Smedley, B. D., & Jenkins, A. (Eds.). (2007). *All things being equal: Instigating opportunity in an inequitable time*. New York, NY: The New Press.

Smedley, B. D., Stith, A. Y., & Nelson, A. R. (2003). *Unequal treatment: Confronting racial and ethnic differences in health care*. Washington, DC: National Academies Press.

Smith, C. (1999). African Americans and the medical establishment. *The Mount Sinai Journal of Medicine, 66*(4), 280–281.

Snowden, L. R., Hastings, J. F., & Alvidrez, J. (2009). Overrepresentation of black Americans in psychiatric inpatient care. *Psychiatric Services, 60*(6), 779–785.

Spurlock, W. R., & Cullins, L. S. (2006). Cancer fatalism and breast cancer screening in African American women. *Journal of the Association of Black Nursing Faculty in Higher Education, 17*(1), 38–43.

Stokes, L. G. (1977). Delivering health services in a Black community. In A. M. Reinhardt & M. D. Quinn (Eds.), *Current practice in family centered community nursing*. St. Louis, MO: Mosby.

Tallant, R. (1994). *Voodoo in New Orleans*. Gretna, LA: Pelican.

Terrazas, A. (2009). *African immigrants in the United States*. Retrieved from http://www .migrationinformation.org/usfocus/display.cfm?ID=719

Terrazas, A. (2010). *Haitian immigrants in the United States*. Retrieved from http://www .migrationinformation.org/feature/display.cfm?ID=770

Thom, D. H., & Campbell, B. (1997). Patient–physician trust: An exploratory study. *Journal of Family Practice, 44*(2), 169–176.

Thomas, E. R. (2007). Phonological and phonetic characteristics of African American Vernacular English. *Language and Linguistics Compass, 1*(5), 450–475.

Todd, K. H., Deaton, C., D'Adamo, A. P., & Goe, L. (2000). Ethnicity and analgesic practice. *Annals of Emergency Medicine, 35*(1), 11–16.

Todd, K. H., Samaroo, N., & Hoffman, J. R. (1993). Ethnicity as a risk factor for inadequate emergency department analgesia. *Journal of the American Medical Association, 269*(12), 1537–1539.

Traylor, A. H., Schmittdiel, J. A., Uratsu, C. S., Mangione, C. M., & Subramanian, U. (2010). Adherence to cardiovascular disease medications: Does patient–provider race/ethnicity and language concordance matter? *Journal of General Internal Medicine, 25*(11), 1172–1177.

Underwood, S. M. (1999). Development of a cancer prevention and early detection program for nurses working with African Americans. *Journal of Continuing Education in Nursing, 30*(1), 30–36.

University of New Castle. (2012). Muslim beliefs about illness and health practices. Retrieved from http://www.newcastle.edu.au/students/current/islaminhealth/health-practices.html

U.S. Census Bureau. (2008). National Sex, Age and Hispanic Origin. *Table 4: Annual estimates of the Black or African American alone or in combination population by sex and age for the United States: April 1, 2000, to July 1, 2007*.

U.S. Census Bureau. (2010). 2010 census data. Retrieved from http://2010.census.gov/ 2010census/data/

Utsey, S. O., Hook, J. N., Fischer, N., & Belvet, B. (2008). Cultural orientation, ego resilience, and optimism as predictors of subjective well-being in African Americans. *The Journal of Positive Psychology, 3*(3), 202–210.

van Ryn, M., Burgess, D., Malat, J., & Griffin, J. (2006). Physicians' perception of patients' social and behavioral characteristics and race disparities in treatment recommendations for men with coronary artery disease. *American Journal of Public Health, 96*(2), 351–357.

van Ryn, M., & Burke, J. (2000). The effect of patient race and socio-economic status on physicians' perceptions of patients. *Social Science & Medicine, 50*(6), 813–828.

Voils, C. I., Oddone, E. Z., Weinfurt, K. P., Friedman, J. Y., Schulman, K. A., & Bosworth, H. B. (2005). For the patient: Who trusts healthcare institutions? Results from a community-based sample. *Ethnicity & Disease, 15*(1), 150.

Wallace, M. P., Weiner, J. S., Pekmezaris, R., Almendral, A., Cosiquien, R., Auerbach, C., & Wolf-Klein, G. (2007). Physician cultural sensitivity in African American advance care planning: A pilot study. *Journal of Palliative Medicine, 10*(3), 721–727.

Wallace, S. P., Levy-Storms, L., Kington, R. S., & Andersen, R. M. (1998). The persistence of race and ethnicity in the use of long-term care. *The Journals of Gerontology Series B, Psychological Sciences and Social Sciences, 53*(2), S104–112.

Welch, M. (2003). Care of Blacks and African Americans. In J. Bigby. *Cross-cultural medicine* (pp. 29–60). Philadelphia, PA: American College of Physicians.

Whaley, A. L. (1998). Cross-cultural perspective on paranoia: A focus on the Black American experience. *The Psychiatric Quarterly, 69*(4), 325–343.

Wolfram, W. A., & Clark, N. H. (Eds.). (1971). *Black-White speech relationships*. Washington, DC: Center for Applied Linguistics.

World Health Organization. (2012). Female genital mutilation (Fact Sheet No. 241). Retrieved from http://www.who.int/mediacentre/factsheets/fs241/en/

For a full suite of assignments and additional learning activities, see the access code at the front of your book.

Hispanics/Latinos

CHAPTER OBJECTIVES

Upon completion of this chapter, the nurse will be able to:

- Define and differentiate between the terms *Hispanic* and *Latino*.
- Plan nursing care for Hispanic/Latino patients that is evidence-based and comprehensive and that incorporates the ethnicity, traditional health beliefs, and biologic variations of these patients.
- Consider the barriers to care that exist and plan for strategies to overcome these barriers when caring for Hispanics/Latinos.

© Feverpitch/ShutterStock, Inc.

INTRODUCTION

The information provided in this chapter is intended to serve as a guide with the intent to help the reader become more aware of the role culture and cultural values can have on individuals and the individual's response to illness. It is essential that the nurse question every patient about the existence of and importance of their individual health beliefs and practices to ensure the provision of culturally appropriate nursing care. It is important for the nurse to remember that not all people within a culture are the same or will respond similarly. The nurse must always consider the uniqueness and individual characteristics of each and every patient and recognize the uniqueness of every medical encounter.

TERMINOLOGY: LATINOS OR HISPANICS?

The terms *Latino* and *Hispanic* are not synonymous. The word *Latin* comes to us from a tribe in early Italy called the Latins. The Latins lived in Latium, whose capital city was Rome. Their language was called Latin as well. As the Roman Empire spread its dominance, the Latin language evolved into several other languages: Italian, Spanish, Portuguese, and French (these are often referred to as the Romance languages). Later, when the Romans invaded the Iberian Peninsula, they found an existing city named Hispalis (Seville). The name *Hispalis* appears to be derived from Greek. The Romans annexed the Iberian Peninsula, naming it Hispania. The Romans spent seven centuries in Hispania, leaving behind an extensive legacy. This legacy tied Hispania to the rest of the Latin world.

The term *Hispano* (*Hispanic*) later was used when referring to Spain; thus, Hispanic refers to people whose culture and heritage have ties to Spain (they may or may not speak Spanish). Hispanic refers not to a race but instead it defines a region of origin. The U.S. Census Bureau (2010b) defined a Hispanic person as any person, regardless of race, creed, or color, whose origins are from Mexico, Puerto Rico, Cuba, Central or South America, or some other Hispanic origin.

Although the term *Hispanic* is prevalent today it was not widely used until the 1970s and 1980s. In the 1950s and 1960s, Hispanics tended to organize around or use the label of their own unique national identity such as Mexican, Mexican American, Puerto Rican, Cuban American, Central American, and South American. The term *Hispanic* has emerged as an inclusive term that refers to all Spanish-speaking ethnic subgroups. It is extremely important for the nurse to remember that Hispanics in the United States can be of any racial background: White, Black, Asian, American Indian, and so on.

In the United States, the federal government uses the term *Hispanic* on all documents and forms, including the 2010 census. Hispanic is not a race but an ethnic distinction and is translated from *Hispania* (Latin) and *Hispano* (Spanish). People from Latin America are all Latin(o), but not all are Hispanics. For example, Brazilians speak Portuguese, which makes Brazilians Latin but not Hispanic. Age of the individual may also play a role in preferred terminology, as younger people tend to prefer the label Hispanic while older people prefer the Latino label. Because it is hard to determine a preference and to ensure inclusiveness, both terms will be used in this chapter. It is also important to state that although Hispanics/Latinos are collectively grouped together in this chapter, each subgroup of Hispanics/Latinos have differing dialects, foods, and traditions that are determined by the original country of origin. Origin can be viewed as heritage, nationality, lineage, or country of birth of the person or person's parents or ancestors before their arrival in the United States. The nurse needs to provide consideration for personal differences, socioeconomic status, migration status, subcultures, and life experiences of his or her patients.

BACKGROUND

The lack of consensus on the label of this group will remain controversial; some individuals prefer to use the term *Latino* because it is inclusive and because it emphasizes geographic area. Others prefer to use the term *Hispanic*, which is consistent with the federal government's documents/forms and its emphasis on the importance of the Spanish heritage. Whichever label is used by the nurse is not as important as the nurse being aware that the label does not refer to one race or racial grouping but instead is an ethnic grouping of people from 20 countries. As a result, many Hispanics/Latinos self-identify with their country of origin or immigrant status, because most Hispanics/Latinos are immigrants to the United States. A few Hispanics/Latinos are exceptions, in that they were granted refugee status (e.g., from Cuba, Columbia, El Salvador, Nicaragua, and Guatemala).

Statistics

Hispanics/Latinos make up the largest minority in the United States, totaling 50.5 million people (16% of the total population), according to 2010 census results (U.S. Census Bureau, 2010a). The vast majority of Hispanics/Latinos in the U.S. identified as White (26.8 million) during the 2010 census. More than half of the total United States population growth that occurred between the years 2000 and 2010 was due to the tremendous growth in the Hispanic/Latino population (the number of Hispanics/Latinos increased by 15.2 million while the total

U.S. population increased by a total of 27.3 million over a 10-year period). It is possible that the change in labels used by the U.S. census (the inclusion of the term *Latino* since 2000) may be responsible for some of the tremendous increase that was seen in the most recent census numbers. The 2010 census revealed that Mexicans account for about three-quarters of the total 15.2 million increase, while Puerto Ricans account for 35% and Cubans 44% of the total population increase. Today, approximately 75% of all Hispanics/Latinos come from one of three countries of origin: Mexico, Puerto Rico, or Cuba. The nurse who strives to develop cultural competence in the Hispanic/Latino population should therefore focus on understanding issues specific to Mexicans, Puerto Ricans, and Cubans. The nurse should also know important demographic characteristics such as that the majority of Hispanic/Latinos are male, three-quarters of the population live in either the West or the South, and the median age for both genders was 27 years of age (U.S. Census Bureau, 2010a). The median age for the U.S. population is older, at 37.3 years of age. Three states in the United States are home to more than 50% of all Hispanic/Latino Americans. Therefore, nurses who practice in California (28% of Hispanic population), Texas (19% of Hispanic population), and Florida (8% of Hispanic population) must develop expertise in providing culturally competent care to Hispanics/Latinos (U.S. Census Bureau, 2010b). Census data is also helpful in identifying the states that have the highest percentage of minorities of all types. Minorities are defined as anyone who is not single-race White and not Hispanic. A population greater than 50% minority is considered "majority minority." Today California, Texas, New Mexico, Hawaii, and Washington, DC, have majority–minority populations. The prevalence of majority-minority states and geographic areas will continue to grow. According to U.S. Census Bureau estimates (2012), for the first time racial and ethnic minorities make up more than half of all children born in the United States (50.4%). Minorities are now estimated by the Census Bureau to account for 36.6% of the total U.S. population.

HISTORY OF HISPANICS IN THE UNITED STATES

Having a historical perspective is helpful for the nurse to develop an understanding of the health status of Hispanics/Latinos. History provides perspective to genetic, biologic, and environmental events and clarifies potential health behaviors that may be seen in practice.

In 1453, Constantinople, the capital of the Byzantine Empire, fell to the Ottoman Turks, cutting off Europe's silk and spice trade with India and Asia (History Scholars, 2009). Thirty-nine years later, an Italian named Christoforo Colombo (Cristobal Colón in Spanish), or Christopher Columbus, sailed west for the Queen of Spain, in search of a new route to the Orient. He instead reached the "New World"; his first landfalls included Juana (Cuba) and the island of Hispaniola (known today as the Dominican Republic and Haiti) (Enchanted Learning, 2010).

The Conquistadors were committed to the expansion of the Spanish empire and recovery of treasure for the crown. Spanish Catholic missions soon followed, with the goal of winning new religious converts. Colonial administrators began spreading Spanish culture from Mexico across Central and South America. Spanish settlement of North America came early and included the first permanent European settlement of the New World at St. Augustine, Florida, in 1565. In 1598, Don Juan de Oñate colonized New Mexico (New Mexico History, 2012).

After the establishment of the United States of America, immigration was impacted by U.S. policies, such as Manifest Destiny and the Monroe Doctrine (Dictionary of American History, 2003). The Spanish–American War brought Cuba and Puerto Rico under U.S. administration in 1898, and various invasions of the Dominican Republic, Nicaragua, Honduras, and other parts of Central America caused waves of immigration following war, rebellion, and occupation. This process has continued as recently as the 1980s, when large numbers of Guatemalans, Nicaraguans, and Salvadorans fled to the United States to escape civil wars. Of the 40 million foreign-born persons in the United States in 2010 of all races/ethnicities, 38% entered the country prior to 1990, 27% entered between 1990 and 1999, and almost 35% entered in 2000 or later. Today, the majority of Hispanic/Latinos are native-born U.S. citizens. In 2010, 47% of the 40 million foreign-born population (about 18.8 million) reported having Hispanic or Latino origins. More specifically, the vast majority of Hispanic/Latino immigrants (29%) were from Mexico (U.S. Census Bureau, 2010b). El Salvador and Cuba each accounted for 3% of all immigrants, while immigrants from the Dominican Republic and Guatemala each accounted for 2% of all foreign-born residing in the United States in 2010.

MEXICAN AMERICANS

The United States is home to the world's second largest Mexican community, second only to the country of Mexico. Mexican Americans compose slightly over 10% of the U.S. population, making them by far the largest group of Hispanics/

Latinos. The number of Mexican Americans grew rapidly between the years 1990 and 2006, but has since stabilized (Pew Hispanic Center, 2009). According to the Census Bureau (2010a), the Mexican origin population in the United States increased by 54% between the years 2000 and 2010, growing from 20.6 million to 31.8 million. Today, Mexican Americans compose approximately 66% of all Hispanic/Latinos living in the United States. Of course, the census numbers do not include all of the undocumented Mexicans in the United States. The undocumented Mexican labor force was estimated at 8.3 million in March of 2008 (Pew Hispanic Center, 2009). The birth rate for unauthorized Mexican immigrants has also contributed to the growth of the number of U.S. citizens. According to the Pew Hispanic Center (2009), 73% of the children of unauthorized immigrant parents were born in this country and are therefore U.S. citizens. The children of both citizens and unauthorized immigrants make up 6.8% of all of the students enrolled in U.S. elementary and secondary schools (Pew Hispanic Center, 2009).

Mexican Americans are also occasionally referred to as *Chicanos*. The term *Chicano* is used solely to refer to people of Mexican descent. The use of the term *Chicano* is controversial. Although it is an old word, many elderly Mexicans do not like the term because in the past it was a derogatory reference to Mexican peasants (peons). In the late 1960s and 1970s, the name *Los Chicanos* was taken by a militant group to make a political statement. For example, the Chicano movement consisted of mass student walkouts in an effort to promote solidarity, unity, and empowerment of the Chicano community.

Mexico, officially called the United Mexican States, is a federal republic located in the southern part of North America. Mexico is the third largest Latin American nation, and it consists of 31 states and a federal district with a country-wide estimated population of over 112 million in 2010 (Nation Master, 2012). Its federal district is Mexico City, a separate entity similar to Washington, DC, in the United States.

In 1821, Mexico fought to win its independence from Spain. The Mexican–American War was fueled by two major factors (History.com, 2012). The first was Manifest Destiny, the belief that America has a God-given right, or destiny, to expand its borders from the Atlantic to the Pacific oceans ("from sea to shining sea"). This desire for expansion resulted in a tremendous negative impact on Mexicans as well as Native Americans and U.S. citizens. The second factor was the Texas War of Independence. In the 1820s and 1830s, Mexico, newly free of Spain, needed settlers in its under-populated northern parts. Anyone agreeing to take an oath of allegiance to Mexico and convert to Catholicism (the national religion) was permitted to settle in this area, which was then known as the Mexican province of Texas. Many settlers became unhappy with the Mexican government and war broke out in 1835 when Texas revolted. In 1836, Santa Anna, the Mexican president, signed the Treaty of Velasco, granting Texas its independence. Many Mexicans refused to see the legality of the treaty because President Santa Anna was a prisoner at the time he signed the treaty. Border fights continued, often with savage fighting. This fighting resulted in some negative stereotypes regarding the Mexican people, some of which have persisted to this day. As the conflict escalated, full war eventually broke out; the Mexican–American War started on April 25, 1846. The war ended in 1848, with Mexico losing half of its northern territory to the United States. This change in the border caused language and cultural obstacles that still exist today (Englekirk & Marin, 2012).

In 1994, the devaluation of the peso (Mexico's money instrument) precipitated a financial crisis from which the country has not yet rebounded. Mexico has been suffering with a significant financial crisis that has resulted in high unemployment and the defaulting of the government in repaying foreign debts. The financial difficulty has been compounded by ongoing governmental and political conflict. These factors have contributed toward many Mexicans deciding to leave Mexico and immigrate to the United States, both legally and illegally. The geographic closeness of Mexico to the United States and an extensive, difficult-to-protect shared border has contributed to the ability of some Mexicans to move illegally between Mexico and United States. It is estimated that approximately one-third of the undocumented aliens in the United States come from Mexico.

The lack of American citizenship presents a significant barrier to Mexicans who are in the United States illegally. Illegal aliens often suffer significant psychological stress caused by fear of discovery and deportation (Sullivan & Rehn, 2005). The implementation of laws requiring employees to present proof of U.S. citizenship to employers often results in illegal immigrants accepting very low-paying day work, such as picking crops. Despite the hardships the illegal immigrant is faced with in the United States, many are motivated to leave Mexico due to the life-threatening poverty and political instability that is prevalent in that country. They hope that immigration into the United States will improve the economic conditions for themselves and their families. Immigration is often in response to the promise of employment, although most of the jobs are in low-paying agricultural and industrial labor positions. Mexican Americans often sacrifice being with their extended family back in Mexico in order to come to the United States with the hope of finding a job to support themselves and their families both in the United States and in Mexico.

There are also Mexican Americans who are descendants of the early Spanish settlers in what is today known as New Mexico. Over time, U.S. citizens also began to settle into this formerly Mexican territory. These early settlers contributed greatly to the development of southwestern cities by sharing and teaching skills in mining, farming, and ranching with the newer settlers (Englekirk & Marin, 2012).

Today, at least 2 million seasonal migratory workers spend part of the year in the United States and the other part in their native Mexico (Pew Hispanic Center, 2005). This population group is least likely to have access to a regular source of healthcare services, most likely to underutilize the available healthcare services, and least likely to have health insurance (Migrant Health Promotion, 2012).

Definitions of Health and Illness

The Hispanic/Latino culture views health from a synergistic point of view through the continuum of the mind, body, and spirit (espiritu); symptoms of health and illness will manifest from the mind, body, and spirit connection (Englekirk & Marin, 2012).

Hispanic/Latinos are emotionally expressive. They expect to be pampered when ill, as it is viewed as the way the family shows love and concern (CultureDiversity .org, 2012). They rely on their families, other relatives, and friends for support and help. They are not likely to accept or request help from social workers or social services. This is a present-oriented society, and as such, they may neglect preventive health care and may also show up late, or not at all, for appointments. Most Hispanics are Catholic, and birth control methods other than the rhythm method

---

Box 6–1 Pertinent Research Studies

1. An older study found that Hispanics who were treated for certain bone fractures at the University of California, Los Angeles (UCLA), Emergency Medicine Center were twice as likely as non-Hispanic Whites to receive no pain medication. The precise reason for this was not specified, but the investigators identified failure on the part of hospital staff to recognize pain in Hispanic patients as a possible reason for the discrepancy. In 2000, the study's lead author and colleagues decided to see if the trauma undertreatment found in the Hispanic population was also true in the Black population. The study found that Black patients with isolated long-bone fractures were less likely than White patients to receive analgesics in this emergency department. No covariate measured in this study could account for this effect. Both of these studies indicate that pain management is a significant healthcare disparity impacting the minority populations of the United States.[1]

Unfortunately the identification of the issue of pain undertreatment has not resulted in any improvement in patient management. A study conducted by Im, Guevara, and Chee (2007) found that Hispanics, due to their marginalized status and cultural factors, could not adequately describe or manage their cancer pain.[2]

2. For Spanish-speaking patients, having a language-concordant physician resulted in better outcomes for well-being and functioning. Monolingual Spanish-speaking patients were more likely to ask more questions and had a better understanding with physicians who also spoke Spanish.[3]

    The negative impact of lack of language concordance during medical encounters has persisted over time. Ferguson and Candib (2002) found that minority patients, especially those not proficient in English, are less likely to experience empathy, establish rapport, or to receive sufficient information from their physician. They also were not encouraged to actively participate in medical decision making, which is the cornerstone of patient-centered health care.[4]

3. According to the National Center for Health Statistics (2011), the 10 leading causes of death for Hispanics/Latinos in 2010 were:

    1. Heart disease
    2. Cancer
    3. Unintentional injuries
    4. CVA/stroke
    5. Diabetes
    6. Chronic liver disease/cirrhosis
    7. Chronic lower respiratory disease
    8. Homicide
    9. Conditions originating in the perinatal period
    10. Influenza and pneumonia

4. Hispanic patients in need of a heart transplant are 50% more likely to die before they get one than White patients. The Hispanic patients who were on the transplantation list had a higher risk of dying while on the waiting list or becoming too ill to receive a transplant compared to the White patients studied.[5]

Notes:

[1]Todd, K. H., Deaton, C., D'Adamo, A. P., & Goe, L. (2000). Ethnicity and analgesic practice. *Annals of Emergency Medicine, 35*(1), 11–16; and Todd, K. H., Samaroo, N., & Hoffman, J. R. (1993). Ethnicity as a risk factor for inadequate emergency department analgesia. *Journal of the American Medical Association, 269*(12), 1537–1539.

[2]Im, E. O., Guevara, E., & Chee, W. (2007). The pain experience of Hispanic patients with cancer in the US. *Oncology Nursing Forum, 34*(4), 861–868.

[3]Pérez-Stable, E. J., Nápoles-Springer, A., & Miramontes, J. M. (1997). The effects of ethnicity and language on medical outcomes of patients with hypertension or diabetes. *Medical Care, 35*(12), 1212–1219.

[4]Ferguson, W. J., & Candib, L. M. (2002). Culture, language and the doctor–patient relationship. *Family Medicine, 34*(5), 353–361.

[5]Singh, T. P., Almond, C. S., Taylor, D. O., Milliren, C. E., & Graham, D. A. (2012). Racial and ethnic differences in wait-list outcomes in patients listed for heart transplantation in the United States. *Circulation, 125*(24), 3022–3030.

are unacceptable. Most Latin Americans see thinness as a problem and plumpness as the ideal. The nurse needs to consider this when counseling the patient or family on weight management issues, as any advice that the patient receives recommending weight loss may not be followed; weight loss would result in a negative body image (CultureDiversity.org, 2012).

Curanderismo is defined as a medical system. It is a coherent view with historical roots that combines Aztec, Spanish, spiritualistic, homeopathic, and scientific elements. The *curandero* is a holistic healer; the people who seek help from him do so for social, physical, and psychological purposes. Because the *curandero* has a religious orientation, much of the treatment includes elements of both the Catholic and Pentecostal rituals and artifacts: offerings of money, penance, confessions, lighting candles, wooden or metal offerings in the shape of the afflicted anatomic part, and laying on of hands (CulturalDiversity.org, 2012).

Privacy is highly valued, as it is felt that personal matters should be handled only within the family. Modesty is valued in Hispanic culture for all, not just for women (Giger, 2013). The nurse should recognize that the area between the waist and knees is considered particularly private. Privacy extends to childbirth. To attend a woman during delivery is viewed as the job of women; ideally, the job of the woman's mother and the midwife. In general, Hispanic/Latina women prefer that their mothers attend them during labor. Cultural tradition dictates that the husband does not see his wife or child until the delivery is over and both have been cleaned and dressed. Postpartum, the custom of lying-in may be followed. The lying-in period is designed to give a woman the period of rest between childbirth and returning to work (traditionally in these cultures, women worked at hard physical jobs and required rest prior to resuming work).

Typically, Hispanics look down on people who are mentally ill. Patients with mental health concerns do not like to share this information with their relatives or friends, and are shy of seeking professional help (Padilla & Villalobos, 2007). Mental health problems and life stressors may appear as chest pain, shortness of breath, abdominal pain, sweats, and/or chronic illness (such as frequent headaches). These symptoms have traditional labels such as *de nervios* (stress). It is felt culturally that each condition has a specific cause and a nonmedical treatment. Mental health problems are often not validated within the culture and may carry the stigma of being a sign of weakness.

Within the last century, health and illness have been approached through a variety of treatments, each with its own philosophical base. Some have been based on empirical science (mainstream medicine), some believe disorders linked to the musculoskeletal system can be corrected by physical manipulations (osteopathy), and some developed treatments based on the belief that minute doses of drugs that mimic diseases can be used to treat diseases (homeopathy). Still other approaches continue to base states of health on a purely spiritual belief system (e.g., Christian Science).

Combining respect for the benefits of mainstream medicine, tradition, and traditional healing, along with a strong religious component from their daily lives, Hispanic patients bring quite a broad definition of health to the medical encounter.

Health promotion and disease prevention strategies that focus on the mind-body-spirit connection would be culturally competent and would be more likely to meet with success. Keep in mind, however, that Hispanics/Latinos do not routinely seek out medical care unless they are ill. Seeking out preventive care is seen as odd or as an unaffordable luxury. It is for this reason that participation in health screening by this population is low (Vega, Rodriquez, & Gruskin, 2009). The nurse should consider this and use the mind-body-spirit focus when planning for and providing all patient education sessions. See **Box 6–4** for more on this.

Traditional Healing Methods

The health and healing philosophy of Hispanics/Latinos is a result of a fusion of cultures. The Central and South American influences include a belief that the natural forces of the sun, moon, and the sea play an important role in an individual's health. Showing respect for these forces was viewed as the key to a healthy life. The Spanish influence is found in the beliefs of the Catholic religion and Hippocrates' humoral theory of health. According to this theory, health is dependent on the proper distribution of the four humors of the body: blood, phlegm, yellow bile, and black bile, which are further classified based on their physical properties as hot, cold, moist (wet), or dry (Eggenberger, Grassley, & Restrepo, 2006). Illness was believed to be caused by an imbalance in the humors, and treatment was geared toward restoring balance.

Religion and faith are also considered important factors in health maintenance for Latinos/Hispanics. Spiritual healing (*curanderismo*), magic (*Santería*), and some herbal remedies were introduced by some African slaves, particularly in Brazil and the Caribbean.

In the Hispanic theory of disease, illness is a result of an imbalance between hot and cold. It is believed that exposure to extreme changes in temperature can cause illness; therefore, one must avoid extremes of hot or cold. Low metabolic diseases are "cold diseases," whereas "hot diseases" are highly metabolic. Specific conditions are classified as either hot or cold and the treatments are also classified as either hot or cold. See **Box 6–5** for classification of common hot and cold disorders. The treatment recommended for any illness would have the opposite property of the illness. This means a *hot* illness would require a *cold* treatment. Because the female in the Hispanic/Latino culture is usually responsible for treating illness, it is usually the female who possesses the knowledge regarding alternative therapies. This information is usually handed down between female relatives. The female will treat an illness until she feels it has progressed outside her area of expertise. Common illness is hardly ever brought into the formal healthcare system. It is at the discretion of the female caregiver if or when the patient will be brought into the formal healthcare system.

There are folk conditions that are culture bound as well. An "evil eye" (*mal de ojo*) is a spell that is cast as a result of someone looking at an infant and complimenting the child without physically touching the child. A *susto* (fright) is described as the experience of the spirit leaving the body as a result of a traumatic event and is associated with panic attacks. *Ataque de nervios* (attack of the nerves) occurs when a person is not able to deal with stress. Families may treat these folk conditions in more than one way. Some may do *promesas* (promises), let the hair grow long, dress the child or themselves in robes or white clothes, kneel-walk to church, or offer extra tidings to a specific church. Others may use amulets for good luck or to keep them healthy.

Although first-generation and new immigrants are more likely to hold traditional health beliefs, a significant number of Hispanics/Latinos utilize at least one complementary/alternative modality either alone or in combination with conventional therapy. Today, there is an extensive practice of traditional medicine carried out by *curanderas, espiritistas,* and healers within the Hispanic/Latino community. In urban barrios, this tradition has been carried on in part by Hispanic pharmacists, familiar with both traditional treatments like *té de manzanilla* (chamomile tea), as well as placing a strong value on the use of modern prescription medicines such as antibiotics.

Alternative/Complementary Folk Medicine

Due to the synergistic health belief of Hispanic/Latinos that recognizes the link between the body, mind, and spirit (*espiritu*) it is very possible that the Hispanic/Latino patient may be utilizing complementary/alternative medicine (CAM), specifically the use of herbal therapies that may be unfamiliar to you. The Hispanic/Latino population does utilize herbs that are unique from other groups. Some commonly used herbs are linden, sapodilla and star anise, brook mint, and passion flower.

CAM modalities are usually used to manage chronic conditions such as diabetes mellitus (DM), asthma, and hypertension. DM is considered a hot disease. Home remedies for diabetes are usually administered in combination with traditional medicine. Nopal (cactus), aloe vera juice, and bitter gourd are three common home remedies that may be unfamiliar to healthcare practitioners (Ortiz, Shields, Clauson, & Clay, 2007). The efficacy of these therapies is yet to be fully elucidated. Some published data suggest that nopal and bitter gourd may be helpful in reduction of blood glucose levels. Nopal may exert its effect as a result of high fiber content or have some insulin-sensitizing properties, and components of bitter gourd may have some insulin-like properties.

Hypertension is also a hot illness according to the Hispanic hot/cold theory. Anger (*corajes*), fear (*susto*), nervousness, and thick blood are thought to be the most common causes of hypertension in this belief system. Cold remedies used to treat this condition include lemon juice, linden (*tila*) tea, passion flower tea (*pasionara*), and sapodilla (*zapote blanco*) tea. Minimal information is available about the safety or efficacy of these products, but all should be treated as pharmacologically active agents (Ortiz et al., 2007).

Asthma is considered a cold disease and remedies with perceived hot properties, such as cod liver oil, oregano, lemon, and castor oil, along with massage, are the most popular modalities used as home remedies (Ortiz et al., 2007). A commercial product, called Siete Jarabes, is often used by Puerto Ricans to treat a cough (Ortiz et al., 2007).

It is important for the nurse to keep an open mind and to demonstrate acceptance toward the use of CAM. Hispanics/Latinos often do not inform healthcare professionals about their use of these practices. If a negative attitude is perceived, they will be even less likely to do so. Lack of knowledge about the use of these agents can put the patient in serious jeopardy. Whenever possible, and of course only if it is safe to do so, the nurse or nurse practitioner should encourage the use of CAM. This will result in improved adherence to conventional treatment and will help to gain the patient's trust. An easy way to do this would be to add the recommendation to a patient who must increase fluids to treat a cold or flu to use a natural tea drink or natural soup to facilitate the replacement of fluids and electrolytes (Ortiz et al., 2007).

Current Healthcare Problems Including Morbidity and Mortality

The use of the U.S. healthcare system has been problematic for Latinos/Hispanics (Englekirk & Marin, 2012). There are several reasons for this. Lack of health insurance is a major problem for this group (Vega et al., 2009). There are many explanations for the lack of insurance, including communication issues and a lack of understanding of a competitive healthcare system with the resultant understanding of the need for health insurance. Illegal or undocumented aliens do not qualify for Medicare or Medicaid, which has contributed to a lack of willingness to treat uninsured, indigent people. Another reason for Latinos/Hispanics not utilizing the U.S. healthcare system is lack of access or transportation concerns. A third reason may be that the Mexican American group strives hard to maintain its cultural uniqueness and resists becoming absorbed into the dominant American culture. This desire to retain a cultural identity is often cited as a reason why Mexican Americans have experienced discrimination in education, jobs, and housing (Englekirk & Marin, 2012).

Impact of Communication

The most common language spoken by Latinos/Hispanics is Spanish. A majority of Hispanics/Latinos in the United States are bilingual and likely to retain their Spanish language skills as their communities are replenished with new Spanish-speaking immigrants. Although only 24% of Hispanics were born outside the United States and the Commonwealth of Puerto Rico, 77% report Spanish as their primary language and the language they speak at home (National Alliance for Hispanic Health, 2001).

Interfacing with Hispanics, appreciation of the Spanish language, and appreciating the different accents, idioms, and meanings within different Spanish-speaking subgroups are crucial to becoming culturally competent. Language is a communication tool by which cultural meaning is transferred and its complexity understood. When understanding language from this perspective, it is important to differentiate its layers. In its simplest form, each word has a meaning. The combination of words within a particular context takes on a specific cultural meaning.

The initial stage of language development is direct translation of words with their literal meaning. However, this level of language may not be effective in communicating health beliefs, core values, or a description of symptoms. As a result, language differences and the width of the gap pose a challenge to both the patient and provider in healthcare communication. To fully understand the complexities of language and culture, one has to examine the layer of language development. Primary language development, the first learned language, provides relational meaning to words and phrases that reflect culture. Secondary language development, or learning a second language, may not provide the speaker with the idiomatic expressions or cultural meanings specific to location and ethnicity. One can learn to speak a language without learning how to use the language to reflect culture. Although it is a difficult proposition, the message is that we should try to bridge any language differences because quality health care can be achieved and language differences overcome, even in the most extreme situations. Cultural competency is *not* necessarily indicated by the nurse's ability to speak the patient's language, but a patient and provider that do not share any language knowledge will have more challenges to quality care than those who have learned the other's language.

Language differences can have a major impact on diagnosis for the nurse practitioner who follows the medical model. Subjective diagnosis or assessing which modality to test for in determining a medical diagnosis is influenced by the patient's description of the symptoms. What the patient says and how they say it is essential to establishing the appropriate diagnosis. Without the element of communication, quality care can be obtained, but it is a challenge. The patient can become frustrated, may not return, or may be unable to comply with treatment. Language discordance can result in misdiagnosis and incorrect patient treatment as well as contribute additional costs to patient care.

There are a growing number of healthcare professionals who care for America's multiethnic, multiracial, and increasingly multilingual society. According to the U.S. Census Bureau (2010a), at least 20% of the nation's population now speaks a language other than English in their home. In fact, the total population speaking a language other than English at home increased by 140% in the past three decades while the overall population grew by 34% (U.S. Census Bureau, 2010a). Spanish is, by far, the main "other language" spoken in the United States. In major cities including New York, Los Angeles, Miami, Honolulu, Newark, and El Paso, Texas, the number of non-English speakers is over 40%. Additionally, there are approximately 7 million persons in the United States who do not speak English well, if at all.

Language diversity in the Spanish language exists in terms of pitch, vocabulary, accent, pronunciation, dialect, and grammar rules, depending on the country of origin. There are over 50 different languages and dialects in Mexico and over 15 in Central and South America. People from the Caribbean have a higher pitch and different accent compared with the people in Central and South America. Puerto Ricans do not pronounce the last "s" and pronounce the double "r" with guttural sounds; Spaniards pronounce the "c" with a "z" sound. One word can be benign in one country and considered rude or offensive in another. The nurse must be careful when using Spanish (if not her first language) when communicating with a patient. Other difficulties are verb tenses and pronoun construction, which are very different than those used in the English language.

Many Hispanics/Latinos speak with their hands and become very animated when expressing emotion or giving emphasis to their words. Nodding the head does not indicate agreement with what was said, just that it was heard. This is a very important concept for the nurse to remember when communicating with Hispanic/Latino patients.

It is important to be aware that not all Latinos/Hispanics are Spanish speakers. Although Brazil, Belize, and Haiti are all considered Latin American countries, the official language of Brazil is Portuguese, English is the official language of Belize, and French or Creole are the primary languages used in Haiti. Literacy, in any language, should not be assumed. It also should never be assumed that all communication between Spanish speakers will be understood by all other Spanish speakers. This is because there are many words and phrases that have different usages and meanings in different countries. This is important for the nurse to consider when dealing with the use of an interpreter who is not of the same ethnic group as the patient.

There have been six identified approaches for bridging language barriers. The six approaches are listed in order from most to least effective (for more information on these seven approaches see **Box 6–2**):

1. Bilingual/bicultural professional staff
2. Interpreters
3. Language skills training for existing staff
4. Internal language banks
5. Phone-based interpreter services
6. Written translator
7. Cultural Mediators

Box 6–2 Seven Approaches for Bridging Language Barriers

1. **Bilingual/Bicultural Professional Staff**
   - Recruit and retain bilingual/bicultural staff at all levels of the organization.
   - Provide significant additional compensation for bilingual ability.

2. **Interpreters**
   - Establish minimum standards for interpreter training, competency, and other continuing education efforts.
   - Make a concerted effort to increase and foster medical interpreter training through national conferences, information clearinghouses, technical assistance, and start-up grants.
   - Provide courses designed to train providers to work with interpreters.
   - Use only trained medical interpreters.
   - Reimburse for interpreter services.

3. **Language Skills Training for Existing Staff**
   - Support the development of bilingual skills for all staff members.
   - Establish clear goals and realistic expectations for Spanish language courses, including idioms.
   - Offer classes in medical Spanish to all staff.
   - Utilize training programs that have a demonstrated track record in increasing the bilingual level or the quality of interpretation services provided.

4. **Internal Language Banks** (Only as a back-up measure)
   - Hire supervisors to assess the language and interpretation capabilities of language bank members, to provide minimal interpreter training, and to regularly assess the quality of the language bank program.
   - List interpretation as a secondary responsibility of language bank members so that supervisors of these staff members understand why they may spend time away from their regular duties.
   - Compensate language bank members who do a significant amount of interpretation.

5. **Phone-Based Interpreter Services** (Emergency back-up measure for brief follow-up questions only)
   - Inform healthcare providers that phone-based interpreters may not be proficient in medical terminology.
   - Use simple or common terms when using phone interpreters.

6. **Written Translators** (Emergency stop-gap measures, never as the sole means of communication)
   - Develop mechanisms to promote the sharing of bilingual written materials, such as consent forms and patient education pamphlets.

7. **Cultural Mediators**
   - In addition to medical interpreting, the cultural mediator interprets the cultural and social circumstances that may affect care.
   - This enables providers to gain a more comprehensive understanding of patients needs and to negotiate culturally appropriate plans of care.

Two common approaches to resolving language differences are so detrimental that they require *Do Not* statements:
- *Do not use the patient's relatives, especially those who are younger in age, as interpreters.*
- *Do not use support staff whose primary job is NOT translation.*

Source: Adapted from: National Alliance for Hispanic Health. (2001). *Quality health services for Hispanics: The cultural competency component.* Washington, DC: U.S. Department of Health and Human Services.

Ten tips that the nurse can follow to have successful patient interactions across cultures are listed in **Box 6–7**. **Box 6–8** includes five tips for working with interpreters. The use of medical interpreters is essential. The use of medical interpreters is associated with improved clinical outcomes. In fact, a systematic review of the literature found that the use of an interpreter when providing care for patients with limited English proficiency raised the quality of medical care to the level of patients who did not have a language barrier (Karliner, Jacobs, Chen, & Mutha, 2007).

Impact of Time

Mexican Americans have a present orientation to time and are often unable or reluctant to consider the future when planning (Giger, 2013; National Alliance for Hispanic Health, 2001). The Mexican custom of the siesta comes from this present orientation to time. It is believed that the present need for rest takes priority over safeguarding the future through the generation of more work/income.

It is felt that a present time orientation, or elasticity, is responsible for the lack of social upward mobility in Mexican Americans as well as a barrier to assimilation and integration into the mainstream American culture. This focus on the present to the exclusion of the future may result in missed appointments or being late for appointments. This is a result of the concern for a present activity and not for the activity of planning ahead to be on time. The concept of elasticity implies that present activities cannot be recovered if lost or missed, whereas future activities can be recovered.

It is important for the nurse to consider the present orientation to time when planning for patient education. Focusing on long-term effects (such as what could occur if medication is missed or discontinued) will not be as beneficial as focusing on any potential short-term problems that could occur.

Impact of Space and Touch

Mexican Americans value physical contact and having a close physical space with family members (National Alliance for Hispanic Health, 2001). As a group, they demonstrate togetherness. A pattern of socialization begins in childhood when parents are permissive, warm, and caring with all of their children. In later years, girls remain much closer to home and are protected and guarded, whereas boys are allowed to be with other boys in informal social groups to develop machismo. Although Mexican Americans are comfortable with physical touching within their social group, a female nurse should always assist a male physician in examining a female client to preserve modesty (Andrews, 2006). Male patients may refuse a complete physical examination because of modesty factors. Females prefer caregivers of the same gender. Nursing care may be resisted if the Mexican American feels that the caregiver is different from the patient. Details are important as both space and touch influence the patient encounter. The nurse should consider maintaining a close personal space—close enough where a handshake would be possible without moving closer (National Alliance for Hispanic Health, 2001).

Eye contact and touching are also important components to an effective interaction. For more on cultural nuances that govern social interactions, see **Box 6–3**.

Impact of Environment

Mexican Americans have an external locus of control (Giger, 2013). This is the belief that the outcome of circumstances is controlled by external forces (Padilla & Villalobus, 2007). They believe that life is under the constant influence of God (or divine will). There is also a reliance on fatalism. This is the belief that one is at the mercy of the environment and has little control over the environment or what occurs. It is felt that personal efforts are unlikely to influence a situation's outcome. This means that Mexican Americans do not believe that they are personally responsible for any future successes or failures (National Alliance for Hispanic Health, 2001). This can be especially impactful when asking the Mexican American patient to participate in screening or health maintenance activities because failing to see any value does not encourage participation.

The environmental health status of Hispanic communities is poor and is a major source of health problems (National Alliance for Hispanic Health, 2001; Vega et al., 2009). Among their high-risk exposures are ambient air pollution, worker exposure to chemicals in industry, pollution indoors, and pollutants in drinking water. In terms of exposure, Hispanics consistently face the worst exposure levels, or levels that represent significant threats to health. Nurse practitioners and nurses should consider environmental sources in diagnosing and treating a variety of conditions that affect their Hispanic/Latino patients.

Biologic Variations

Several diseases occur with high incidence in Mexican Americans (Vega et al., 2009). Hispanic/Latinos are almost twice as likely to be diagnosed with diabetes than whites (Office of Minority Health, 2012); 13.3% of Mexican Americans have diabetes (National Diabetes Fact Sheet, 2011). There is an increased tendency toward decreased insulin action in peripheral tissues, skeletal muscle, and also in the liver. The incidence may also be a result of increased abdominal obesity, and there may also be abnormalities in beta-cell function (this is not yet well understood), which, in combination, may lead to more problems. Forty-three percent of Hispanic women are obese and 34% of Hispanic men are obese (BMI = or > than 30) (National Health and Nutrition Examination Survey [NHANES], 2008).

There are cultural aspects that influence diabetes care that are specific for the Hispanic/Latino population. The following have been identified as factors that may influence diabetes care: family orientation, fatalism, faith/religion, body image, nutrition/physical activity, acculturation, language, and myths (National Alliance for Hispanic Health, 2001; Vega et al., 2009). In the Hispanic/Latino culture, the family is the primary unit—this is referred to as *familisimo*. (Padilla & Villalobus, 2007). The family's needs are placed above an individual's needs. They also place a strong emphasis on respect (Padilla & Villalobus, 2007). *Respecto* dictates deferential behavior toward others based on their position of authority, social position, gender, and economic status. Hispanic/Latino patients expect their healthcare providers to engage in non–health-related conversation. The attitude of the healthcare provider is also analyzed by the patient. It is important for the nurse to realize that a neutral attitude can be perceived as negative by the Hispanic/Latino patient.

When caring for Hispanic/Latino patients, it is important to try to win their *confianza* (trust). (National Alliance for Hispanic Health, 2001). This is done by showing a respect for their culture. Being open and warm with the patient will help to develop *confianza*. The development of a therapeutic relationship will be difficult, if not impossible, if *confianza* has not been achieved. *Fatilismo* is a significant threat to providing effective nursing care. *Fatilismo* is the belief that you cannot change your destiny or fate. Thus, fatalismo acts as a barrier to self-care, something that is held in high esteem by nurses and all healthcare professionals who are trained in the Western Biomedical Model.

When providing for patient education regarding DM with the Hispanic/Latino patient, the nurse should recognize that a preference has been found for listening to stories over reading printed materials. In a study conducted at the Latino Diabetes Initiative at the Joslin Diabetes Center by Dr. Caballero (2005), patients learned more and retained more information when it was presented in an audio-based manner rather than with printed material. Culturally appropriate resources are available from the American Diabetes Association, National Diabetes Education Program, and the National Institutes of Health. Nutritional information is available from the National Dietetics Organization. The Joslin Diabetes Center website (http://www.joslin.org) is an excellent resource because it has initiatives for the Black American, Asian American, and Hispanic/Latino cultural groups. Another study by Caballero (2006) found that one out of three Hispanics/Latinos believe that insulin causes blindness. The belief in this myth was found to be highly correlated with decreased adherence to the diabetes management plan and highlights the need to address pertinent myths such as this when providing patient education.

Hypertension is also found with an increased prevalence among Mexican Americans, as this group is slightly more likely to have high blood pressure than non-Hispanic Whites. The onset of pernicious anemia, which is most often seen in the elderly, has been shown to occur in those of Latin American origin at a younger age than in White patients.

Approximately 85% of the health problems common to Mexican Americans involve communicable diseases, including respiratory tract infections, diarrhea, and skin disorders (National Center for Health Statistics, 2002). The risk of contracting tuberculosis (TB) among Hispanics/Latinos is more than four times the risk among non-Hispanic Whites. Among Hispanics, TB is most prevalent in young adults aged 25 to 44 years. Evidence suggests that the HIV epidemic is, in part, responsible for the recent increases in TB. TB also appears to be a significant problem for migrant workers. This is a group that would benefit from TB screening.

The prevalence of HIV is a major concern. By 1997, Hispanics/Latinos made up 12% of the total U.S. population, yet they accounted for 21% of the new AIDS cases. HIV diagnoses have gone up 10% in this group, whereas other ethnic groups, such as Black Americans, have seen a decline. The primary mode of exposure is heterosexual sexual activity with an intravenous drug abuser.

AIDS strikes Puerto Ricans the hardest, followed by Cubans, probably, in part, because Puerto Ricans and Cubans are concentrated in East Coast cities where AIDS has taken a high toll. Mexican Americans seem less affected by the epidemic. Overall, Hispanic men are nearly twice as likely as White non-Hispanic men to die from AIDS, and Hispanic women are nearly five times as likely to die from the disease as White non-Hispanic Women (National Alliance for Hispanic Health, 2001).

Malignant neoplasms are the second leading cause of death in the United States among both Hispanics and non-Hispanic Whites, although Hispanics have a slightly lower rate. This trend continues with cardiovascular disease. Although it is the leading cause of death for Hispanic/Latinos, the incidence is less than found in Whites or Black Americans, despite the fact that Hispanics/Latinos have a higher prevalence of conditions that increase the risk for coronary heart disease, such as obesity and DM.

Hispanic/Latino men are more likely to have undiagnosed and untreated hypertension than the national average. Although Hispanic/Latina women are more likely than men to be aware of the diagnosis, they are more unlikely to have it be controlled or treated. It appears that race is a significant factor in hypertension. There also appears to be a genetic link to DM as the incidence of non-insulin-dependent DM appears to be highest in Mexican Americans who have a substantial Pima Indian heritage.

Impact of Social Organization

It is not possible to make accurate generalizations about an area as large and diverse as Latin America. There are many different kinds of Latinos/Hispanics. The intent of this section of this chapter is to provide some background on Latino/Hispanic family life and to acknowledge the impact of the struggle for economic survival on many in this group. The prevalence of economic hardship and the increased number of children in this group has resulted in poverty being the way of life for most Latino/Hispanic children (Tienda & Mitchell, 2006). High costs place marriage out of reach for many poor, and for those who are unhappily married, divorce is often financially out of reach.

According to the National Women's Law Center (2012), the poverty rate for Hispanic women (as well as for Black women) rose even more than the poverty rate for all women. It rose for Hispanic women to 25% in 2010 from 23.8% in 2009. Seventy percent of Mexican American families were married couple families, whereas 21% were female-headed households. Thirty-one percent of Mexican American households had five or more people making up the household, compared with 12% among non-Hispanic Whites. Latinos/Hispanics are a rapidly growing group. They are a younger population, with 35.7% aged 18 years old or younger. The mean age for Hispanic/Latinos is 27.4 years (compared with 36.8 years for the population as a whole), and Mexican Americans are the youngest group among all Latinos/Hispanics (U.S. Census Bureau, 2010b).

The family is the most valued institution and the main focus for social identification. Elders have a prestigious status in the Hispanic family because of their experience. Family members look to elders for advice. An individual who becomes sick will turn first to family members, especially elders, for support, comfort, and advice. They may recommend safe, simple home remedies.

In the traditional household, the man is the head of the family and makes all major decisions. There is a strong sense of paternalism—what most Westerners call "male dominance"—but the female's role is equivalent and she is the maternal powerhouse in her home. The truth is that the female is sacred and revered, often protected, not because she cannot handle herself or has no voice, but because the solidarity of the family unit depends on her well-being. The nuclear family is strong, but there also commonly exists many extended families of three or more generations. Men are the authority figure and women tend to maintain traditional roles. The Hispanic/Latino family is usually patriarchal; however, the mother cares for the children and older relatives and possesses power within the family. Mothers within the Mexican American community enjoy a high social status. Mexican

American women consider motherhood a desirable role and are likely to leave a career during pregnancy to care for self and the pregnancy and to remain out of work to care for their children as they grow. Many Mexican American mothers rate their role as a mother as second in importance only to God. It is felt that personal behavior has the potential for increasing community respect for the family.

An important concept for Mexican Americans is familism (Tienda & Mitchell, 2006). Familism is a model of social organization, based on the prevalence of the family group and its well-being being placed against the interest and necessities of each one of its individual members. It is part of a traditional view of society and highlights loyalty, trust, and cooperative attitudes within the family group. There are positives and negatives associated with familism (Eggenberger et al., 2006). Familism provides a source of collective pride, which is a strong positive. Familism has also been identified as a major cause of resistance to change and it is felt to be a contributor to the lack of collective and individual progress found in this group.

Impact of Faith and Spirituality

The vast majority of Latinos/Hispanics are Catholic, with an increasing presence of Pentecostals (Pew Research Center, 2007). In addition to spirituality, the Catholic religion also has a powerful influence on the perceptions of norms and behaviors, beliefs about social interaction, and spiritual ideas regarding fate and faith. The Catholic Church and Catholic religion provide a powerful source of support, hope, and strength within the Latino/Hispanic community (Pew Research Center, 2007).

Box 6–3 Common Cultural Nuances for Hispanics in the United States and Their Impact on Nursing Care

Disclaimer: It is always important to note that there can be individual variation from any cultural norm.

La Familia (Family)
Large in size and scope: Hispanics include many members in their extended family. Family is considerd critical to health care. Often the patient will be accompanied by several family members of varying ages who will be very actively involved in the healthcare encounter (commadres, compadres, or *padrinos* [godparents]). The nurse may have to handle institutional policy violations related to the number of hospital visitors permitted at any one time.

Emphasis on interdependence and cooperation: Hispanic families also traditionally emphasize interdependence over independence and cooperation over

(Continues)

Box 6–3 *Continued*

competition, and extended family are likely to be involved in the decision-making process. Family involvement should be encouraged and supported by the nurse whenever possible or feasible. Flexibility is required of the nurse. The patient may not be the one responding to the provider's questions or even the one asking questions because he or she may defer to someone in the familial group. The person conversing with the provider may be a spouse, the eldest family member, son or daughter, or friend. Often, the spokesperson will be the person who has the most respect and power in the family. Most often, the speaker is the matriarch/patriarch or, in many cases in the United States, it is the more acculturated children.

Recognize the family hierarchy and its cultural implications: A nurse relying on a child to provide input into the patient's health care in any way can cause a disruption in family dynamics. The nurse must be respectful and inclusive of family elders when younger family members are the key communicators. Encouraging the whole family to be on board with any treatment decisions offers the best chance for a positive patient outcome.

Respeto (Respect)

Respect determines behaviors: Respect is determined by many factors including age, sex, social position, economic status, and authority. This means that elders expect respect from younger people, men expect it from women, and employers expect it from their employees. Nurses are held in high esteem and are given much respect from Hispanic/Latino patients. Body language has cultural overtones and therefore can be misinterpreted. For example, a sign of respect from a Hispanic/Latino patient to the nurse would be the avoidance of eye contact by virtue of the nurse's authority position over the patient. On the other hand, it would be considered disrespectful for the nurse not to maintain eye contact with the patient, even if another is translating for the patient. This is important for the nurse to remember because the nurse may exclude the patient or focus on the translator during the encounter, which will be viewed as disrespectful by the patient.

Consequences of a breach in respect: If the patient feels that the nurse is being disrespectful, they may terminate the therapeutic relationship. Always be sensitive and respectful, especially when data collecting. Avoid asking direct questions about things that would be considered too personal or requesting information that should stay within the family (such as alcohol intake, incidence of domestic or substance abuse, sexual activity, or family history of mental illness). Directly asking for this information may be viewed as challenging and disrespectful to the practice of keeping such things within the family. A better approach is to ask for the essential information in a more nondirect manner.

Pearls for the nurse to follow to maintain respect from Hispanic/Latino patients:

1. If the nurse is younger than the patient: Use formal titles and more formality when communicating with the patient to convey respect to the patient. The formal title can be spoken in either English or Spanish. The Spanish terms are *señor* (Mister), *don* (Sir), *señora* (Missus), or *doña* (Madam).

2. Incorporate at least some Spanish into the encounter: Even if you do not speak Spanish you should include some basic Spanish in your communication. Offering an opening Spanish phrase at the beginning of the interaction (such as *buenos dias*, which means good morning) suggests that you have respect for the Spanish language and the patient.

3. Encourage patient questions: Hispanic/Latino patients often avoid asking questions as a sign of respect. This is even more likely if the question appears to be challenging. The end result is the patient will often not follow the treatment plan or discontinue therapy entirely. There is a cultural taboo against expressing negative feelings directly. Nurses need to take seriously the responsibility and *respeto* (respect) conferred on them by many Hispanic patients. The nurse needs to explain all medical procedures and treatments thoroughly and ascertain through careful indirect questioning whether the patient has understanding or if outstanding questions remain.

Personalismo (Personal)

Provision of personalized patient care is preferred: Hispanics expect all healthcare providers to be warm, friendly, and personable. The nurse should begin every encounter by offering a personal greeting, which will put the patient at ease prior to any needed intervention. The Hispanic/Latino patient often develops loyalty to their primary care provider and other regular caregivers, which can have significant implications for continuity of care. When assigning nursing staff to care for a Hispanic/Latino patient and his or her family, keeping the same nursing assignment (if at all possible) during the course of the admission will be very helpful toward establishing *personalismo*.

Utilize appropriate body language and personal space: The nurse should know that Hispanics/Latinos prefer a close personal space during encounters. The standard 2-ft-away space traditionally utilized during history taking can be perceived as the nurse being uncaring, uninterested, or detached from the patient. This perception can be overcome if the nurse leans forward, sits closer, or uses other body language cues (such as patting the patient's hand) that indicate the nurse has a personal interest in the patient as a human being.

Confianza (Trust)

Attaining trust is rare but extremely valuable: Respecting the patient's culture and showing interest in the patient can, over time, result in the development of trust. This means that the patient believes that the nurse has the patient's best interest at heart. Our busy healthcare system with limited time makes it difficult for trust to be achieved. The nurse should still strive to establish trust because it will result in increased compliance on the patient's part, which will improve the patient's health outcome.

Source: National Alliance for Hispanic Health. (2001). *A primer for cultural proficiency: Towards quality health services for Hispanics*. Retrieved from http://www.hispanichealth.arizona.edu/ primer%20for%20culural%20proficiency%20nahh.pdf; and Salimbene, S. (2000). *What language does your patient hurt in? A practical guide to culturally competent patient care*. Amherst, MA: Diversity Resources.

The Catholic Church teaches that the soul is eternal and continues on after the physical body has died (Pew Research Center, 2007). The faith also holds that all life as sacred. Pain and illness may be viewed as a "test." This faith may interfere with the patient agreeing to the use of comfort measures, such as the use of pain medication. Health is a gift from God and should not be taken for granted. The prevention of illness is an accepted practice that is accomplished with prayer, the wearing of religious medals or amulets, and keeping relics in the home. Visiting shrines, offering medals and candles, offering prayers, and the lighting of candles is a frequently observed practice. Many homes have shrines with statues and pictures

---

Box 6–4 The Synergy of the Body-Mind-Spirit Continuum in Hispanics/Latinos as a Focus for Patient Education

The nurse should use a holistic approach when assessing a Hispanic/Latino patient's learning needs. Utilizing a body-mind-spirit approach will ensure that the patient will receive comprehensive and effective patient education.

Body

1. Encourage smoking cessation in smokers. Encourage nonsmokers not to smoke.
2. Inform patients of the risks of excessive alcohol intake and the gender differences associated with safer alcohol intake.
3. Eat and prepare healthy meals.
4. Avoid a sedentary lifestyle through regular exercise.
5. Listen to your body.

Mind

1. Encourage rest and relaxation as a component of a healthy lifestyle.
2. Emphasize the importance of stress reduction to good health.
3. Encourage participation in pleasurable and healthy activities.
4. Establish and nurture close relationships with family and friends.

Spirit

1. Contribute to society through the provision of good deeds.
2. Maintain a positive attitude and think good thoughts.
3. Establish time for reflection through "quiet time" or time for oneself.
4. Utilize prayer and/or meditation. Participate in activities related to the church if pertinent.
5. Keep communication open with family and friends. Encourage frequent visitation.

Source: Adapted from: National Alliance for Hispanic Health. (2001). *Quality health services for Hispanics: The cultural competency component.* Washington, DC: U.S. Department of Health and Human Services.

of saints. The candles are lit here and prayers are recited. Many believe that illness is a result of God's will and that fate controls life and health (Eggenberger et al., 2006). Spirituality can be manifested as a fatalistic feeling in which individuals are seen as having little control over their lives and health or by the optimistic belief that divine faith and trust can overcome any possible adverse event. Family and faith are the two most important sources of strength to Hispanics/Latinos. Most will not have living wills or advance directives due to the belief that it is God's decision as to when it is one's time to die, and that no one should make that decision on their own. They believe that they possess a spirit and a soul and that their spiritual needs must be given attention (Pew Research Center, 2007).

The Protestant religion is gaining some Latino/Hispanic followers. The grass root efforts of the Protestant Evangelical Movement are making inroads as an organizing force for Latinos/Hispanics (Pew Research Center, 2007).

Many Mexican Americans (as high as 72% in a study by Kalish and Reynolds, 1981) believe that whatever the cause of death, it is God's will. Death also offers a release from the troubles of life and passage to a new eternal life. This belief is shared by just 56% of Anglo Americans (Kalish & Reynolds, 1981).

PUERTO RICANS

Puerto Ricans are the second largest Hispanic/Latino group in the United States (Pew Hispanic Center, 2012). Puerto Ricans are American citizens who possess a different language and culture. The island of Puerto Rico is located about 1,000 miles east-southeast of Miami. The geography of the island, which encompasses 3,425 square miles, is diverse and includes a central mountain range, northern coastal plains, low eastern mountains, and the El Yunque rain forest (Buffington, 2012c).

The island was claimed for Spain by Christopher Columbus in 1493. Columbus found the island was populated by Taino Indians who were living in small villages. The Spanish colonizers who arrived in 1508 were welcomed by the Taino. The port of San Juan (today the capital of Puerto Rico) became a very important military outpost in the Caribbean for Spain (Buffington, 2012c). Under the leadership of Governor Juan Ponce de Leon, extremely brutal treatment came to the Taino Indians. A fixed number of Indians were distributed to officials and colonists to provide forced (wage-free) labor.

Puerto Ricans that come to the mainland are in a unique position; they are technically neither natives nor immigrants (Green, 2012). Despite the fact that Puerto Ricans are American citizens, there is a general lack of knowledge that it is a poor island and the culture is also not well known or understood by the many Americans. When many Puerto Ricans come to the mainland, they bring with them problems from the island such as poor health and poor socioeconomic status. Most migrate to the East Coast, with the largest number living in New York City and New Jersey. They come to the mainland in search of a better life or to join family members already here. Unemployment is very high on the island.

According to the U.S. Census Bureau, there are 3 million people of Puerto Rican descent living on the U.S. mainland and 3.2 million living on the island of Puerto Rico. Nine percent of the Hispanic population is made up of Puerto Ricans (U.S. Census Bureau, 2008).

As mentioned above, Puerto Rico was discovered by Columbus in 1492 and conquered by Ponce de Leon in 1508. The natives who lived there, the Taino and Arawak Indians, were killed off through starvation and forced labor. Yoruba African slaves were then brought to the island to work in the sugar cane fields. Eventually, the slaves were freed and intermarried, which resulted in the two cultures and beliefs being incorporated into a new culture. In 1815, more Spanish settlers came to the island and attempted to establish themselves as an elite population, which caused tension between the groups. In 1897, Puerto Rican nationalists declared themselves independent from Spain. A year later, during the Spanish–American War, U.S. troops landed in Puerto Rico and maintained their claim to the island. In 1917, Puerto Ricans were made U.S. citizens under the Jones Act. In 1952, Puerto Rico was declared a commonwealth of the United States (Buffington, 2012c).

Economic underdevelopment on the island has resulted in a large number of Puerto Ricans coming to the mainland of the United States, which has resulted in large Puerto Rican communities in New York and throughout the Northeast and Chicago. Because of the relationship between the United States and Puerto Rico, Puerto Ricans can easily and freely move back and forth between the mainland and the island. It is for this reason that they are unlike other Hispanics/Latinos; they can maintain many cultural, family, and social connections with their island home even after many years of living on the mainland of the United States (Green, 2012).

Traditional Health Beliefs

Many people from Puerto Rico share similar health beliefs with other Hispanics/Latinos, especially those beliefs held by Mexican Americans (Buffington, 2012c).

Box 6–5 Disease Classification Based on the Hot/Cold Theory

Disease or Condition	Classification
Arthritis	Cold
Common cold	Cold
Constipation	Hot
Diarrhea	Hot
Fever	Hot
Indigestion	Cold
Menstrual pain	Cold
Muscle spasm	Cold
Pregnancy	Hot
Rash/hives	Hot
Stomachache	Cold
Ulcer	Hot

Sources:
Centers for Disease Control and Prevention (CDC). (n.d.). *Cultural insights: Communicating with Hispanics/Latinos.* Retrieved from http://www.cdc.gov/healthcommunication/Audience/AudienceInsight_Cultural Insights.pdf; Ortiz, B. I., Shields, K. M., Clauson, K. A., & Clay, P. G. (2007). Complementary and alternative medicine use among Hispanics in the United States. *The Annals of Pharmacotherapy, 41,* 6, 994-1004; and Salimbene, S. (2000). *What language does your patient hurt in? A practical guide to culturally competent care.* Amherst, MA: Diversity Resources.

There are, however, important differences in how health and illness are perceived by Mexicans and Puerto Ricans. Puerto Ricans classify their diseases as hot or cold, like the Mexicans, but they have three categories for treatments: hot (*caliente*), cold (*frío*), and cool (*fresco*) (Harwood, 1971). Cold illnesses are treated with hot treatments, and hot diseases are treated with either cold or cool remedies. The goal is to maintain the proper hot–cold balance in the body. In addition, some Puerto Ricans also practice *Santería* (Buffington, 2012c).

Santería is a form of magic that has a very structured system (Buffington, 2012c). It was first practiced in Nigeria by the Yorubas. Many Yorubas were brought to America as slaves, and in time, the practice has been handed down through the generations. The practice includes a reliance on storytelling to promote coping with life. The traditional religion brought from Nigeria was, over time, combined with Catholicism. The Yoruba gods (*orishas*) were identified with Christian saints, so the saints were invested with supernatural God-like powers.

There is a hierarchy in *Santería*. Certain people claim to have *facultades* that provide them with the ability to practice. It is believed that the *facultades* were given to the healer from the Catholic saints. The head is a man, the *babalow*; second is the *presidente*, who is the head medium; and third are the *santeros*. Novices to *Santería* are called believers. *Santería* can be and is practiced anywhere—even

---

Box 6-6 Pain Response in Hispanics/Latinos

To most Hispanics/Latinos, pain is accepted as part of life, a fate that one is obligated to endure. Accepting pain without complaint is a sign of courage and strength. Men who strive for machismo will be reluctant to acknowledge or succumb to pain. The nurse should reinforce to the male patient, that even though they may require assistance or help, they are still strong and courageous men.

Some Hispanic/Latinos view pain as an act from "God" that must therefore be endured (Lipson & Dibble, 2005, 330). Pain may also be viewed as a punishment or a consequence to bad behavior that must be endured as a type of penance. Others may be open to pain management due to the philosophy that pain is not a punishment but a consequence of disharmony between the person and the environment. Pain must be managed to restore balance. Pain is subjective and requires proper description by the patient. Hispanic/Latinos often use emotional terms when describing or quantifying the pain or its intensity.

The nurse must educate the patient and family about the need for pain to be properly managed and the consequences associated with inadequate pain management. Due to the cultural fear of drug addiction associated with the use of prescribed pain agents, patient education must stress that the pain medication for true physiologic pain will not result in addiction and that the benefits of pain management significantly outweigh the risks associated with pain management.

Although the pain response differs based on culture it is an important issues when dealing with Hispanic/Latinos because many studies have shown that this population are less likely to receive pain medication or to have their pain acknowledged by medical staff than Caucasian or White ethnic groups members.

Sources:

Lipson, G. J., & Dibble, S. T. (Eds.). (2005). Culture & clinical care. San Francisco, CA: UCSF Nursing Press.

Lovering, S. (2006). Cultural attitudes and beliefs about pain. Journal of Transcultural Nursing, 17(4), 389–395.

Purnell, L. & Paulanka, L. (2008). Transcultural Health Care: A Culturally Competent Approach (3rd ed.) Philadelphia, PA: F.A. Davis.

Box 6–7 Ten Tips for Improving the Cross-Cultural Patient Interaction

1. Let the culture of the patient determine how you treat the patient.
   "Do unto others," which is often referred to as the Golden Rule, does NOT apply to all cultures. Because we are all not the same, our responses will be unique and individualized. Culture determines the rules for what is considered appropriate behavior as well as what constitutes appropriate nursing care.

2. Formality is best.
   The use of first names as a means of communicating respect and equality is unique to the United States. In most countries, a respectful distance is maintained between patient and nurse. Unless the patient is a child or young adult, it is best to use the patient's last name when addressing the patient, unless told otherwise.

3. Be aware of how the patient may be showing you respect as it may be negatively impacting him or her.
   Our cultural group determines how we show respect. Patients want to show you, as the nurse, respect for your knowledge and position. In many countries, it is disrespectful to look directly at another person (especially one in authority) or to contribute to the authority figure losing face by asking questions. Encourage the patient to ask any questions that he or she may have.

4. Determine the patient's views on how they maintain health, causes of illness, and methods to prevent or cure illness. Do not assume.
   Perform a cultural assessment by asking questions that will help you determine the patient's beliefs about health and illness.

5. Do not discount your patient's beliefs.
   Allow the patient to be open and honest with you with regard to his or her traditional health beliefs or the use of alternative or complementary medicine practices.

6. Consider that the patient may have supernatural beliefs.
   The Hispanic patient may believe that their illness is caused by bewitchment (English translation for *embrujado*) or the casting of a spell or the evil eye as a punishment for something they may have done. Ask the patient about his or her beliefs.

7. Use indirect questioning when asking about supernatural beliefs.
   An indirect approach is more likely to be successful, as will letting the patient know you are aware of health beliefs common to the Hispanic/Latino culture.

8. Determine the value of including the entire family in the treatment plan.
   In many cultures, medical decisions are made by the entire family. Inclusion of the family increases the likelihood of gaining patient compliance.

9. Use restraint when discussing bad news or potential complications—do not exceed the amount of information that the patient can handle.
   The "need to know it all" is an American custom. In some cultures, placing yourself in your provider's hands is the ultimate sign of trust. The nurse should watch for signs that the patient has learned as much as he or she is able to deal with.

10. If not contraindicated, incorporate the patient's traditional health beliefs into the plan of care.

The inclusion of the patient's health beliefs (that are positive or neutral) will increase the likelihood of compliance and will foster the establishment of trust between the patient and nurse.

Source: Salimbene, S. (2000). Providing culture-sensitive care to African Americans. In *What language does your patient hurt in? A practical guide to culturally competent patient care.* Amherst, MA: Diversity Resources.

in some college dormitories. *Santeros* wear special beaded bracelets so they can be identified by other believers. They wear white robes during the conduction of ceremonies.

Mental health is also viewed somewhat differently by Puerto Ricans (Rojas-Vilches, Negy, & Reig-Ferrar, 2011). They have a higher tolerance for what others may consider odd or unique behaviors. They make a very sharp distinction between what would be odd behavior versus being *loco*. To be *loco* is considered to be dangerous or evil and will result in the loss of all social status. As such, Puerto Ricans who seek mental health treatment are ostracized and criticized by their community. It is acceptable to seek help from a *santero*; the symptoms are accepted because they are not attributed to the patient but to spirits outside the body that are causing the mental illness. The *santero* also will maintain confidentiality so the patient has no worry about being labeled or judged—or more importantly, worry that his confidence will be violated. Culturally competent mental health providers need to recognize the prevalence of *santero* when dealing with the mentally ill Puerto Rican, as the reliance on *santero* in that situation can be frequent. The inclusion of a belief in God and the benefit of prayer will also be an important cultural component of the treatment plan.

Impact of Communication

Spanish and English are the two official languages of Puerto Rico, despite the fact that many Puerto Ricans do not speak English well or at all. An attempt was made, because of political pressure, to pass a bill to make Spanish the only official language of the island. Equal status was restored to both languages shortly thereafter, and today, Spanish tends to be the language spoken at home and in schools, whereas English is used for all federal matters, is spoken in major Puerto Rican tourist sites, and is taught as a second language in most schools. Puerto Ricans from large cities are more likely to read, understand, and speak at least some English.

Puerto Rican Spanish is unique and differs from the Spanish from other cultures, which may present a problem when the use of an interpreter is required. When an interpreter lacks the cultural and linguistic background in Puerto Rican Spanish, the meaning of the words may change from one culture to the next and the translation may be inaccurate. Nonverbal communication and symbolism are conveyed with hand gestures and facial expressions and are a critical component of the message being sent. A close distance is maintained by Puerto Ricans when talking, and they may feel slighted if the nurse were to move away, even slightly, during a clinical encounter. The use of titles to show respect is also valued, as is saving face. A Puerto Rican patient who speaks limited English may be hesitant to ask the nurse for even basic clarification or to slow down the speed of her speech. They have a tendency to be sensitive, especially if they interpret an action as being a rejection of them. In addition, tone of voice is unique in that it is typically melodic and peaceful. A tone of voice that is considered high in pitch and inflection may be perceived as confrontational and the nurse should consider this when communicating with Puerto Rican patients.

Impact of Social Organization

For Puerto Ricans, the family, and especially children, is highly valued, and the patient may rely on the advice and guidance of older adults and elders. In some families, it is the eldest son or daughter who has the final decision-making authority for health-related matters; if the patient is married, the wife will typically consult her husband. This may vary depending on the age of the family members and the patient, so the nurse should establish who has decision-making authority on an individual basis.

Impact of Faith and Spirituality

The vast majority of Puerto Ricans are Catholic (estimated at 85%), and the remainder are made up of Protestants and agnostics/atheists (Pew Hispanic Center, 2012). Despite the separation of church and state in Puerto Rico, religion plays a highly public role. Many Christians may also practice *espiritismo* (spiritualism) which is a blend of Indian, African, and Catholic beliefs. This is the belief that both good and bad spirits are present and can be influenced through the use of herbs and rituals.

Others practice some version of *Santería* which is fairly common in Caribbean nations; it has had an impact on the Catholic practices of some Puerto Ricans (Green, 2012).

There are important cultural beliefs related to death and dying for this cultural group that the nurse must be aware of. In some Hispanic families, there is a code of silence, which means the patients are not informed that they are terminally ill. The family may rely on one designated member to make treatment and end-of-life decisions (Giger, 2013). In this situation, the family will wish to provide a constant vigil and the family's spiritual leader should be with the patient at the time of death (National Alliance for Hispanic Health, 2001). The nurse should then notify the appointed family spokesperson for the news to then be communicated to the rest of the family members. The family may wish private time to say final goodbyes and this may include touching and kissing of the loved one's body. Organ donation is often supported in this culture as a way to help others, but the nurse must handle this matter very delicately. On the other hand, autopsies are not supported, as it is viewed as invasive and a violation to the body. If an autopsy is required, the reason must be clearly communicated to the family spokesperson and consent obtained.

Biologic Variations

It appears that health and quality of life for Puerto Ricans are affected by a multifaceted combination of biology, demographics, and socioeconomic status (Green, 2012). Lower income is associated with decreased quality of life and increased illness, whereas the opposite is true with a higher income (Green, 2012). When counseling patients about a healthy body, it is important to recognize the value that is placed on excessive body weight in the Puerto Rican culture (Lopez, 2007). Being thin or underweight is viewed negatively as it is associated with poor health and illness, whereas being overweight is associated with good health and an economic advantage. This belief must be considered and incorporated into the nurse's patient teaching plan. This is especially important when providing nutritional counseling for the diabetic Puerto Rican patient. As with other Hispanic/Latino groups, type 2 diabetes is a major health problem.

CUBAN AMERICANS

Cuban Americans make up about 4% of the Hispanic/Latino population in the United States (U.S. Census Bureau, 2011). The island of Cuba is only 90 miles from Key West, Florida. It was colonized by Spain in 1511 and all of its native people were killed. Cuba and its capital port of Havana became a major shipping and transportation hub. It was a key port in the trade of rum, sugar, cod, and slaves. Because all of its native people were killed, Cuba's population was made up of European settlers and African slave laborers. In 1902, the United States granted Cuba its independence but maintained a major influence over the island, which became a popular resort destination for the next 50 years until the Cuban Revolution of 1959 (Sierra, 2011).

The Cuban Revolution of 1959 that overthrew the regime of Fulgencio Batista and brought Fidel Castro to power drove close to half a million upper- and middle-class refugees to south Florida (Siera, 2011). Between 1965 and 1978, many Cuban immigrants came directly from Cuba, whereas others came through Spain, Mexico, and Jamaica, to the United States. In the late 1970s and early 1980s, Cubans came to America when Castro allowed political prisoners to join their families. The last large group arrived in the early 1980s and was referred to as the *Marielitos*, because they left from the Mariel port in Havana, Cuba. This group of immigrants was of a lower socioeconomic status, some had criminal records, some were less educated, and they all were more likely to live in poverty (Buffington, 2012a).

CENTRAL AMERICANS

Since its early settlement, Central America has had a history of turmoil. People from Central and South American countries including Colombia, Nicaragua, Guatemala, and Venezuela, have come to the United States over the last 25 years because of political instability, civil wars, and natural disasters such as landslides, earthquakes, and tropical storms (Rosenblum & Brick, 2011). The economies of Central American countries tend to be unstable because of their dependence on a few agricultural export crops, such as coffee, sugar, bananas, and cotton, that are owned by a very small segment of society. Because of the political and economic struggles that the nations of this region have endured, many Central Americans have immigrated to the United States, often in search of refuge from violence and economic instability created by civil wars and other conflicts.

Central Americans have settled in different parts of the country (Brick, Challinor, & Rosenblum, 2011). Salvadorans have settled mainly in Los Angeles and Washington, DC; Guatemalans in Los Angeles, San Francisco, and Houston; and Nicaraguans in San Francisco and Miami. Many suffer from posttraumatic stress problems relating to their countries' civil wars. Communication can be complicated by the large number of languages and dialects spoken in both Central and South America (estimated to be over 15). Diseases that are endemic to Central and South America include leprosy, cholera, yellow fever, and malaria.

DOMINICAN AMERICANS

Discovered by Columbus in 1492, the island of Hispaniola later divided following a slave rebellion leading to the establishment of the independent nation of Haiti. The remaining eastern two-thirds of the island eventually became the Dominican Republic, a predominantly agricultural, Spanish-speaking nation (Buffington, 2012b).

Since the U.S. invasion of the Dominican Republic during a period of civil unrest in 1965, over half a million Dominicans and their descendants have settled in the United States, 70% of whom are located in New York City and adjacent parts of New Jersey (Buffington, 2012b).

SOUTH AMERICANS

The number of South Americans born in the United States make up about 6% of the foreign-born population (Dixon & Gellat, 2006). Although the overall number is low, the number of immigrants born in South America has been growing continuously over the past 30 years (Dixon & Gellat, 2006). The top five states with residents from South America are New York, Florida, New Jersey, California, and Massachusetts (Dixon & Gellat, 2006). Although there are various reasons for South American immigration to the United States, two key causes include political instability and the search for economic opportunity or prosperity.

CONSEQUENCES OF IMMIGRATION TO THE UNITED STATES FOR HISPANICS

When dealing with the Hispanic/Latino group, it is important for the nurse to recognize the tremendous range of historical experiences that exist within this group. Each nationality has its own perspective on how they view themselves within the context of living in the United States and how they have been treated as an immigrant in this country. How they entered the country (whether legally or illegally, as a refugee, or for economic reasons) will impact them as well.

SUMMARY

Hispanics/Latinos are a heterogeneous group with many similarities but also many differences. Each patient must be assessed within the context of their unique circumstances, the role of their family, and membership in subgroups or subcultures. The degree of acculturation exhibited, along with the level of education, socioeconomic status, and country of origin, must all be considered when planning for care delivery to the Hispanic/Latino patient population.

CASE STUDY 6–1

www

Hispanic/Latino Patient in Pain

Tomas is a 42-year-old Hispanic male construction worker who presents to the emergency room with sudden onset low back pain for the past 2 days. Tomas is slightly obese and developed sharp, right-sided low back pain that has worsened over the last 2 days. The pain began immediately after Tomas tried to lift a 50-pound bag of concrete. He has no paresthesia or bowel or bladder dysfunction. His past medical history is negative, he has no known drug allergies, and he is not taking any medication other than the occasional over-the-counter acetaminophen for the back pain. Family history is positive for type 2 DM in his mother and hypertension in his father. He is a nonsmoker and does not drink alcohol. Tomas denies any substance abuse. Physical examination is within normal limits except that the flexion of the right great toe is weaker than on the left side. Radiograph reveals slight narrowing of the L5–S1 disc space. He is diagnosed with lumbar disk herniation impinging on the L5 nerve root. Because this is a relatively recent onset, and the patient does not demonstrate any muscle weakness or loss of bowel or bladder control, a conservative treatment course is warranted. In the acute phase, the patient will benefit from a combination of physical and pharmacologic treatment. Bed rest for 24 hours only (because there is a disk herniation); a course of physical therapy modalities such as moist heat, ice, and massage; attendance at "back school" once he is stable is also appropriate. For pain management, a nonsteroidal anti-inflammatory drug (NSAID) was prescribed. The patient was also counseled on the benefits of weight loss for back health.

The nurse questions the order for the NSAID for pain management. The nurse is concerned because earlier in the same day, the same physician prescribed an opiate pain medication for a patient with the same diagnosis, the only difference being that the previous patient was a 48-year-old White male. She is aware of the study (Pletcher, Kertesz, Kohn, & Gonzales, 2008) that examined treatments for more than 150,000 pain-related visits to U.S. hospitals between 1993 and 2005. This study found that 31% of Whites received opioid drugs compared with only 23% of Blacks and 24% of Hispanics. About 28% of Asians received opioids. In contrast, nonopioid pain relievers (such as was the case with Tomas) such as ibuprofen were prescribed much more often to non-Whites (36%) than to Whites (26%). According to Dr. Mark Pletcher, the study's lead author, "studies in the 1990s showed a disturbing racial or ethnic disparity in the use of these potent pain relievers, but we had hoped that the recent national efforts at improving pain management in emergency departments would shrink this disparity; unfortunately, this is not the case." Based on the results of this study, the nurse feels empowered to advocate on behalf of Tomas and discusses Tomas' need for pain management with the emergency department attending physician.

REVIEW QUESTIONS

1. Should the nurse question the NSAID order?
2. What if any evidence/research studies would inform the nurse on how to provide effective pain management to the Hispanic/Latino patient?

CASE STUDY 6–2

The Use of a Family Member as an Interpreter for a Female Hispanic/Latino Patient

The importance of the use of a qualified interpreter and the need to avoid the use of family members as interpreters is quite clear from this case study.

Gabrielle is a 36-year-old Hispanic woman who was asked to sign an informed consent for a hysterectomy. Gabrielle only speaks Spanish but she was accompanied by her bilingual son, Jose, who is an adult aged 18 years old. The hospital was not able to find a qualified interpreter, so the son was asked to serve in that role. When the son explained the procedure to his mother, he appeared to be translating accurately and indicating the proper body parts. His mother signed the consent form willingly. The next day, after the surgery was completed, when she learned that her uterus had been removed and she could no longer bear children, she became very angry and threatened to sue the hospital.

What went wrong? Because it is inappropriate for a Hispanic male to discuss his mother's private parts with her, the embarrassed son had explained that a tumor would be removed from her abdomen and pointed to the general area. He did not tell her that her uterus would be removed as he was uncomfortable to discussing or describing the sexual organ with his mother. Gabrielle became quite angry and upset because a Hispanic woman's status is derived, in large part, from the number of children she produces. She was very upset because she was not yet finished with childbearing.

REVIEW QUESTIONS

1. What may have gone wrong with the communication process in this case study?
2. Are there any concerns with the use of a family member to serve as an interpreter?
3. Can the gender of the patient and the interpreter have any impact on the outcome of the communication/interpretation process?

When selecting an interpreter, it is always best to avoid the use of family members. Even if a potential interpreter can speak the same language, it is not always sufficient. Cultural rules often dictate who can discuss what and with whom. In general, it is best to use a same-sex interpreter when translating matters of a sexual or private nature with this cultural group.

Box 6–8 Five Tips for Improving the Effectiveness of the Use of Interpreters

---

1. Brief the interpreter in advance. Summarize the key information that needs to be communicated. Do not be afraid to repeat yourself or to restate important information.
2. Keep it short. Avoid long or complicated sentences.
3. Do not interrupt and do not be impatient. Take as much time as is needed.
4. Position yourself so that you, the patient, and the interpreter are visible to each other. Look for signs of comprehension or confusion.
5. Do not underestimate the impact of culture.
6. Culture may cause even a professional interpreter to modify what the nurse or the patient may say. The nurse should clarify with the interpreter whether it is appropriate or comfortable to discuss sexual or other delicate subjects and ask for input from the interpreter on the best approach to increase patient comfort during interpretation.

Source: Salimbene, S. (2000). Providing culture-sensitive care to African Americans. In *What language does your patient hurt in? A practical guide to culturally competent patient care*. Amherst, MA: Diversity Resources.

REFERENCES

Andrews, C. (2006). Modesty and healthcare for women: Understanding cultural sensitivities. *Community Oncology, 3*(7), 443–445.

Brick, K., Challinor, A. E. & Rosenblum, M. R. (2011). *Mexican and Central American immigrants in the U.S.* Retrieved from http://www.migrationpolicy.org/pubs/MexCentAmimmigrants.pdf

Buffington, S. (2012a). *Cuban Americans.* Retrieved from http://www.everyculture.com/multi/Bu-Dr/Cuban-Americans.html

Buffington, S. (2012b). *Dominican Americans.* Retrieved from http://www.everyculture.com/multi/Bu-Dr/Dominican-Americans.html

Buffington, S. (2012c). *Puerto Rican Americans.* Retrieved from http://www.everyculture.com/multi/Pa-Sp/Puerto-Rican-Americans.html

Caballero, A. E. (2005). Diabetes in the Hispanic or Latino population: Genes, environment, culture, and more. *Current Diabetes Reports, 5*(3), 217–225.

Caballero, A. E. (2006). Building cultural bridges: Understanding ethnicity to improve acceptance of insulin therapy in patients with type 2 diabetes. *Ethnicity & Disease, 16*(2), 559–568.

CultureDiversity.org. (2012). *The Hispanic American community.* Retrieved from http://www.culturediversity.org/hisp.htm

Dictionary of American History. (2003). *Manifest Destiny.* Retrieved from http://www.encyclopedia.com/topic/manifest_destiny.aspx

Dixon, D., & Gellat, J. (2006). *Detailed characteristics of the South American born in the United States.* Retrieved from http://www.migrationinformation.org/usfocus/display.cfm?ID=400

Eggenberger, S. K., Grassley, J., & Restrepo, E. (2006). Culturally competent nursing care for families: Listening to the voices of Mexican American women. *The Online Journal of Issues in Nursing, 11*(33). Retrieved from http://www.nursingworld.org/MainMenuCategories/ANAMarketplace/ANAPeriodicals/OJIN/TableofContents/Volume112006/No3Sept06/ArticlePreviousTopics/CulturallyCompetentNursingCare.html

Enchanted Learning. (2010). *Christopher Columbus: Explorer.* Retrieved from http://www.enchantedlearning.com/explorers/page/c/columbus.shtml

Englekirk, A., & Marin, M. (2012). *Mexican Americans.* Retrieved from http://www.everyculture.com/multi/Le-Pa/Mexican-Americans.html

Ferguson, W. J., & Candib, L. M. (2002). Culture, language and the doctor–patient relationship. *Family Medicine, 34*(5), 353–361.

Giger, J. N. (2013). *Transcultural nursing: Assessment and intervention* (6th ed.). Philadelphia, PA: Elsevier.

Green, D. (2012). *Puerto Rican Americans.* Retrieved from http://www.everyculture.com/multi/Pa-Sp/Puerto-Rican-Americans.html

Harwood, A. (1971). The hot-cold theory of disease. Implications for treatment of Puerto Rican patients. *JAMA, 216*(7), 1153–1158.

History.com. (2012). *Mexican-American War.* Retrieved from http://www.history.com/topics/mexican-american-war

History Scholars. (2009). *The rise and fall of the Ottoman Empire.* Retrieved from http://historyscholars.weebly.com/uploads/1/4/7/8/1478974/theottomanempire_pp_notes.pdf

Im, E. O., Guevara, E., & Chee, W. (2007). The pain experience of Hispanic patients with cancer in the U.S. *Oncology Nursing Forum, 34*(4), 861–868.

Kalish, R. A., & Reynolds, D. K. (1981). *Death and ethnicity: A psychocultural study* (2nd ed.). New York, NY: Baywood.

Karliner, L. S., Jacobs, E. A., Chen, A. H., & Mutha, S. (2007). Do professional interpreters improve clinical care for patients with limited English proficiency? A systematic review of the literature. *Health Services Research, 42*(2), 727–754.

Lopez, G. (2007). "Why are we so fat?" Mexican immigrant perceptions of obesity in California's central valley. Proceedings of the Southwestern Anthropological Association, *1*, 47–59. Retrieved from http://www.academia.edu/353488/_Why_are_we_so_Fat_Mexican_Immigrant_Perceptions_of_Obesity_in_Californias_Central_Valley

Migrant Health Promotion. (2012). *Farmworkers in the United States*. Retrieved from http://www.migranthealth.org/index.php?option=com_content&view=article&id=38&Itemid=30

Nation Master. (2012). Mexico: Government. Retrieved from http://www.nationmaster.com/country/mx-mexico/gov-government

National Alliance for Hispanic Health. (2001). *Quality health services for Hispanics: The cultural competency component*. Washington, DC: U.S. Department of Health and Human Services.

National Center for Health Statistics. (2002). *Health, United States, 2002: With chartbook on trends in the health of Americans*. Retrieved from http://www.cdc.gov/nchs/data/hus/hus02.pdf

National Center for Health Statistics. (2011). Table 26: Leading causes of death by race/ethnicity. *Health, United States, 2010: With special feature on death and dying*. Hyattsville, MD: Author.

National Health and Nutrition Examination Survey (NHANES). (2008). Overweight and obesity statistics. Retrieved from http://win.niddk.nih.gov/statistics/index.htm

National Women's Law Center. (2012). *Analysis of new 2010 census poverty data—September 2011*. Retrieved from http://www.nwlc.org/analysis-new-2010-census-poverty-data-%E2%80%93-september-2011

New Mexico History. (2012). Retrieved from http://www.newmexicohistory.org/filedetails.php?fileID=312

Ortiz, B. I., Shields, K. M., Clauson, K. A., & Clay, P. G. (2007). Complementary and alternative medicine use among Hispanics in the United States. *The Annals of Pharmacotherapy, 41*(6), 994–1004.

Padilla, Y. C., & Villalobus, G. (2007). Cultural responses to health among Mexican American women and their families. *Family & Community Health, 30*(1), s24–s33.

Pérez-Stable, E. J., Nápoles-Springer, A., & Miramontes, J. M. (1997). The effects of ethnicity and language on medical outcomes of patients with hypertension or diabetes. *Medical Care, 35*(12), 1212–1219.

Pew Hispanic Center. (2005). *Survey of Mexican migrants*. Retrieved from http://www.pewhispanic.org/files/reports/58.pdf

Pew Hispanic Center. (2009). *A portrait of unauthorized immigrants in the United States*. Retrieved from http://pewhispanic.org/files/reports/107.pdf

Pew Hispanic Center. (2012). *The 10 largest Hispanic origin groups: Characteristics, rankings, top counties*. Retrieved from http://www.pewhispanic.org/2012/06/27/the-10-largest-hispanic-origin-groups-characteristics-rankings-top-counties/

Pew Research Center. (2007). *Changing faiths: Latinos and the transformation of American religion*. Retrieved from http://www.pewhispanic.org/2007/04/25/changing-faiths-latinos-and-the-transformation-of-american-religion/

Pletcher, M. J., Kertesz, S. G., Kohn, M. A., & Gonzales, R. (2008). Trends in opioid prescribing by race/ethnicity for patients seeking care in US emergency departments. *Journal of the American Medical Association, 299*(1), 70–78.

Rojas-Vilches, A., Negy, C., & Reig-Ferrar, A. (2011). Attitudes toward seeking therapy among Puerto Rican and Cuban American young adults and their parents. *International journal of clinical and health psychology, 1*(2), 313–341.

Rosenblum, M. R., & Brick, K. (2011). *U.S. immigration policy and Mexican/Central American migration flows: Then and now.* Retrieved from http://www.migrationpolicy.org/pubs/RMSG-regionalflows.pdf

Salimbene, S. (2000). *What language does your patient hurt in? A practical guide to culturally competent patient care.* Amherst, MA: Diversity Resources.

Sierra, J. A. (2011). *The struggle for Cuban identity and independence: An introduction.* Retrieved from http://www.historyofcuba.com/history/havana/struggle.htm.

Singh, T. P., Almond, C. S., Taylor, D. O., Milliren, C. E., & Graham, D. A. (2012). Racial and ethnic differences in wait-list outcomes in patients listed for heart transplantation in the United States. *Circulation, 125*(24), 3022–3030. Retrieved from http://circ.ahajournals.org/content/early/2012/05/14/CIRCULATIONAHA.112.092643

Sullivan, M. M., & Rehm, R. (2005). Mental health of undocumented Mexican immigrants. *Advances in Nursing Science, 28*(5), 240–255.

Tienda, M., & Mitchell, F. (2006). *Hispanics and the future of America.* National Research Council (US) Panel on Hispanics in the United States. Washington, DC: National Academic Press.

Todd, K. H., Deaton, C., D'Adamo, A. P., & Goe, L. (2000). Ethnicity and analgesic practice. *Annals of Emergency Medicine, 35*(1), 11–16.

Todd, K. H., Samaroo, N., & Hoffman, J. R. (1993). Ethnicity as a risk factor for inadequate emergency department analgesia. *Journal of the American Medical Association, 269*(12), 1537–1539.

U.S. Census Bureau. (2008). *Table 4: Annual estimates of the Black or African American alone or in combination population by sex and age for the United States: April 1, 2000, to July 1, 2007.*

U.S. Census Bureau. (2010a). *Overview of census data.* Retrieved from http://2010.census.gov/2010census/data/

U.S. Census Bureau. (2010b). *Overview of race and Hispanic origin: 2010. 2010 census briefs.* Retrieved from http://www.census.gov/prod/cen2010/briefs/c2010br-02.pdf

U.S. Census Bureau. (2011). 2010 *Census shows nation's Hispanic population grew four times faster than total U.S. population.* Retrieved from http://2010.census.gov/news/releases/operations/cb11-cn146.html

U.S. Census Bureau. (2012). *Minorities constitute 37 percent of U.S. population.* Retrieved from http://www.nationaljournal.com/thenextamerica/demographics/census-minorities-constitute-37-percent-of-u-s-population-20120517

Vega, W. A., Rodriquez, M. A., & Gruskin, E. (2009). Health disparities in the Latino population. *Epidemiology Review, 31*(1), 99–112.

www For a full suite of assignments and additional learning activities, see the access code at the front of your book.

CHAPTER 7

Asians/Pacific Islanders

CHAPTER OBJECTIVES

Upon completion of this chapter, the nurse will be able to:

- Describe the illness behaviors of Asian Americans (Chinese, Japanese, Korean, Vietnamese, Cambodian, Laotian, and Filipino) and Pacific Islanders.
- Provide a plan of care that considers the cultural needs of Asians/Pacific Islanders.
- Identify the associated biologic variations of Asians/Pacific Islanders.

© Digital Vision/Photodisc/Thinkstock

INTRODUCTION

Remember to use the information contained in this chapter as a guide only, as all people within a culture are not the same. Developing awareness and an understanding of Asian American/Pacific Islander (AAPI) cultures provides a starting point to help the nurse establish a therapeutic relationship and deliver more effective, individualized nursing care.

BACKGROUND

The 2010 census revealed that members of the AAPI groups made up 3.6% of the population of the United States (U.S. Census Bureau, 2010b), with Asians numbering 18.2 million. The 2010 U.S. census data reveals that the AAPI population is the second fastest growing of all of America's ethnic groups. Hawaii is currently the only majority-Asian state (57.1% of Hawaiians are Asian). Currently the AAPI population makes up about 4% of the total U.S. population, and AAPIs are projected to reach 41 million U.S. residents (11% of the total U.S. population) by the year 2050 (Ghosh, 2003).

AAPIs have roots in at least 29 Asian countries and 20 Pacific Islander cultures. Members of this group speak over 100 languages and belong to numerous religions; most (95%) are of Asian origin, whereas the rest (5%) are Pacific Islanders. According to the Office of Management and Budget (1997), Asians are persons having origins in any of the original people of the Far East, Southeast Asia, or the Indian subcontinent, including China, India, and the Islands of the Philippines. Native Hawaiians and other Pacific Islanders include people who have origins in any of the original peoples of Hawaii, Guam, Samoa, or other Pacific Islands.

The ranks of Asians are rapidly growing, and they represent the third largest minority group. According to the 2012 census data, Chinese Americans are the largest Asian American group (almost 3.8 million), followed by Filipinos (3.4 million), and then Asian Indians (3.2 million). As of 2010, immigrants composed 13% (40 million). of the total U.S. population. China (including Hong Kong but excluding Taiwan) accounted for 5% of all foreign born, while India and the Philippines each contributed approximately 4% of the immigrant population. Vietnam and Korea each contributed another approximate 3% of the immigrant population.

There are more than 30 different languages spoken by AAPIs and many unique cultures exist. It is helpful to note that many of the health and illness beliefs and practices of AAPIs are derived from Chinese traditions. Having a strong

Figure 7–1 Population percentage breakdown for Asians/Pacific Islanders, 2003.

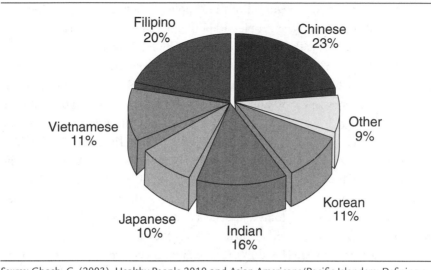

Source: Ghosh, C. (2003). Healthy People 2010 and Asian Americans/Pacific Islanders: Defining a baseline of information. *American Journal of Public Health, 93*(12), 2093–2098.

understanding of Chinese health and illness beliefs will provide a foundation or starting point when striving to provide health care for AAPIs. The nurse should consider utilizing a Chinese frame of reference when planning for or providing care to Pacific Islanders because less is known about this group. This is because this group is so small that health data is not reported separately. It is for these reasons that AAPIs will be discussed as one grouping in this chapter.

Statistics

The largest group of Asians is Chinese with a total of 3.8 million, closely followed by Filipinos, at 3.4 million. Close to half of the Asian-born population in the United States lives in one of three metropolitan areas: Los Angeles, New York, or San Francisco (U.S. Census Bureau, 2012).

CHINESE AMERICANS

The People's Republic of China has the world's oldest continuous civilization, extending more than 5,000 years (Szczepanski, 2012). The People's Republic of China is often referred to as mainland China or Communist China. Taiwan became a Chinese province in the mid-1680s and was annexed to the Japanese in 1895. After World War II, Taiwan again came under the control of China in the form of a noncommunist government, which is still in effect today. Hong Kong was returned to the control of the People's Republic of China after 150 years of British control. The People's Republic of China is the most populated nation in the world, with over 1.3 billion inhabitants, yet slightly under 50% of its people live in urban areas (CIA World Factbook, 2012). Chinese immigration to the United States began in the 1800s. A rapid increase in immigration occurred between 1850 and 1880 (from 1,000 to over 100,000) due to the California gold rush, which resulted in a need for cheap labor to build the transcontinental railroads (Library of Congress, 2012). The boom in the West was in stark contrast to a significant period of poverty that was occurring at the same time in China. The Chinese who came to the United States intended to stay for a short time as temporary workers. Most of the immigrants were men and they clung to their customs and beliefs and stayed close to their communities. Life was difficult and, other than work on the railroads, jobs were hard to find—in fact, many were closed to them because they were not White (Library of Congress, 2012). There was a significant nativist movement in the United States at this time in response to Chinese immigration. Chinese immigrants were faced with hatred and outright violence. The violence, in fact, was horrific, and included burnings, hangings, and lynchings. Many decades of racism and hostility culminated with the passage of the Chinese Exclusion Act, enacted in 1882. Initially, this was to be a 10-year policy, but it was extended indefinitely and became permanent in 1902 (U.S. News and World Report, 2012). The act prohibited the further entry of additional Chinese people into the United States, and was not repealed until 1943, when China had become an important ally to the United States against the Japanese in World War II. The racism and hostility caused a large number of immigrant workers and their families to return to China before 1930. Overall there was a 20% decline in the population of Chinese living in America between 1880 and 1930. The Chinese that remained in the United States left the West and moved eastward to cities where there were more employment opportunities, such as running laundries and restaurants (Herbert Hoover Presidential Library, 2012). The Chinese settled in tight-knit groups in urban neighborhoods called Chinatowns. In Chinatowns, they were able to maintain their ancient traditions. Due to their commitment to a strong work ethic and because of hard work, many were able to survive on menial jobs (Herbert Hoover Presidential Library, 2012).

U.S. immigration laws and political problems in China have greatly impacted the Chinese population in the United States. Many men were left alone without the possibility of their family ever joining them. By 1965, a large number of refugees who had relatives in the United States were able to come here to join them, causing the Chinese population to grow (Herbert Hoover Library, 2012). The new immigrants joined their relatives in the urban Chinatowns. Since 1965, the population rate of increase for Chinese Americans has been 10% per year. The newer immigrants were better-educated professionals and specialists. This change in the type of immigrants coming from China has resulted in a great deal of cultural and linguistic diversity among Chinese Americans. The majority of Chinese Americans today are immigrants from Taiwan, Hong Kong, and mainland China. A total of 66% of Chinese Americans live in five states: California, New York, Hawaii, Illinois, and Texas (Harris & Jones, 2005).

Chinese Americans maintain high educational standards but have a poverty rate of 14% (compare this with 13% for the general U.S. population). The majority (65.9%) participate in the workforce (Harris & Jones, 2005). In the United States, the educational levels of Chinese are divided between the highly educated and the poorly educated. It is important to recognize that not all Chinese Americans are poorly educated or have service-oriented occupations (e.g., garment industry, restaurant work). The failure of Chinese Americans to return to China once they have been educated in the United States has been viewed as a detriment to China and has resulted in much tighter control over immigration by the Chinese government.

As noted previously, the majority of Chinese Americans are immigrants from Taiwan, Hong Kong, and mainland China. Chinese Americans are the majority group of Asian Americans. The population saw a 47.5% growth rate from 1980 to 1990, and now Chinese Americans residing in the United States represent 0.7% of the total U.S. population (Harris & Jones, 2005).

Chinese culture is dominated by Confucianism (Herbert Hoover Presidential Library, 2012). This encourages people to strive for piety, righteousness, decorum, and wealth. A harmonious relationship with nature and other people is stressed. The emphasis is on accommodation and not confrontation; if conflict is present, the individual should submit to the interest of the group. Public debate is not socially acceptable and a person is expected to be very sensitive and gracious to others, so as not to make them "lose face."

As we shall see, Chinese Americans are a very diverse group in terms of economics, healthcare behaviors, and modernization. As always, a disclaimer is important: while possessing knowledge of the dominant Chinese values (and of all of the AAPI values and culture) is extremely helpful, it should only be used as a guide.

Chinese Definitions of Health and Illness

Health is a state of spiritual and physical harmony with nature. Most beliefs come from old philosophies, most especially Taoism (Herbert Hoover Presidential Library, 2012). To live according to the Tao, one must adapt to the order of nature. In Chinese culture, physical problems are hard to distinguish from psychological or spiritual concerns. Illness may be attributed to typical scientific causes, but it may also be seen as being caused by spirits, emotions, or taboo behaviors. Disability carries a stigma in Chinese culture, although this has been slowly changing over time, especially since 1980 (Weiss, 2010). At a minimum, the onset of disability may be seen as bad luck, or it may be seen as a result of inappropriate behavior by the birth mother if disability occurs in the newborn (Weiss, 2010).

The Chinese believe that each being has a function within the universe. No one thing can exist without the others; the goal is to achieve harmonious balance. Violation of harmony results in illness. The underlying belief is that people must adjust themselves within the environment, and that five elements can both create and destroy each other. The five elements are wood, fire, metal, water, and earth.

The holistic concept is an important idea for preventing and treating disease. A holistic view is one that considers pathologic changes in conjunction with other organs of the body, and integrates the human body with the environment.

The Chinese have made tremendous contributions to medicine. The first known description of how blood circulates, including the oxygen-carrying powers of blood, was contained in Huang-ti Nei Ching's *Yellow Emperor's Book of Internal Medicine*, which was published in the 1200s. This book also defined the basic principles of yin and yang, powers that regulate the universe and human beings. Yin represents the female, a negative energy such as the force of darkness, cold, or emptiness. Yang represents the male, a positive energy source that produces light, warmth, and fullness.

According to the yin and yang theory, everything in the universe contains these two aspects, which are both in opposition and in union. When yin and yang are in disharmony, illness will result. The pulse is controlled by both yin and yang. If yin and yang are not balanced, the person's life will be short. Half of the yin force is depleted by age 40, and for this reason it is believed that a person becomes sluggish at age 40. At age 60, the yin is totally depleted and the body then begins to deteriorate. See **Table 7–1** for more on yin and yang.

It is felt that alertness at the time near death is important for spiritual reasons. It is for this reason that the patient or family may refuse medications that may impair consciousness. As a general rule, the Chinese do not report discomfort. Death is a topic that is not readily discussed. Family members may not tell the patient that he or she is dying, and they also may not discuss it among themselves.

Table 7–1 Components of Yin and Yang

Yin	Yang
Inside of the body	Outside of the body
Front part of the body	Back of the body
Gall bladder, stomach, large intestine, small intestine, bladder, lymphatic system	Liver, heart, spleen, lungs, kidneys
Diseases of winter and spring	Diseases of summer and fall
Stores the vital strength of life	Protects the body from outside forces

Source: Ody, P. (2000). *Practical Chinese medicine: Understanding the principles and practice of traditonal Chinese medicine and making them work for you.* Berkshire, UK: Sterling.

This is less common in younger generations of Chinese Americans; they may be more open to talking about the illness and the patient's prognosis. A great deal of importance is placed by the family on being present with the loved one at the time of death. There is also ritual associated with the care of the body and how the body is dressed. The women in the family prepare special funeral clothing. Funerals are carried out in an extremely traditional manner.

Food, illness, and medications are classified as "hot" or "cold," according to the perceived effects on the body. Health is believed to be a balance of positive (yang) and negative (yin) energy in the body. Many Chinese people will assume a "sick role" when they are ill, depending heavily on others. A demanding healthcare provider may be viewed as uncaring by the Chinese patient. To appear caring, the nurse should speak sympathetically, take an interest in the patient, and verbally encourage them.

The use of hospitals and healthcare professionals is avoided in the Chinese culture. When health care is sought, a doctor of the same sex is preferred, especially by female patients. Most Chinese people will expect to be given a prescription when they go to the doctor; going to the doctor when they are not sick, such as for health prevention or health promotion, might be considered strange. Keep in mind the Chinese cultural norms of lack of eye contact, shyness, and passivity. Assertiveness may be mistaken or interpreted by the Chinese patient as aggressive or even hostile behavior. Because of the cultural norm of shyness, it is important for the nurse to realize that the Chinese will be reluctant to talk to them—an outsider—about their health and psychosocial problems. Finally, many Chinese believe that saying no is impolite, so the nurse must be cautious not to mistake silence for agreement.

Traditional Healing Methods

Nutrition is essential to health. There are strict rules within Chinese culture governing food combinations and timing of ingestion, especially in relation to monumental life events such as childbirth or surgery. Daily exercise is important and many Chinese participate in tai chi.

Congee is a rice porridge often given to sick children. The nurse should consider that many Western foods may be foreign to the patient, as the Chinese prefer to eat traditional foods.

Acupuncture is an ancient practice, older than 5,000 years, that is believed to cure disease or relieve pain (Xinnong, 1987). The practice, considered a "cold" treatment, involves puncturing the body with special needles at precisely predetermined sites known as meridians. Acupuncture is used when there is an excess of yang (Xinnong, 1987).

According to traditional Chinese medicine, health is achieved by maintaining the body in a balanced state; disease is caused by an internal imbalance of yin and yang. This imbalance leads to blockage in the flow of qi along pathways known as meridians. Qi can be unblocked by using acupuncture at certain points on the body that connect with these meridians. Sources vary on the number of meridians, ranging from 14 to 20. One commonly cited source describes meridians as 14 main channels "connecting the body in a web-like interconnecting matrix" of at least 2,000 acupuncture points (Acupuncture, 2009). It is believed that the way to treat internal problems is to puncture the meridians, which are also categorized as yin or yang, with the goal of treatment being restoration of yin and yang. Through the years, acupuncture has gained some legitimacy within Western medicine, and non-Asians are seeking treatment. According to the 2002 National Health Interview Survey—the largest and most comprehensive survey of complementary and alternative medicine (CAM) use by American adults to date—an estimated 8.2 million U.S. adults had ever used acupuncture, and 2.1 million U.S. adults had used acupuncture in the previous year (Barnes, Powell-Griner, McFann, & Nahin, 2004). Relatively few complications from the use of acupuncture have been reported to the U.S. Food and Drug Administration, considering that millions of people are treated each year and the high number of acupuncture needles used. Still, complications have resulted from inadequate sterilization of needles and from improper delivery of treatments. Practitioners should use a new set of disposable needles taken from a sealed package for each patient and should swab treatment sites with alcohol or another disinfectant before inserting needles. When not delivered properly, acupuncture can cause serious adverse effects including infections and, rarely, punctured organs (Medical News Today, 2009).

Moxibustion is another ancient treatment. Moxibustion is a traditional Chinese medicine technique that involves the burning of mugwort, a small, spongy herb, to facilitate healing (Wong, 2012). Moxibustion has been used throughout Asia for thousands of years; in fact, the actual Chinese character for acupuncture, translated literally, means "acupuncture-moxibustion." The purpose of moxibustion, as with most forms of traditional Chinese medicine, is to strengthen the blood, stimulate the flow of qi, and maintain general health. It is used in diseases in which there is an excess of yin. It is considered unsafe for use in diabetics (Wong, 2012). It is performed by applying it directly to the skin along certain meridians, although it cannot be applied to all of the meridians that are used for acupuncture. Mugwort, also known as *Artemisia vulgaris* or *ai ye* in Chinese, has a long history of use in folk medicine. Research has shown that it acts as an emmenagogue, that is, an agent that increases blood circulation to the pelvic area and uterus and stimulates menstruation. This could explain its use in treating breech births and menstrual cramps. Moxibustion is most commonly used during labor and delivery. In Western medicine, moxibustion has successfully been used to turn breech babies into a normal head-down position prior to childbirth. A study published in the *Journal of the American Medical Association* in 1998 found that up to 75% of women suffering from breech presentations before childbirth had fetuses that rotated to the normal position after receiving moxibustion at an acupuncture point on the bladder meridian, compared to 48% in the control group ($N = 260$) (Cardini & Weixin, 1998).

Other studies have shown that moxibustion increases the movement of the fetus in pregnant women, and may reduce the symptoms of menstrual cramps when used in conjunction with traditional acupuncture. A Cochrane review published in 2005 found that there is evidence, although limited, suggesting that moxibustion may be useful for turning babies from breech presentation (bottom first) to a cephalic presentation (head first) for labor (Coyle, Smith, & Peat, 2005).

Cupping refers to an ancient Chinese practice (over 3,000 years old) in which a cup is applied to the skin and the air pressure in the cup is reduced (by using change in heat or by suctioning out air), so that the skin and superficial muscle layer is drawn into and held in the cup (Dharmananda, 1999). In some cases, the cup may be moved while the suction of skin is active, causing a regional pulling of the skin and muscle (the technique is called "gliding cupping"). Cupping is applied by acupuncturists to certain acupuncture points, as well as to regions of the body that are affected by pain (where the pain is deeper than the tissues to be pulled). In ancient times, cups were made of animal horn, bamboo, or, for the wealthy, brass. According to Dharmananda (1999), since the 20th century, the cups have been made of glass (**Figure 7–2**). In ancient times, the name for cupping was horning. When the cups are moved along the surface of the skin, the treatment is somewhat like *guasha* (literally, "sand scraping"), a folk remedy of Southeast Asia that is often carried out by scraping the skin with a coin or other object with the intention of breaking up stagnation. Movement of the cups is a gentler technique than *guasha*, as a lubricant allows the cup to slide without causing as much of the subcutaneous bruising that is an objective of *guasha*. Still, a certain amount of bruising is expected both from fixed-position cupping (especially at the site of the cup rim) and with movement of the cups. In some cases, a small amount of

Figure 7–2 A. Three types of cups. B. Flash-fire cupping.

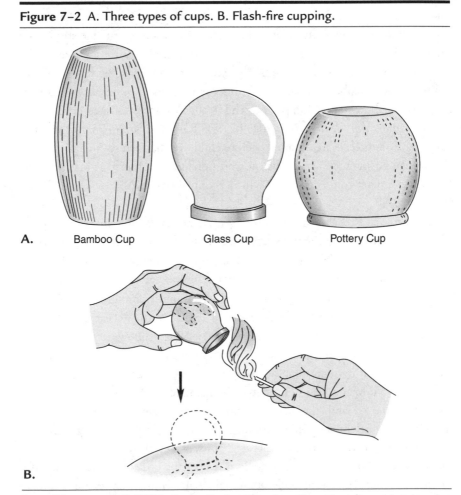

Source: Dharmananda, S. (1999). *Cupping.* Retrieved from http://www.itmonline.org/arts/cupping .htm

blood letting (*luoci,* or vein pricking) is first done, using a pricking needle, and then the cup is applied over the site. The pricking is usually done with a three-edged needle that is applied to a vein, and it typically draws 3 to 4 drops of blood (sometimes the skin on either side is squeezed to aid release of blood). A standard thick-gauge acupuncture needle or plum blossom needle may be used instead. Generally, the cup is left in place for about 10 minutes (typical range is 5 to 15 minutes). The skin becomes reddened because of the congestion of blood flow. The cup is removed by pressing the skin alongside it to allow some outside air to leak into it, thus equalizing the pressure and releasing it.

Today, cupping is mainly recommended for the treatment of pain, gastrointestinal disorders, lung diseases (especially chronic cough and asthma), and paralysis, although it can be used for other disorders as well. It is frequently used to treat lung congestion. The areas of the body that are fleshy are preferred sites for cupping. Contraindications for cupping include areas of skin that are inflamed; cases of high fever, convulsions or cramping, or easy bleeding (i.e., pathologic level of low platelets); or the abdominal area or lower back during pregnancy. Movement of the cups is limited to fleshy areas; the movement should not cross bony ridges, such as the spine (Dharmananda, 1999).

Cupping is said to promote blood circulation, remove stasis, and alleviate swelling and pain. It is employed especially when there is a toxic heat syndrome as well as for a variety of acute ailments. Cupping is used to draw blood and lymph to the body's surface that is under the cup, which increases the local circulation. Cupping is used to remove cold and damp from the body and to assist with blood circulation. Cupping is also frequently applied after treatment by acupuncture, bloodletting, or plum blossom treatment (Dharmananda, 1999). Cupping is not only traditionally practiced in China and Japan; it is also a traditional healing method in Arab cultures, where it is called Al-hijamah (Benlafquih, 2009).

Is it very important for the nurse to be aware that dermabrasion and cupping, both of which can leave marks or bruising, can easily be mistaken as signs of physical abuse.

Alternative and Complementary Folk Medicine

CAM represents a group of diverse medical and healthcare systems, practices, and products that are not presently considered to be part of conventional medicine (National Center for Complementary and Alternative Medicine, 2011). It has been estimated that 38% of Americans use CAM (National Center for Complementary and Alternative Medicine, 2011). Complementary medicine is used together with conventional medicine, and alternative medicine is used in place of conventional medicine. In the United States, where practitioners incorporate healing traditions from China, Japan, Korea, and other countries, acupuncture is considered part of CAM.

Some Chinese prepare amulets that are used to protect health by preventing harm from evil spirits. The amulet is hung over a door or on a curtain or wall, worn in the hair, pinned on clothing, or carried in a red bag (Varner, 2008). Jade is considered the most precious of all stones and when worn it is believed to bring health. Jade is so valued that in Chinese contests, jade is awarded for first place, followed by gold for second, and ivory for third place. Jade is believed to be the closest mineral form of the yin and yang, and it is used to speak to heaven. It is also believed that the jade stone can prevent harm and accidents and can keep children safe. Jade is also seen as the "giver" of children, health, immortality, wisdom, power, victory, growth, and food. It is important that the jade stone be maintained, for it is believed that if the stone turns dull or breaks, the wearer will have misfortune.

Medicinal herbs are still widely used in the practice of Chinese healing. Herbs used in Chinese medicine are derived from plant, animal, and mineral substances. Although plant-derived herbs, such as ginseng and ginger, are the most common, minerals and animal parts such as oyster shells, deer antlers, and bear gallbladder are also prescribed. In China, herbs in powder form are boiled and made into a tea. In the West, traditional Chinese medicine practitioners often premix the herbal remedy or supply the herb in pill form, especially for those patients who find the bitter taste intolerable. Herbs have four basic qualities and properties: nature, taste, affinity, and its primary action. See **Table 7–2** for more on herbal therapy.

Table 7–2 Herbal Therapy

Nature: An herb's nature is often described as cooling or heating, but it can also be described as moistening, relaxing, or energizing. The peppermint herb, for example, has a cooling energy, and is used to lower the metabolism or reduce gas and bloating.
Taste: Herbs are categorized by five tastes—sour, bitter, sweet or bland, spicy, and salty. Herbs representing different tastes are used to treat different conditions. Dandelion and goldenseal are two bitter herbs used for their drying properties in treating upper respiratory conditions.
Affinity: This property refers to the affinity that an herb has for a particular organ network.
Primary action: This property refers to the effect of a particular herb. An herb may be used to dispel (move), astringe (restrain), purge (expel), or tonify (strengthen).

Source: Ergil K. V., Kramer, E. J., Ng, A. T. (2002). *Chinese herbal medicines. Western Journal of Medicine, 176,* 275–279; Xie, Z. (2000). *Practical traditional Chinese medicine.* Beijing, China: Foreign Languages Press.

Table 7–3 Comparison of Health Beliefs Among Asians/Pacific Islanders

Group	Health Beliefs	Traditional Healing Methods
Cambodian	Comfortable with Western medicine but will resort to traditional healing first. They are reluctant to complain. Tend to focus on symptoms, not on the cause. May view symptom remission as a cure and stop medications too early.	Coin rubbing Cupping Massage Herbs
Korean	The kior chi force is the life force of the body. Withdrawing blood, sweating, and sex reduce the kior chi force. Illness is often seen as fate. Hospitalization is seen as a sign of impending death. Illness is attributed to disharmony. Illness can have spiritual causes. Treatment is through the use of the opposite force to achieve balance. Traditional healing can be provided by family members or healers. They do believe in do not resuscitate (DNR) orders. They do not wish to discuss terminal status, as it is viewed as unacceptable. Organ donation and transplantation are seen as a disturbance in integrity of the body. Most patient care is provided by the family. Physician is seen as powerful and trustworthy.	Herbs Acupuncture Cupping Moxibustion
Vietnamese	Expect to be cured immediately. Seek out Western medicine to relieve symptoms. May view symptom remission as a cure and stop medications too early. Feel medicines are too powerful for them and may adjust dosage down. Fear loss of blood to lab studies is harmful to health.	Coining Cupping Balm Acupuncture Massage Herbs

(Continues)

Table 7–3 *Continued*

Group	Health Beliefs	Traditional Healing Methods
Laotian	Illness may be attributed to the loss of one of the 32 spirits thought to inhabit the body and maintain health.	Coining
		Pinching—rubbing the temples, pulling forward to the eyebrow and nose and pinching the nose—is used to relieve headache
	Health is related to ability to eat and sleep.	Cupping
	Will look to family and community for treatment first.	Massage
		Traditional Chinese medicine
	Traditional treatments may be tried first—Western medicine is last resort.	Ceremony—if the cause of illness is thought to be a result of a spirit, a special ceremony may be performed
	Often will continue traditional healing with Western medicine in combination.	Mental illness is attributed to spirit loss. In Laos, if a person exhibits symptoms that we may think of as mental illness, such as hallucinations, they will simply be left alone as long as they are viewed as not dangerous to others. If they consider mental health a problem, they are more likely to go to a monk for a ceremony to treat it.
	Obtaining a health history is difficult because of desire for privacy. Patient is concerned about confidentiality and will benefit from reassurance that confidentiality will be maintained.	
	The entire family will want to be present for a patient's last days.	Here in the United States, some Laotians have learned about the value of treatment for mental health problems and will accept help. They are not likely to understand, however, why some medications have side effects that sometimes make a person feel worse. Laotians are not likely to seek treatment from a traditional mental health source unless there is a long-standing or very serious problem, or unless specifically referred for treatment.
	Respect for the patient and his culture is essential.	
	The head of the body is sacred.	
	Avoid touching the head and the shoulder unless absolutely essential.	
	Modesty is highly valued, especially among women.	
Japanese	Believe body is as holy as the mind. View the mind and body as one.	
	Concerns with medical diagnosis of brain death and organ donation. Organ donation violates oneness of body and soul, and receipt of organs can cause anxiety in Japanese recipient.	
	Individual assertion is highly discouraged, so the patient may not ask questions during health teaching.	

Group	Health Beliefs	Traditional Healing Methods
Japanese (*cont.*)	Silence may be a way of avoiding conflict. Healthcare providers should avoid prolonged eye contact to show respect. Patience is an important skill when dealing with Japanese. Avoid physical touching, which can cause anxiety.	
Asian Indians	Most Indians in the United States accept and understand Western medicine. The traditional philosophy and science of medicine in India is called Ayurveda. *Ayur* means longevity and *veda* means science. This promotes a routine where one's health and daily routine, body, and the five elements of the universe are in sync. The five elements are water, fire, earth, wind, and ether. When elements are in balance, the body is healthy, and imbalance results in illness. Foods have properties that determine if they are "hot" or "cold" (it is not based on temperature or the spiciness of the food) and it is believed that proper food balance is essential for temperature regulation. Consuming certain foods can cause a temperature imbalance. Examples of cold foods are yogurt, fruit, and rice; hot foods are teas, chicken, garlic, and cloves.	Most Indians feel that blood is precious and not to be wasted. Expect reluctance on the patient's part for any blood drawing. Colostrum is perceived as bad for newborns. Newborns are fed sugar water until the third day postpartum. On the third postpartum day, the new mother has a ritual bath and then will commence breastfeeding. Honey is often given to newborns, which is potentially dangerous because of bacterial contamination. Smiling is only done in informal situations and then only shared between people of an equal social status. Although there is a public health system in India, Indians who can afford it will use a fee-for-service private system. There is no health insurance in India. Three of the five elements correspond to the human body. Bile corresponds to fire, phlegm to water, and gas to wind. Balance equates with health. Most Indians are vegetarians. Most Hindus follow dietary restrictions, which prohibits ingestion of beef. Muslims do not ingest pork or pork products. Second-generation Asian Indians may not follow these food taboos. Fasting is common with Hindus and Muslims during certain times of the year.

Source: Adapted from: Blanchette, P. L. (2001). Health and healthcare for Asians and Pacific Islander American elders. Retrieved from http://www.stanford.edu/group/ethnoger/apiaintroduction.html

Chinese medicine is successfully used for a very wide range of conditions. The more commonly treated disorders are listed in **Table 7–4**.

More than 300 herbs that are commonly used today have a history of use that goes back at least 2,000 years. Over that time, a vast amount of experience has been gained, which has gone toward perfecting their clinical applications. According to Chinese clinical studies, these herbs and others that have been added to the list of useful items over the centuries can greatly increase the effectiveness of modern drug treatments, reduce their side effects, and sometimes replace them completely.

In China, the two most common methods of applying herb therapies are to make a decoction (a strong tea that must be simmered for an hour or more) and to make large honey-bound pills. Both of these forms meet with considerable resistance in Western countries. The teas are deemed too time-consuming, smelly, and awful tasting to justify their use, and the honey pills (boluses) are sticky, difficult to chew, and bad tasting. Thus, modern forms that are more acceptable have been developed for most applications.

The two popular forms to replace the standard Chinese preparations are extract powders (or granules) and smooth, easy-to-swallow tablets or capsules. The extracts are made by producing a large batch of tea and then removing the water and producing a powder or tiny pellets; the resulting material is swallowed down with some water or mixed with hot water to make a tea. Tablets and capsules contain either powdered herbs or dried extracts or a combination of the two.

Table 7–4 Systems and Disorders Treated with Chinese Herbs

System	Associated Disorders
Integumentary	Eczema, psoriasis, acne, rosacea, urticaria
Respiratory	Asthma, bronchitis, chronic coughs, allergic and perennial rhinitis and sinusitis
Gastrointestinal	Irritable bowel syndrome, chronic constipation, ulcerative colitis, hepatitis C
Gynecologic/genitourinary	Premenstrual syndrome and dysmenorrhea, endometriosis, infertility, chronic cystitis
Endocrine	Diabetes (treatment and prevention)
Psychological	Anxiety, depression
Rheumatologic	Osteoarthritis, rheumatoid arthritis, chronic fatigue syndrome

Source: Ergil K. V., Kramer, E. J., Ng, A. T. (2002). Chinese herbal medicines. *Western Journal of Medicine, 176,* 275–279.

Arguably, the most important Chinese herb is ginseng. Ginseng (*renshen*) has long been valued as a disease-preventive herb. It is purported to calm the spirit and help one gain wisdom. Modern usages include normalizing blood pressure, regulating blood sugar, resisting fatigue, increasing oxygen utilization, and enhancing immune functions. Traditionally, the root is cooked in a double boiler to make a tea, used either alone or with several other herbs. Today, ginseng is much easier to ingest. A tea can be made quickly and there are tablets and other formulations to ease consumption. Typical ginseng dosage is 0.5 to 3.0 grams (g). Higher doses may be used over the short term for specific therapeutic actions: in China, 30 g is recommended to treat shock (sudden hypotension). As with all herbs, there is concern that they are not regulated by the U.S. Food and Drug Administration; purity of herbs can be an issue as well. Use caution when recommending the use of herbal preparations for yourself or your patients. Although herbs such as ginseng are considered safe, be aware that excessive consumption of ginseng can lead to nervousness and may produce hormonal imbalances in women.

Current Healthcare Problems Including Mortality and Morbidity

The four leading causes of death for Chinese Americans are identical to those for White Americans. They are heart disease, cerebral vascular disease, cancer, and chronic respiratory disorders (National Center for Health Statistics, 2002). The fifth leading cause of death is pneumonia. The rate of suicide found in Chinese Americans, especially females, is an area that is under further investigation. Suicide ranks ninth as a cause of death for Chinese Americans and eleventh for White Americans (National Center for Health Statistics, 2002). Mortality data reveals that the four leading causes of death for Chinese Americans are the same as those for European Americans.

There is a stigma among the Chinese and Chinese Americans regarding mental illness. Many believe that mental illness indicates inability to solve problems or out-of-control behavior, and that it brings shame to the individual and the family. Further study is required to determine if the lower rates of psychiatric hospitalization among AAPIs is caused by this stigma or prevalence.

Impact of Communication

In China and Taiwan, the official language is Mandarin, which is based on the northern Beijing dialect and is spoken by more than 70% of the population. Nearly all Chinese are bilingual, speaking the national language as well as a native dialect. The major dialects are Cantonese and Shanghaiese. Chinese who immigrated from Hong Kong and southeast China speak Cantonese. Because these native dialects are so different, many groups cannot understand one another verbally, although the written language is the same. It is important for the nurse to recognize that all dialects of spoken Chinese share the same written language of Mandarin. Mandarin in the written form can be used as a way to ensure effective communication among all Chinese patients. Written Chinese consists of characters that represent an object or idea. Each Chinese character consists of only one syllable. Tones within the language change the meaning of a syllable or word. The Chinese language has a limited number of verbs, does not have tenses, and does not use plurals. The Chinese rely on a highly contextualized language where the nonverbal communication is just as important as the verbal. Eye contact is minimal, as too much eye contact is viewed as rude. Few words are used to express a thought; they value silence highly and strive for intuitive understanding. Individuals endeavor to conduct themselves with restraint and speak in a moderate-to-low volume of voice. To raise one's voice is viewed as a loss of control.

Also of note is the avoidance of the use of the word *no*. In China, one usually avoids saying "no" out of respect to the other person. Remember that the Chinese typically communicate more with the use of nonverbal language and may be saying "yes" when they really mean "no." Do not forget to ask for assistance from an interpreter, especially if you note a disconnect between the verbal and nonverbal communication. An interpreter is also very helpful in interpreting the meaning of silence during a conversation. Silence in Chinese culture can mean respect, interest, anger, or even disagreement, so clarification of the meaning of the silence is very important. The Chinese American may also be uncomfortable with discussing family-related problems with strangers as it is viewed as disrespectful. Rapport building by the healthcare provider is essential.

Impact of Time and Space

Asians typically prefer a greater amount of physical space than we may be accustomed to. Physical touching or displays of affection are uncommon (Giger, 2013). The nurse should consider carefully the appropriateness of touching an Asian patient, as it would be considered inappropriate to hug or console a Chinese adult or child with touch.

Timing may be an issue with appointments. Chinese Americans are often polychromic (adhering less rigidly to time as a distinct and linear entity, focusing on the completion of the present, and performing more than one activity at the same time) (Hall, 1963). The U.S. healthcare system has a monochromic orientation, which emphasizes schedules, being on time, synchronization with clocks, and standardization of activities (Hall, 1963), which can cause clashes. Some Chinese Americans have a more modern view of time, especially if they have been in the United States for a prolonged period of time, or are a second-generation immigrant. This modern view emphasizes the importance of being on time, and lateness is viewed as a serious act of disrespect. These Chinese Americans will arrive on time and will expect others to do the same. It is important for the nurse to not cause the Chinese American to lose face: in Chinese culture if you make a high-ranking person wait for you, both of you have then lost face. Chinese Americans value the past as evidenced by the value placed on elders and also an appreciation for the future by stressing education in the younger generation.

Impact of Environment

Harmony with nature is stressed in Chinese culture. Some Chinese Americans ascribe to feng shui (wind and water). Feng shui is an effort to achieve harmony and balance through the art of location and design of physical structures (Rossbach, 2000). Positive feng shui wards off evil spirits, promotes good health, and brings prosperity. Others have beliefs related to colors and numbers. Certain numbers are considered to bring good or bad luck (Chinese Historical and Cultural Project, 2002). The number four is bad luck, whereas the number eight is good luck. The birth date of the patient can be perceived as being either lucky or unlucky depending on the numbers utilized. A person born in August (the eighth month) on the eighth day of the month in a year beginning or ending in eight would be considered extremely lucky. Colors also are lucky or unlucky. White, the color of mourning, is considered bad luck. This can be upsetting to the Chinese American when dealing with many members of the healthcare team, who traditionally wear white coats, scrubs, or uniforms.

Biologic Variations

The Chinese are more prone to fractures and osteoporosis because their bone density is lower than White Americans (Wang, Tao, Hyman, Li, & Chen, 2009). Most Chinese do not have much facial or body hair and the hair on the head is usually black and straight (Hays, 2011).

There are three genetic diseases found in the Chinese: adult lactose intolerance, alpha-thalassemia, and glucose-6-phosphate dehydrogenase (G-6-PD) deficiency. Lactose intolerance causes gastrointestinal disturbances after milk or dairy products containing the sugar lactose are ingested (cheese is often tolerated) (Hays, 2011). There are two types of thalassemia, which is a hemoglobin abnormality characterized by a high rate of red blood cell destruction. The first type usually does not have a major effect on health status and is characterized by an increase in red blood cells. The second type is more serious as it is associated with an early death and requires frequent blood transfusions. G-6-PD also causes fragility of the red blood cells and makes patients prone to anemia (Hays, 2011).

Drug metabolism is an issue with this group. Studies have revealed that Asians require lower dosages than Whites for several psychiatric medications (antidepressants, lithium, neuroleptics). There is an increased sensitivity to alcohol; often, Chinese demonstrate facial flushing and vasomotor responses when drinking, which may explain the low alcoholism rate among the Chinese (Overfield, 1995). The nurse should be aware that Chinese Americans born in the United States consume more alcohol than immigrant Chinese Americans (Huff & Kline, 1999). Some Chinese believe that medications are too potent for them and, while this may be true of some medications (such as the psychotropic agents), it is important that the patient not self-adjust medications but have an open dialogue with their prescriber.

Infectious diseases, including tuberculosis (TB), are a major health threat to the Chinese immigrant. Complicating the diagnosis of authentic TB from false-positive on the Mantoux test is the widespread exposure of Southeast Asians to the bacilli-Calmette-Guérin vaccine against TB in childhood. Other infection risks include parasites, hepatitis, and malaria.

Cancer is a major burden for all AAPIs. Cancer is the leading cause of death for AAPIs aged 25 to 64 years. This is startling because cancer does not become a leading cause of death for Whites until they reach the age range of 45 to 64 (Chen, 2000). Cancer death rates have increased at much higher rates for AAPIs than for any other racial or ethnic group (Chen, 2000). Part of the blame may be a result of the high rate of cigarette smoking among male AAPIs (U.S. Department of Health and Human Services, 1998). Smoking is the single most important preventable cause of death, including death from cancer.

Diabetes is an emerging disease in Asian Americans, particularly those who have lived in the United States for several years. Comparing the prevalence of diabetes for Japanese living in Tokyo with Japanese Americans living in Seattle, Washington, the rates for diabetes are four or five times higher for that population in the United States. The data are similar for Chinese in China versus Chinese Americans, and for Vietnamese in Vietnam versus Vietnamese Americans. Reliance on the use of body mass index (BMI) as a screening tool to identify patients at risk for diabetes has not been found to be effective, as there is difficulty in defining obesity in this population using BMI. People in the Asian American population may develop insulin resistance and type 2 diabetes at much lower BMI levels than would be found in other population groups. BMI criteria for being overweight are between 25 and 30 kg/m², whereas a BMI above 30 kg/m² is considered obese. For the Asian American population, the numbers need to be lower: probably between 23 and 25 kg/m² to be considered overweight, and anything above 25 kg/m² as obese. Another screening tool is waist circumference, but this also must be modified based on population group. The International Diabetes Foundation (IDF) has suggested that for Caucasians, the waist circumference should be less than 37 inches in men and 31.5 inches in women. For South Asians (Chinese and Asian Indian populations), the waist circumference in men should be less than 35 inches and less than 31.5 inches in women. In the Japanese, the waist circumference should be less than 35 inches in men and in women, it should be less than 33.5 inches. According to the IDF, when dealing with sub-Saharan Africans, eastern Mediterranean, and Middle East (Arab) populations, it is acceptable to use the Caucasian data for now. For South Americans and Central Americans, use the South Asian recommendations for now.

Impact of Social Organization

Family is the foundation of Chinese society (Gailliard, 2011). The family includes multiple generations and also includes ancestors in daily life. The most treasured values of Chinese society are family relationships, loyalty, obligation, obedience, cooperation, interdependence, and reciprocity. The father is typically the family spokesperson and decision maker, whereas the mother is the manager of the house and finances and is responsible for childrearing (Gailliard, 2011). There is frequent use of the "family bed" as children may sleep with their parents in one bed until school age. Early toilet training is valued (and is often completed by age 1) (Chou, 2009), but breastfeeding is continued until age 2 or even longer.

Maintaining face is very important to the Chinese and is accomplished by adhering to the rules of society. Chinese believe in status and do not feel that true equality is possible based on Chinese history. Decisions are made based on group consensus, with deferral usually given to the oldest members. The individual must strive not to bring shame and not cause another to lose face. Status is acquired through age, job, marriage, and wealth. The concept of privacy is negatively viewed. Privacy is not highly valued or viewed as a luxury by the Chinese people. This is helpful because the majority of Chinese reside in urban areas where privacy is difficult to achieve.

Impact of Faith and Spirituality

Older generations of Chinese may be influenced by a blend of Buddhism, Taoism, and Confucianism (Herbert Hoover Presidential Library, 2012). A small minority of Chinese are Muslim or Christian. Many Chinese state that they have no particular religious affiliation or tradition, although they may be very active spiritually.

KOREAN AMERICANS

Prior to World War II, Korea was impacted by Japanese culture during the 35 years the country was under Japan's control (Lee, 2006). During World War II, Japan sided with Nazi Germany, and the Japanese government forced the Koreans to support the war effort. When Japan attacked Pearl Harbor, Hawaii, on December 7, 1941, bringing the United States into World War II, the Korean provisional government finally had an opportunity to take a stand against Japan. The provisional government declared war on Japan and formed the Restoration Army to fight alongside the Allies in the Pacific theater.

At the end of World War II in 1945, the United States and the Soviet Union divided the peninsula along the 38th parallel into two zones of occupation—a Soviet-controlled region in the north and an American-controlled one in the south (Lee, 2006). The peace that Koreans envisioned did not come, however. The Soviets occupied the north and the United States stationed troops in the south. In the months that followed the end of World War II, postwar international decisions were made without the consent of the Korean people. The Soviet Union set up a provisional Communist government in northern Korea, and the United States created a provisional Republican government in the south. In 1948, the Republic of Korea was founded south of the 38th parallel, followed by the establishment of the Democratic People's Republic of Korea in the north. Both governments claimed authority over the entire peninsula and tempted fate by crossing the border at various points along the 38th parallel.

On June 25, 1950, North Korea launched a surprise attack on South Korea, beginning a costly, bloody, 3-year struggle known as the Korean War (Kraig, 2011). It was perhaps the most tragic period in modern history for the Korean people. In the end, neither side achieved victory. On July 27, 1953, in the town of Panmunjom, the two sides signed an armistice designating a cease-fire line along the 38th parallel and establishing a surrounding 2.5-mile-wide (4-kilometer-wide) demilitarized zone, which remains the boundary between the two Koreas (BBC. com, 2012). The war left the peninsula a wasteland and a divided country that still exists in the 21st century.

Emigration was discouraged by the South Korean government after World War II, and North Korea forbade any kind of emigration. The quota system created by the United States Office of Immigration in the 1940s allowed between

105 and 150 immigrants from each of the Asian nations into the country (U.S. Department of State, Office of the Historian, 2012). This law favored immigrants with postsecondary education, technical training, and specialized skills. Most of the Koreans allowed to immigrate were women with nursing training. The War Brides Act of 1945 also helped women and children obtain papers to immigrate.

More women who had married American soldiers were allowed into the United States after the Korean War. By this time, Koreans and all Asians in America were able to acquire citizenship through naturalization as a result of the McCarran-Walter Act of 1952 (U.S. Department of State, Office of the Historian, 2012). Foreign adoption of Korean babies also began at the end of the Korean War. The war had left thousands of children orphaned in Korea. Over 100,000 South Korean children were adopted abroad since the war, and roughly two-thirds of these children have to adopted by American families. An estimated 10,000 Korean children have been adopted by Minnesota families alone (Nash, 2012). Criticized by other countries for running a "baby mill," the South Korean government began to phase out the practice in the 1990s. Although adopting children is traditionally frowned upon in Korean society, social workers are attempting to encourage domestic adoption.

In 1965, the U.S. Congress passed the Immigration and Naturalization Act (Nash, 2012). The quota system was replaced with a preference system that gave priority to immigration applications from relatives of U.S. citizens and from professionals with skills needed by the United States. Thousands of South Korean doctors and nurses took advantage of the new law. They moved to America and took jobs in understaffed, inner-city hospitals. Koreans with science and technology backgrounds also were encouraged to immigrate. These new immigrants came from middle- and upper-class families, unlike the earlier immigrants. The portion of the law informally known as the Brothers and Sisters Act has also been a factor in the dramatic increase in the Korean American population. In 1960, 10,000 Koreans were living in the United States. The number of Korean immigrants in the United States grew 27-fold between 1970 and 2007, from 38,711 to 1.0 million, making them the 7th largest immigrant group in the United States (Terrazas, 2009).

Statistics

Despite the changes in immigration law that permitted educated Koreans to enter the United States, problems with language have consequences. In 2007, 57% of Korean immigrants were limited English proficient (Terrazas, 2009).

A lack of command of English remains a major setback in the work and social arenas. It is for this reason that some Koreans choose to work in family-owned businesses, which permits them to hold on to their customs and native language (Nash, 2012). There is a strong desire to maintain a sense of community. Korean culture is maintained within Korean American communities through church organizations, Korean schools, and Korean culture camps (Nash, 2012). Most Korean immigrants are active Christians and that connection has held strong during migration to the United States. Since the beginning of this century, Korean Protestant churches have offered classes in Korean culture and language. This link between the church and the community has resulted in an easier acculturation for Korean Americans compared to other Asian Americans. Today, approximately 1 million Korean Americans live in the United States, and 50% of them live in California, New York, New Jersey, and Virginia (Terrazas, 2009).

Korean Traditional Health Beliefs

Koreans often avoid entering the U.S. healthcare system because they fear being a burden because of language difficulties. They also fear the unknown, being taken advantage of, or accruing a large medical bill due to a lack of health insurance.

Koreans are very private people who do not like to seek medical attention and their focus is on curative measures and not on preventive health care (Beller, Pinker, Snapka, & Van Dusen, 2012). The language barrier also impacts the seeking out of traditional health care. The act of asking for help from a stranger is considered bold in the Korean culture. The desire to stay within their own cultural group is another barrier, as Koreans prefer to seek help only from members of their own social group. Self-expression is not counted as a virtue among Koreans and, therefore, many Koreans feel that medical problems should be kept to oneself. Furthermore, Koreans do not like to discuss things that are distressful in nature; they would prefer to go without necessary health care. Illness is often attributed to fate and hospitalization may often be viewed as a sign of impending death for the patient (Beller et al., 2012).

Endurance of pain without complaint is a measure of a person's maturity, and emotions are not freely expressed (Beller et al., 2012). Although it is not culturally acceptable to complain of sadness or emotional pain, it is acceptable to utter somatic complaints and seek treatment for indigestion, insomnia, or abdominal pain. Women are more likely to complain of physical symptoms and seek care; men are more likely to seek relief in alcohol.

In general, no restrictions exist that prevent healthcare providers from delivering care to the opposite gender. However, some women may prefer a female physician for gynecologic and obstetric problems.

Impact of Communication

The Korean alphabet consists of 14 consonants and 10 vowels (Nash, 2012). The degree of formality that exists during communication is dependent on social status and age. In order to gauge a person's age during conversation, the Korean American may ask questions (such as what year did you graduate from high school) to help determine the age of the person with whom they are communicating, and hence the degree of formality that is required. Age is the most important factor in determining the degree of respect a person should be given. It is traditional to bow when greeting elders and to use titles such as "Nurse" in greetings and communication to convey respect (Beller et al., 2012). Men may shake hands in greeting but the shake will be done lightly with eyes averted.

Gestures and nonverbal methods of communication are very important in Korean culture (Beller et al., 2012). Eye contact is minimal, as prolonged eye contact is considered to be rude. Koreans, when needing to point to an object, will use the entire hand or the middle finger—not the index finger. Men do not shake hands with women, and women will usually offer a nod in greeting. Any public displays of affection between genders, such as hugging and kissing, are considered inappropriate. It would be considered appropriate for two members of the same gender to walk down the street holding hands, but not for a male and female couple to do so. It is considered impolite to enter a home or room without knocking or removing one's shoes.

Impact of Time and Space

Time is a loose construct in Korean culture (Beller et al., 2012). Even in the school setting, the submission of assignments or schoolwork is not guided by a deadline. The priority is on work completion, not its timeliness. Education is highly valued, however. Korea has the world's highest ratio of PhDs to the general population, as well as one of the lowest illiteracy rates. Parents will often significantly sacrifice to ensure the most prestigious education possible for their children (Beller et al., 2012).

Impact of Environment

Food is very important to this culture. Korean food is very unique and highly valued. Garlic is the primary flavoring utilized along with ginger, black and red pepper, and soy sauce (Beller et al., 2012). Because there are generally far fewer Korean restaurants than Chinese or Japanese in the United States, many Koreans eat in those restaurants, or they prepare their own food at home. Larger cities that have a Koreatown or a high number of Korean immigrants may have some Korean restaurants. Korean cuisine is similar to that of the Chinese and Japanese.

While it is a common practice to offer a guest food or drink, the visitor should not accept the first offer made; respect is shown by allowing several offers before finally accepting the food or drink (Beller et al., 2012).

Biologic Variations

In the Korean culture, a son or daughter of a cancer survivor or patient might be considered less marriageable because of the concern that there is an "inferior" gene in the family. Children with disabilities are viewed as a punishment from family ancestors on the parents (Beller et al., 2012). Mental illness also carries a stigma in Korean culture and should be approached with sensitivity (Beller et al., 2012). Koreans are reluctant to talk about psychological issues or share emotion-laden issues. Stress and depression can affect older Korean immigrants who are isolated by the language barrier and insulated by social customs.

Impact of Social Organization

Family provides a very important social structure in Korean culture (Shin, Shin, & Blanchette, 2012). The family is male led, as the male is the decision maker for the family unit (Beller et al., 2012). Individualism is not considered a virtue, and discipline of children within the family may be considered strict when evaluated by other cultures. Education is highly valued and no expense is spared for this. A Korean child's first birthday is considered an event of great importance. Until recently, the infant mortality rate for children younger than the age of 1 was very high in Korean children (University of North Carolina, 2012). As a result, the first birthday is celebrated with prayers and feasts. This celebration, a major milestone in a child's life, is called *Tol* (Sophia, 2003).

Korean social class is determined by educational level, family background, and financial status. There are a large number of Korean American business owners. Koreans have enjoyed the highest level of entrepreneurial success of any ethnic group and they often pool their resources to help other Koreans in their community to start or expand their business (Reference for Business, 2012). Although business people may have a higher income than professionals (physicians, attorneys, etc.), the professional, based on his educational level, would be considered to possess the higher social status in the Korean culture.

Korean culture is based on a vertical concept of respect, which is different from the horizontal concept found in the United States. Koreans adhere to a vertical concept of respect in which hierarchical relationships determine to whom you give respect. The mannerisms used and the formality of the language are all based on this vertical concept of respect (University of North Carolina, 2012).

Impact of Faith and Spirituality

Ethnic churches serve as social networks and opportunities for healthcare professionals to provide education and programs relating to physical and mental health. Although many Koreans have a Buddhist heritage, Christianity has become very popular and most Korean immigrants to the Unites States are Protestant (Beller et al., 2012).

CAMBODIAN AMERICANS

Cambodia is part of Southeast Asia. Although mainly known as a small agricultural country, Cambodia has a rich artistic and musical tradition (Bankston, 2012a). Cambodia was deeply affected by the conflict in Vietnam and was the target of many attacks. The conflict forced many Cambodians to escape to refugee camps in Thailand, and many have made their way to the United States. In addition, there was a terrible genocide in Cambodia called the Khmer Rouge Holocaust. This occurred in the 1970s after the U.S.-supported government in Cambodia was overturned in 1975 (Bankston, 2012). The Khmer Rouge slaughtered millions of Cambodians in an attempt to establish a new government. Former supporters of the United States within Cambodia were targeted for elimination, as were intellectuals and the upper classes. Others, such as rice farmers once driven from the land, made their way to refugee camps in nearby countries and then eventually to the United States.

This forced immigration caused a tremendous amount of stress, which led to psychological and physical problems in many immigrants (Bankston, 2012). Also, because many Cambodian immigrants were rice farmers with limited education and financial resources, employment opportunities were and continue to be severely limited. Some have found work in factories or have developed trades, such as jewelers or mechanics. With the recent downturn in the U.S. economy, many have lost their positions and are having difficulty finding a new job that would permit reentry into the U.S. workforce.

Cambodian Traditional Health Beliefs

Cambodians believe that imbalance can cause illness (Curran, 2002). This imbalance may be caused by natural forces or changes in the environment. Cambodians also believe that illness can have spiritual causes (Curran, 2002). They are likely to use traditional herbs that they purchase at Asian markets, and the traditional Khmer rely on spiritual healing practices.

Traditional healing is preferred and may be performed by family members or traditional healers. Cambodians are fairly comfortable with Western medicine, but they are likely to try more traditional methods of healing first (Curran, 2002). This means Cambodians are not likely to enter the healthcare system for most illnesses, and they practice few if any preventive measures. Normally, they will only seek treatment when experiencing serious injury or illness. Cambodians are usually reluctant to complain or express negative feelings, so it may be difficult for a physician to identify the problem. There is acceptance within the culture of illness and discomfort. Because the illness or discomfort is accepted, the result may be not to seek out care or it can result in a delay in seeking treatment. Cambodians traditionally tend to focus on the symptoms rather than the cause of an illness or disease and, therefore, may stop using medicines after symptoms disappear. They do not place an emphasis on preventive health. Cambodians do not normally value adult immunizations, early disease detection, or health screenings, but they do believe in childhood immunizations. One practice that may be employed is coining. Coining is the practice of firmly rubbing a coin repeatedly on an ill person. The nurse should be careful to consider this healing practice as a possibility when suspecting abuse or physical punishment. Coining has been mistaken for child abuse in some instances.

Impact of Communication

Khmer is the ethnic term for most people from Cambodia, as well as the name of their most commonly spoken language. The Cambodian alphabet has 47 letters (Bankston, 2012). Other languages, such as English, French, Thai, and Chinese, are also sometimes utilized in schools and business settings. Immigration to the United States has resulted in most second-generation Cambodians being fluent in English. Some first-generation Cambodians may only speak Khmer and require the use of an interpreter.

Impact of Time and Space

Because most Cambodian refugees were farmers, time orientation has its roots in an agricultural paradigm. In the morning, they would head to the fields to work, and they would stay until the sun went down. This lack of reliance on the use of a clock has resulted in many Cambodian immigrants missing or being late for scheduled appointments (University of North Carolina, 2012).

Be mindful of spacing and avoid prolonged eye contact (CultureCrossing. net, 2012). It is considered highly inappropriate to stare. Children and youth are expected to approach adults with respect. If an elderly person is seated, children should not walk in front of them or stand up higher than them without bowing the head. Girls should not whistle and must sit with their legs tightly closed. It is considered very disrespectful for a male to approach a female to start a conversation.

Impact of Environment

Cambodians choose to live in close proximity or to have several generations of family all under one roof. The traditional Cambodian diet is naturally healthy and nutritious; it consists of seafood, rice and vegetables (Stockton, 2001). Some immigrants have adapted their diet to be more American (including fast foods), which has resulted in the development of preventable diseases such as diabetes mellitus and obesity.

Biologic Variations

Excessive alcohol ingestion is becoming a problem with the Cambodian immigrant population. Drinking alcohol is viewed as a very American activity. The use of alcohol is frowned upon in Buddhist tradition and access to alcohol in Cambodia was nearly impossible (University of North Carolina, 2012). Many drink in excess because the lack of access to alcohol has not permitted them the ability to drink moderately or to become social drinkers.

Excessive alcohol use may be in response to the tremendous stress that the Cambodian immigrant is experiencing. There is a very high incidence of mental health issues, especially posttraumatic stress disorder (University of North Carolina, 2012). Although many Cambodian immigrants have been exposed to traumatic situations prior to entering the United States, which has resulted in significant mental health issues, there is a tremendous reluctance to seek help from Western mental health services.

Impact of Social Organization

A high value is placed on the family unit (Bankston, 2012). Elderly family members are cared for in the home (placement of an elderly family member in a nursing home or assisted living facility is extremely rare) (University of North Carolina, 2012). Family needs always take top priority. The male is the head of the household, providing income and making the important decisions. The female is to keep house and rear the children. Because of the Khmer Rouge holocaust, there are more females than males. This has resulted in the development of some female-headed households (where the female is separated from her spouse or widowed). The shortage of Cambodian men has resulted in some

Table 7–5 Cultural Nursing Implications When Caring for Asian/Pacific Islander Patients

Group	Nursing Implications
Laotians	Avoid touching the head or shoulders during assessment.
	Always provide for modesty, especially with female patients.
	Respect for the patient, family, and culture is essential.
	Ensure confidentiality. Remember the patient will be reluctant to share health information. It may take some time to establish a rapport before the patient feels comfortable sharing personal or health information.
	Laotians, in general, prefer to avoid conflict and are unlikely to show signs of anger even when displeased or annoyed.
	If they are not satisfied with their nursing or health care, they will not complain but will go elsewhere.
	When asked a question or given a command to follow, they may say "yes" even if they really mean "no."
	It is helpful to use open-ended questions that cannot be answered with a simple "yes" or "no" in order to ensure accuracy.
	One of the most important things that the nurse must do is always offer respect. This is demonstrated by being polite, courteous, and friendly, and having good manners.
Japanese	The patient will listen attentively to patient education but will not ask clarifying questions.
	Remember that silence does not mean agreement.
	When providing education, remember that the Japanese believe that illness is out of their control. Therefore, they do not place an emphasis on personal control and may not be open to lifestyle modification for disease prevention.
	They greatly value guidance from the nurse and other healthcare team members regarding health-related issues; in general they are not proponents of patient autonomy.
	Avoid physical touch as it may result in role confusion and cause the patient anxiety.
	They prefer formality and structure. The nurse should keep this in mind when planning for nursing interventions.
	Avoid intense or prolonged eye contact. Patience is an important skill to utilize when providing nursing care.
Vietnamese	Ensure that patient education stresses the importance of compliance with all prescribed interventions, especially with medications and antibiotic therapy as the patient may not complete the dose and may store the medication for later use.
	They may also self-adjust medication doses because of the belief that the medications are "too strong" for their body build.
	There is the concern that oral medications can throw the body out of "balance."

Anticipate fear and resistance to cooperating with laboratory and diagnostic testing. They believe blood loss can exacerbate the illness and cannot be replaced because of the illness.

Surgery is particularly feared and will only be considered as a last resort.

Koreans	Prolonging life is seen as unacceptable, so DNR orders are not considered.
	Discussing terminal status is unacceptable.
	Organ donation and transplantation are seen as a disturbance in the integrity of the body.
	Kimchi is considered the national dish and is served at virtually every meal. Made from cabbage, turnips, radishes, or cucumber, kimchi can be prepared many ways, from mild to very spicy. If dietary restrictions permit, allow the patient's family to bring this to the patient.
	Korean Americans are often comfortable with silence, according to Confucius's belief that "silence is golden." Small talk could appear senseless and insincere.
	In the Korean culture, the physician's social role can be extremely powerful. Families trust the physician and do not question other options.
	The sharing of thoughts, feelings, and ideas is very much based on age, gender, and status in the Korean society. The Korean American community might value age over youth, men over women, and the group over the individual.
Chinese	The patient may be reluctant to disclose the use of alternative treatments.
	Many Chinese will assume the "sick role" and rely on others for care/assistance.
	To appear caring, the nurse should stand close to the patient, speak sympathetically, take an interest in the patient, and verbally encourage them.
	Do not mistake silence for agreement. There is a reluctance to say "no."
	The Chinese are shy and will be reluctant to talk to an outsider about their health or psychosocial problems.
	Try not to be too assertive. Assertiveness can be interpreted as aggressive or even hostile.
	Avoid touching the head unless absolutely essential. If it must be done, inform the patient first and ask for permission. Avoid touching children, as "careless" touching is believed to be damaging. Again, the nurse should request permission and explain the reason why touch is required.

Source: Adapted from: Blanchette, P. L. (2001). Health and healthcare for Asians and Pacific Islander American elders. Retrieved from http://www.stanford.edu/group/ethnoger/apiaintroduction.html

cross-cultural arranged marriages, but this is not generally accepted within the majority Cambodian culture. Children are treated differently based on gender. The role of the girl child is to stay home and help her mother, whereas boys are allowed more freedom and can participate in activities outside the home. Marriages are generally arranged but disagreement over this practice is causing conflict among second- and third-generation Cambodian immigrants and their families. Gambling and betting are activities that traditionally have been enjoyed (University of North Carolina, 2012).

Impact of Faith and Spirituality

The primary religion in Cambodia is Buddhism (Bankston, 2012). There are a small number of Cambodians who are Muslim or Christian. Most Cambodian immigrants follow Buddhist practices, recognize Buddhist holidays, and actively participate in Buddhist rituals.

VIETNAMESE AMERICANS

Vietnam is a part of Southeast Asia, making up approximately half of the Malay Peninsula. There was a protracted military conflict in Vietnam. In 1975, the communist troops invaded most of Southeast Asia (Vietnam, Cambodia, and Laos). The United States began to admit refugees from these three countries. The need to depart suddenly may have resulted in psychological stress, trauma, and physical complaints. The Vietnamese compose the largest population of Southeast Asian refugees that have settled in the United States. There was a large influx of Vietnamese "boat people" in the late 1970s, which resulted in the passage of the Refugee Resettlement Act of 1980 (InfoPlease.com, 2012).

It is interesting to note that there are cultural differences between North and South Vietnam. A region of Vietnam was once part of Cambodia, so many of its inhabitants are ethnic Cambodian and speak Khmer. Other ethnic identities exist, including the Cham, a Muslim group, and the tribal people of the southern highlands (the Montagnards), who maintain a separate cultural identity from the Vietnamese.

Vietnamese Traditional Health Beliefs

The diagnosis of illness is frequently attributed to three different models. The Vietnamese believe illness can come from spiritual causes, an imbalance (similar to the yin and yang in Chinese culture), and Western medicine (concept of diseases being caused by germs) (Gordon, Bernadett, & Evans, 2012). Traditional

Vietnamese medicine is based on the elements of air, fire, water, earth, and metal, with associated characteristics of cold, hot, wet, and dry. Elements must be kept in balance, similar to Chinese traditions of yin/yang and hot/cold. A sweet rice porridge is often given to the ill. Dermabrasion is often used to treat a cough. Cupping is used as a treatment for fever reduction and balance, and it may leave marks on the skin that can be mistaken as abuse (Gordon et al., 2012).

The Vietnamese view Western medicine or American health care as a way to relieve symptoms. When seeking medical care, the expectation is that they will be prescribed something to cure their illness immediately. The Vietnamese frequently discontinue medicines after their symptoms disappear because they feel that if they do not experience any symptoms, there is no illness (Gordon et al., 2012). This can make chronic disease management very difficult. Patient education must place an emphasis on the need to continue therapy, stressing that chronic disease requires long-term medication management and that symptom remission is not equivalent to a cure. Another safety concern is the fact that it is quite common for Vietnamese patients to save large quantities of half-used prescription drugs for another use. This can be extremely dangerous with infection management. Patient education must stress the importance of completing the full course of prescribed antibiotics.

Medicines are viewed as causing imbalance, which may also be another barrier to compliance. The Vietnamese prefer traditional alternatives, such as a balm, which may better meet the patient's needs while incorporating their cultural values (Gordon et al., 2012). The Vietnamese have concerns about Western medicine, believing that it was developed for Americans and Europeans and not Asians. They feel the dosages are too strong and often will self-adjust the prescribed dosage to compensate for this belief.

The Vietnamese hold great respect for those with education, and this is especially true of physicians. The physician is considered the expert on health. The expectations of health restoration are difficult to achieve because they desire a diagnosis and treatment to require just one visit, and they do not want much time spent on physical examination, or any time spent on laboratory or other diagnostic procedures. Laboratory procedures involving the drawing of blood are feared and even resisted by Vietnamese, who believe that blood loss will exacerbate their illness and that their body cannot replace what was lost (La Borde, 1996). Surgery is particularly feared for this reason and will be agreed to only as a last resort (Gordon et al., 2012).

In conclusion, Vietnamese people will combine all treatment elements—both traditional healing and Western medicine—in order to achieve maximum benefit. The culture is strongly influenced by China.

Impact of Communication

The Vietnamese language is shared by most people from Vietnam except for isolated minorities such as Montagnards. Dialects vary between north and south and also between rural and urban areas (Bankston, 2012).

Communication is subtle and repetitive. Courtesy is important, and smiling is common. Smiling, therefore, should not indicate to the nurse that the patient is happy or in agreement with what is being said (La Borde, 1996). The Vietnamese American may laugh at things that may be deemed inappropriate by other cultures, because laughing is not reflective of something being funny or humorous but rather a reflection of disharmony or conflict (La Borde, 1996). Pointing and gesturing can be interpreted as rude.

It is important to not publicly criticize or correct a Vietnamese American as this can cause them to lose face.

Impact of Environment

Many distinguishing cultural factors have been lost to the passage of time since the huge influx of Vietnamese refugees in the 1970s. Today, some Vietnamese Americans are third generation. Earlier immigrants were factory workers but since then, many Vietnamese have moved into technology, education, and business (Bankston, 2012). Prevalent Vietnamese businesses include restaurants, grocery stores, video stores, nail salons, and gift shops.

Biologic Variations

Many Vietnamese Americans are Amerasians, children born in Vietnam to Vietnamese women and American men during the Vietnam War. More than 100,000 immigrants were Amerasians. There is not much focus on exercise, but a healthy diet is the norm. A large part of the diet consists of meat, fish, vegetables, and rice (Gordon et al., 2012).

Impact of Social Organization

Family is the primary social organization (La Borde, 1996). Families often live in multigenerational or extended housing and great respect is provided to the elders. The eldest male is the head of the household. While handshaking is acceptable, elder Vietnamese prefer to bow the head.

Impact of Faith and Spirituality

Many of the early Vietnamese refugees were Roman Catholic and well educated because they worked closely with the government of the United States (Bankston, 2012). Later refugees were more diverse.

Buddhism, especially Mahayana Buddhism, which is heavily influenced by Chinese tradition, is the prevalent religion of the country (Bankston, 2012). The Buddhism of the Khmer is different and is part of the Theravada tradition connected to India. Roman Catholicism, although a minority religion, has also been influential because of the history of colonialism by the French and the political structures that grew out of that. Another popular religion is Cao Dai, prevalent primarily in regions of South Vietnam.

The Lunar New Year is known as *Tet Nguyen Dan*. It occurs at the beginning of the year between January and February, and it is usually treated as a community celebration regardless of religious affiliation or faith commitment. Another important celebration is *Tet Moon*. It is usually celebrated around September and its significance is to remind children to be obedient and honest.

ASIAN INDIAN AMERICANS

India is a peninsula and is the most populous country in south Asia. The population of approximately 1.22 billion is second only to China (IndiaOnline.com, 2012). It is populated by a diverse group of ethnicities, languages, and religions.

Most Asian Indians migrated to the United States for educational or economic reasons. In general, the more educated or affluent Indians are the ones that visit or emmigrate to the United States. Effort is spent on maintaining close ties with family and loved ones who remain in India.

Impact of Communication

The Indian government recognizes 15 national languages (Gordon et al., 2012). The most common is Hindi, followed by English (Gordon et al., 2012). There are hundreds of dialects in India. The English language is commonly used for national and commercial needs. Because India was ruled by Great Britain for more than 100 years (British control was relinquished in 1947), the English spoken is "British English." Some of the vocabulary is different from "American English." India is a multilingual country with over 300 dialects. About 24 of these dialects are spoken by over 1 million people. This diversity is reflected in the Asian Indian community in America. First-generation Indians continue to speak their native language within the family—with spouses, members of the extended family, and friends within the community. Most also speak English fluently, which has made the transition to American society easier for many Indian immigrants.

Regional differences are prevalent. Hindi is spoken mostly by immigrants from northern India and is generally not spoken by Indians from the south. Immigrants from the states of southern India speak regional languages like Tamil, Telegu, or

Malayalam. A substantial number of immigrants from western India, particularly those from the state of Gujarat, continue to speak Gujarati, whereas those from the region of Bengal speak Bengali. Most second- and third-generation Asian Indians understand the language spoken by their parents and extended family, but tend not to speak it themselves. Many Indians are multilingual and speak several Indian languages.

Impact of Faith and Spirituality

Two sovereign nations developed at the end of British rule of British India: India and Pakistan. This was a result of the irreconcilable differences between the Hindu and Muslim religions. India became the land of the Hindus and Pakistan the land of the Muslims. Today's India is a secular nation, although there is growing political unrest and a push to restore India as the land of the Hindus (Pavri, 2000).

The two primary religions of Indian Americans are Hinduism (approximately 80%) (Gordon et al., 2012) and Muslim (approximately 12%), with a small number of followers of Christianity, Sikhism, Buddhism, Jainism, Zoroastrianism, and Judaism. Jains follow the doctrine of *ahimsa* (nonviolence); they are vegetarian because of their refusal to kill animals. For more on traits of the different religions of Asian Indians, see **Box 7–1**.

Religion plays a part in burial and funeral rites. There is a preference for Hindus to die at home and many prefer to return to India while dying (Gordon et al., 2012). After priests offer prayers, the Hindu dead are cremated (Gordon et al., 2012). In India, the cremation traditionally takes place on a wooden pyre, and the body, which is often dressed in gold-ornamented clothing, burns over several hours. This is in contrast to electric cremation in the United States. Asian Indian Muslims are buried in cemeteries according to Islamic tradition and Christians are buried in accordance with Christian tradition.

Impact of Social Organization

Family is an important construct, and Indian families tend to be large and multi-generational (Gordon et al., 2012). Extended family may all live together in the same house or in close proximity and rely on each other for childcare. Public displays of affection are avoided as love and affection are only expressed in private. Problems in communication can occur because Indians may shake their head from side to side (usually indicating "no" in Western culture) to mean "yes." Other body language of interest is that pointing is considered rude, and to beckon someone, the palm should be turned down.

Box 7–1 Characteristics of the Religions of Asian Indians

Religion	Characteristics
Hinduism	Functionally polytheistic, but philosophically monotheistic.
	Less formally organized than other religions, as prayer meetings can be held in individual homes.
Islam	*Islam* means "submission to God."
	One who adheres to Islam is called a Muslim.
	Belief in the prophet Muhammad, whom the angel Gabriel ordered to spread the word of God in 610 AD.
	Muhammad recorded the revelations in the holy book, the Koran.
	There are five pillars (requirements) of Islam: (1) confess that there is "no god but God," and that Muhammad is the messenger of God; (2) pray five times daily; (3) give of alms; (4) fast in daylight hours for the Muhammadan month of Ramadan; and (5) pilgrimage to Mecca at least once in a lifetime.
Sikhism	Sikhism is different from Hinduism in its belief in one God.
	Sikhs follow the teachings of Guru Nanak, the founder of the religion, and worship in temples called Gurudwaras (Gurudwaaras). Services in Gurudwaras are held about once a week, as well as on religious occasions. Tenets of Sikhism include wearing a turban on the head for males and a symbolic bangle called a *Kara* around their wrists. In addition, Sikh males are required to not cut their hair or beards. This custom is still followed by many in the community; others choose to give up the wearing of the turban and cut their hair.

Source: Adapted from: The Pew Forum on Religion and Public Life. Retrieved from http://www.pewforum.org/Asian-Americans-A-Mosaic-of-Faiths-overview.aspx

---

Asians Indians are divided into castes, and a child belongs to the caste of his parents (EveryCulture.com, 2012). The caste placement has implications for everything: social standing, education, career, and marriage. Marriage is influenced by region and religion in addition to the caste system and is often arranged. Despite the discrimination associated with a caste system, tolerance and diversity are central to Indian culture. India is considered the largest democracy in the world.

Asian Indians are an extremely ethnically diverse group. The subgroups trace their roots to different regions or states within India, each of which speak different languages, eat different diets, and follow unique customs. On festive occasions, you may expect to see female Asian Indians wearing the traditional sari (yards of colorfully embroidered or printed silk or cotton wrapped around the body) or a bindi (a dot placed on the forehead), which may indicate that the woman is married but may also be worn at celebrations. Jewelry is also valued in the culture. Indians are very fond of gold jewelry, and many women wear simple gold ornaments like rings, earrings, bangles, and necklaces daily, and more elaborate ones at special occasions. Jewelry is often passed down through the generations from mother to daughter or daughter-in-law.

Asian Indian Traditional Health Beliefs

Most Asian Indians accept the role of Western medicine and pay careful attention to health matters. Despite this, ayurvedic medicine continues to have many adherents.

Ayurveda emphasizes spiritual healing as an essential component of physical healing and bases its cures on herbs and natural ingredients such as raw garlic and ginger (Gordon et al., 2012). Ayurveda also focuses on preventive healing. Homeopathic medicine also has adherents among Asian Indians in the United States. Some members of the Asian Indian American community practice yoga. The ancient practice of yoga dates back several thousand years. It combines a routine of exercise and meditation to maintain the balance between body and mind.

There is a stigma associated with mental health disorders, and Asian Indians are less inclined to seek out assistance for mental health problems than they are for physical health problems (Leung, Cheung, & Tsui, 2011). The traditional Indian belief has been that mental problems will eventually take care of themselves, and that the family rather than outside experts should take care of the mentally ill.

JAPANESE AMERICANS

Japan is a country of islands located in the Pacific Ocean. Japan is composed of four large islands and approximately 4,000 small islands (Easton & Ellington, 2000). In addition to the ban on immigration for all Asians between 1924 and 1950, there was a tremendous injustice perpetrated against Japanese Americans as a result of World War II. In 1942, anyone of Japanese ancestry living on the Pacific Coast was placed in a relocation camp (Easton & Ellington, 2000). Descendents of the survivors of this internment may have psychological issues. Many Japanese who seek out health care may be in the United States temporarily, studying or working for Japanese-owned corporations.

Japanese Traditional Health Beliefs

The Japanese believe that the body is as holy as the mind. In fact, Japanese tradition views the mind and body as one. Japanese people are very reluctant to accept the diagnosis of being brain dead (Haldane, 2006). Stating that the person is "dead" could be viewed as disrespectful.

Organ donation can be a very difficult topic to broach because many Japanese are unwilling to alter the dead body of a person who they feel could influence their lives in the future (Haldane, 2006). Agreeing to donate one's organs could cause concern that the oneness of body and soul might be destroyed. The issues are not only related to donation of the organs but also to accepting a transplant (Haldane, 2006). There is also concern about whether the patient would benefit from organ transplantation. Accepting the organs of a dead person could be seen as disrespectful by some Japanese and could trigger anxiety.

Japanese individuals will probably listen well during health education, but they may be reluctant to ask a question or add a comment, because individual assertion is highly discouraged in their culture. They may be reluctant to bring up anything they believe would cause a conflict and would not share a differing opinion. Be careful not to assume that silence means agreement with the plan of care, as it may just be the patient's way of avoiding a conflict.

Japanese culture does not place an emphasis on personal control, so they may be more likely to view an illness as something outside their own control (McLaughlin & Braun, 1998). Therefore, healthcare providers will need to keep this in mind when educating Japanese Americans about risk factors for a particular disease (such as a fatty diet being a risk factor for heart disease).

U.S. healthcare delivery is based on the premise of patient autonomy and patient choice. Patient choice is not a value of the Japanese. It is for this reason that the Japanese patient will greatly require and appreciate guidance from physicians, nurses, and other healthcare team members.

Impact of Touch

Nurses and other healthcare professionals should avoid physical touching, which may cause anxiety in the Japanese (McLaughlin & Braun, 1998). Because the Japanese view health professionals as authority figures, physical touching may cause role confusion. Careful explanation of all interventions, especially when touch is required, should always be provided. The nurse should also consider the amount of eye contact they are providing. To show respect, the nurse should avoid intense or long-term eye contact. Patience is an important skill and will be helpful when dealing with the Japanese.

FILIPINO AMERICANS

Filipino Americans now rank as the second largest Asian group in the United States, with over 3.4 million individuals reported in the 2010 census. The current census reveals a tremendous growth in the Filipino American population from earlier census studies. It is felt that this tremendous growth is caused by the search of Filipinos for economic opportunity and the political relationship between the governments of the United States and the Philippines (U.S. Census Bureau, 2010).

Emmigration from the Philippines to the American continent began with the Manila–Acapulco Galleon Trade. From 1565 to 1815, Filipinos were forced to work as navigators and sailors on Spanish ships (NationsOnline.org, 2012). In 1587, Filipino sailors claimed Morro Bay, California, for the Spanish king. In 1763, the first permanent settlement occurred in the bayous of Louisiana. These early settlers, called "Manilamen," settled in Louisiana after jumping ship to escape the brutality they had experienced from their Spanish masters. They built houses on stilts along the gulf ports of New Orleans, Louisiana (NationsOnline.org, 2012).

Today, one in five foreign-born Filipinos arrived in the United States in the year 2000 or later (Terrazas, 2009). In addition, Filipinos are most likely to become naturalized citizens of the United States than any other minority group; with 62.8% compared to 42.1% (Terrazas, 2008).

In Philippine society, Pilipino or Tagalog is the national language, and English is the second official language (McBride, 2012). Although 80 to 100 ethnic languages are spoken in this country of 7,000 islands, English is used to conduct internal and global business. Among Filipino Americans, a combination of English/Tagalog, or "Tag-Lish," a hybrid language, is spoken by many and is used extensively. More than two-thirds of households speak a non-English language.

Health Status

It is difficult to determine the health status of Filipinos because of the limited number of studies that have been conducted. Often, Asians are grouped together or there are other inconsistencies in coding for race or ethnicity. Therefore, it is not always possible to distinguish Filipinos from the rest of the AAPI sample. Moreover, it is difficult to generalize research findings because the sample size is too small, few studies have been done, or the only populations studied are in California or Hawaii. Finally, in some cases, data are just not available. For these reasons, the information contained in this section of the chapter is based on an estimate of Filipino American health status based on the limited data available.

The National Health Interview Survey (conducted between 1992 and 1994) revealed that 37% of the Filipino respondents described their health as excellent, 32% as very good, 24% as good, and 7% as fair or poor. These results are very similar to those for other APPIs (Kuo & Porter, 1997).

It does appear that high blood pressure is an issue for Filipino Americans, as Filipinos living in the Philippines tend to have lower blood pressure. It appears that the excessive sodium intake associated with the American diet may be responsible. In addition to hypertension, Filipino immigrants are also considered at high risk for coronary artery disease, adult-onset diabetes mellitus, gout, and cancer. High rates of hyperuricemia and gout are found among men, particularly in low- to middle-income groups in the Philippines.

Filipino women have been shown to have a high rate of gestational diabetes. Filipino mothers born outside of the United States are significantly more likely to have diabetes during pregnancy. Very low birth weight (500–1499 g) and moderately low birth weight (1500–2499 g) was more likely among Filipino women than Whites.

Cancer is the second leading cause of death among Filipino Americans (Hoyert & Kung, 1997). The prevalence of some cancers seems to vary depending on place of birth. Rates of primary liver cancer were higher for foreign-born Filipino men than American-born Filipino men (11% to 7%), and both were higher than Whites (3%).

Filipino women born in the Philippines had 3.2 times the rate of thyroid cancer of U.S.-born White women, whereas U.S.-born Filipino women were not at any increased risk compared to White women. For other cancers, prevalence does not seem to depend on place of birth.

Ovarian cancer incidence among U.S.-born Filipino women is comparable to foreign-born Filipino women (8.1 versus 11.0 per 100,000), and lower than in White women (15.6 per 100,000). Breast cancer incidence was the same for U.S.- and foreign-born Filipino women, and 40% lower than breast cancer incidence of U.S.-born Whites.

There are other disparities in cancer prevalence. The incidence of liver cancer in Filipino populations is higher than among Caucasians.

Filipino men born in the Philippines had 2.6 times the rate of thyroid cancer of U.S.-born White men, whereas U.S.-born Filipino men had 1.5 times the risk of White men.

Breast cancer is a concern and there appear to be regional differences in incidence. Filipino women in Hawaii had the lowest risk at 29 per 100,000 (Goodman & Segal, 1991), whereas women 40 years and older in the San Francisco Bay Area had an age-adjusted risk of 119 per 100,000, much higher than Black, Chinese, and Japanese women, but lower than Whites (Northern California Cancer Center [NCCC], 1993b). Filipino women had the lowest survival rate of the five groups except Blacks. Bay Area Filipino women had higher overall age-adjusted cancer incidence for all sites than the other groups except Whites (NCCC, 1993b). Rates in the Bay Area Filipino men for age-adjusted incidence of cancer in all sites are lower than most of the five groups compared, but higher than Chinese and Japanese (NCCC, 1993a). Liver cancer among Filipino men and women was second only to the Chinese and three times higher than among Whites (NCCC, 1993a, 1993b).

The Philippines is reported to have the highest incidence of TB in the world (McBride, 2012). Filipino World War II veterans were permitted a rapid entry into the United States in the 1990s, which waived the need for a physical examination. It is felt that this may explain the increased incidence of TB in this population. Infectious diseases are a major health issues for AAPIs as AAPIs have greater incidence rates of TB and hepatitis B than any other ethnic or racial group.

Impact of Social Organization

The Filipino values of interdependence and social cohesiveness may have evolved from the group orientation necessary to live in an archipelago of 7,000 islands located in the ring of fire, where only 1,000 islands are habitable (McBride, 2012). This may partly explain the existence of hundreds of Filipino American organizations across the United States.

Impact of Faith and Spirituality

An estimated 92.5% are Christians, of which 80% are Catholics (Stanford. edu, 2012). The remainder are made up of members of Protestant churches; the Aglipay, a church whose origin is in the Philippines; and Filipino Muslims, who originate primarily from Mindanao and Sulu, the southernmost region of the country, where successful resistance to Spanish colonization led to preservation of their culture and traditions (Stanford.edu, 2012). Collectively, the sociocultural, psychological, economic, and political legacy of the precolonial Filipino tribes was congruent with those of Islander people in the Pacific Rim.

PACIFIC ISLANDER AMERICANS

In reality, there is no such thing as one AAPI composite, especially when there are more differences than similarities among the many groups designated by the federally defined categories of Asian American and Pacific Islander. Although there are varied and historical reasons for reporting these groups under one umbrella, it is critical for nurses to recognize that there are numerous AAPI ethnicities, many historical backgrounds, and a full range of socioeconomic spectra, from the poor and underprivileged to the affluent and highly educated. There is no simple description that can characterize AAPI patients or communities as a whole.

Statistics

In the 2010 census, a total of 540,000 people, or 0.2% of the total population, reported that they belonged to the Native Hawaiian and other Pacific Islander population (U.S. Census Bureau, 2012). More than half of the Native Hawaiian and other Pacific Islanders identified as belonging to multiple races (U.S. Census Bureau, 2012). Over half of all Native Hawaiian and other Pacific Islanders live in two states: Hawaii and California (U.S. Census Bureau, 2012).

SUMMARY

AAPIs are one of the fastest growing ethnic groups. The nurse will encounter patients from this group. Because of the variety and complexity of cultural values and health beliefs, the nurse must strive to learn about these values and beliefs and then strive to provide individualized patient care. The nursing care should be formulated to consider the impact of barriers to care such as communication, time and space, social organization, and biologic variations. Comprehensive and holistic care can only be delivered when the cultural values and beliefs of the patient are incorporated and considered.

CASE STUDY 7–1

Vietnamese Woman with Complaint of Dizziness

A 70-year-old Vietnamese woman accompanied by her two adult children presented to the emergency room with a complaint of dizziness. During the examination, emergency room physician noted deep red welts running up both of the patient's arms. Alarmed, the physician requested that the nurse contact social services with a suspicion of elder abuse. Luckily, the nurse had had cultural competency training and was familiar with the Vietnamese custom of coin rubbing. When the nurse questioned the patient's son, he told the nurse that he had rubbed his mother's body with a coin in an attempt to heal her. The woman was properly diagnosed with labyrinthitis, and because coin rubbing is not harmful to the patient, it was included in the treatment plan. The patient was discharged home, where she recovered.

REVIEW QUESTIONS

1. What should the nurse know about coin rubbing to prevent an incorrect accusation of abuse?
2. Should coin rubbing be included in a culturally competent plan of nursing care for the Vietnamese or Asian patient?

Rationale: The patient's family was practicing a traditional form of healing known as coin rubbing. There are several variations, including heating the coin, but they all involve vigorously rubbing the body with a coin. This produces red welts, which can distract medical staff from the real problem or be mistaken for elder or child abuse. It is important for the nurse to recognize and become familiar with this practice, and not to be distracted from the real problem or mistakenly make accusations of abuse.

Asians rubbing their children, their elders, or themselves with coins is not abuse as it is an attempt to heal an illness, and it is often effective.

CASE STUDY 7–2

Critically Ill Korean Patient

A 27-year-old Korean man was visiting extended family in the United States when he became very ill. He was brought to the emergency room by his concerned family. The patient was diagnosed with renal and respiratory failure and an order was written for strict bed rest to limit his exertion. The patient speaks very little English and the family speaks only a minimal amount of English. This made communication difficult for all involved. Frequently, conflict would erupt when a staff member would find the patient, with assistance from his family, standing over a bedpan attempting bowel elimination. The staff would interrupt and tell the patient and his family that the patient was not permitted out of bed and that the bedpan was to be used in the bed. This was difficult to convey because of the language barrier and the patient and his family would become very upset. The nurse educator for the hospital was consulted as she had expertise in cultural competency. She explained to the staff that the patient was using the bedpan in the only way that he knew because in most Asian countries, toilets are holes in the ground. To eliminate from the bowels, the Asian squats over the hole, just like the patient was attempting to do with the bedpan. The nurse called the nurse practitioner who changed the order to permit the patient out of bed for bathroom privileges as needed with assistance. The patient and his family were much happier and more cooperative as a result.

REVIEW QUESTIONS

1. Develop a culturally competent plan of care for the Korean/Asian patient that supports ADLs and cultural beliefs while maintaining patient safety.

Rationale: In Asian culture, bowel elimination is unclean and should not be done in bed. The patient and his family were trying to maintain standards of cleanliness and decency. Knowledge of cultural practices permitted the treatment plan to be safely modified so that the patient and his family could manage this bodily function in an appropriate manner.

REFERENCES

Acupuncture. (2009). In *Natural Standard Database*. Retrieved from http://www.natural standard.com

Bankston, C. (2012a). *Cambodian Americans*. Retrieved from http://www.everyculture.com/multi/Bu-Dr/Cambodian-Americans.html

Bankston, C. (2012b). *Vietnamese Americans*. Retrieved from http://www.everyculture.com/multi/Sr-Z/Vietnamese-Americans.html

Barnes, P. M., Powell-Griner, E., McFann, K., & Nahin, R. L. (2004). Complementary and alternative medicine use among adults: United States, 2002. *Advance data from vital and health statistics, no. 343*. Hyattsville, MD: National Center for Health Statistics.

BBC.com. (2012). *North Korea profile*. Retrieved from http://www.bbc.co.uk/news/world-asia-pacific-15278612

Beller, T., Pinker, M., Snapka, S., & Van Dusen, D. (2012). *Koreans*. Retrieved from https://bearspace.baylor.edu/Charles_Kemp/www/korean_health.htm

Benlafquih, C. (2009). *Al-Hijaham: Cupping and bloodletting in Islam*. Retrieved from http://suite101.com/article/alhijamah-cupping-and-bloodletting-in-islam-a109197

Cardini, F., & Weixin, H. (1998). Moxibustion for correction of breech presentation: A randomized controlled trial. *Journal of the American Medical Association, 280*(18), 1580–1584.

Chen, M. S. (2000). Launching of the Asian American Network for Cancer Awareness, Research and Training (AANCART). *Asian American and Pacific Islander Journal of Health, 8*(1), 1–3.

Chinese Historical and Cultural Project. (2002). *Chinese numerology*. Retrieved from http://www.chcp.org/numbers.html

Chou, F. (2009). *Potty-training infants: An ancient Chinese secret*. Retrieved from http://nacd.org/newsletter/0409_pottytraining.php

CIA World Factbook. (2012). China demographics profile 2012. Retrieved from http://www.indexmundi.com/china/demographics_profile.html

Coyle, M. E., Smith, C. A., & Peat, B. (2005). Cephalic version by moxibustion for breech presentation. *Cochrane Database of Systematic Reviews, 2*, CD003928.

CultureCrossing.net. (2012). *Cambodia*. Retrieved from http://www.culturecrossing.net/basics_business_student_details.php?Id=9&CID=35

Curran, M. A. (2002). *Cambodian Americans*. Retrieved from http://personal.uncc.edu/macurran/2002/webproject/asi.htm

Dharmananda, S. (1999). *Cupping*. Retrieved from Institute for Traditional Medicine website: http://www.itmonline.org/arts/cupping.htm

Ergil K. V., Kramer, E. J., Ng, A. T. (2002). *Chinese herbal medicines. Western Journal of Medicine, 176,* 275–279; Xie, Z. (2000). *Practical traditional Chinese medicine.* Beijing, China: Foreign Languages Press.

Easton, S. E., & Ellington, L. (2000). Japanese Americans. *Gale Encyclopedia of Multicultural America.* Retrieved from Encyclopedia.com: http://www.encyclopedia.com/doc/1G2-3405800094.html

EveryCulture.com. (2012). *Countries and their culture: India.* Retrieved from http://www.everyculture.com/Ge-It/India.html

Gailliard, T. (2011). *Role of family in Chinese culture.* Retrieved from http://www.ehow.com/about_6426341_role-family-chinese-culture.html

Ghosh, C. (2003). Healthy People 2010 and Asian Americans/Pacific Islanders: Defining a baseline of information. *American Journal of Public Health, 93*(12), 2093–2098.

Giger, J. N. (2013). *Transcultural nursing: Assessment and intervention* (6th ed.). Salt Lake City, UT: Elsevier.

Goodman, D. S., & Segal, G. (Eds.). (1991). *China in the nineties: Crisis management and beyond.* New York, NY: Oxford University Press.

Gordon, S., Bernadett, M., Evans, D., Bernadett Shapiro, N., & Patel, U. (2012). *Vietnamese culture: Influences and implications for health care.* Retrieved from http://www.molinahealthcare.com/medicaid/providers/common/pdf/vietnamese%20culture%20-%20influences%20and%20implications%20for%20health%20care_material%20and%20test.pdf?E=true

Haldane, M. (2006). *Cultural concepts of brain death and transplants.* Retrieved from http://www.mcgill.ca/reporter/34/09/lock/

Hall, E. T. (1963). A system for the notation of proxemic behavior. *American Anthropologist, 65*(5), 1003–1026.

Harris, P. M., & Jones, N. A. (2005). *We the people: Pacific Islanders in the United States. Census 2000 special reports.* Washington, DC: U.S. Census Bureau.

Hays, J. (2011). *Chinese people and DNA.* Retrieved from http://factsanddetails.com/china.php?itemid=118&catid=4&subcatid=18

Herbert Hoover Presidential Library. (2012). *Chinese Americans.* Retrieved from http://hoover.archives.gov/exhibits/China/Chinese_Americans/index.html

Hoyert, D. L., & Kung, H. C. (1997). Asian or Pacific Islander mortality, selected states, 1992. *Monthly Vital Statistics Report, 46*(1 Suppl.). Hyattsville, MD: National Center for Health Statistics.

Huff, R., & Kline, M. (1999). *Promoting health in multicultural populations: A handbook for practitioners.* Thousand Oaks, CA: Sage.

Indiaonline.com. (2012). India's population 2012. Retrieved from http://www.indiaonlinepages.com/population/india-current-population.html

InfoPlease.com. (2012). Vietnam. Retrieved from http://www.infoplease.com/ipa/A0108144.html

International Diabetes Foundation. (IDF). Retrieved from www.idf.org

Kraig, B. (2011). Hidden Korea. Retrieved from http://www.pbs.org/hiddenkorea/history.htm

Kuo, J., & Porter, K. (1997). Health Status of Asian Americans: United States, 1992–1994. *Advance data from vital and health statistics, no. 298.* Hyattsville, MD: National Center for Health Statistics.

La Borde, P. (1996, updated 2010). *Vietnamese cultural profile.* Retrieved from http://ethnomed.org/culture/vietnamese/vietnamese-cultural-profile

Lee, J. J. (2006). *The partition of Korea after World War II: A global history.* New York, NY: Palgrave MacMillan.

Leung, P., Cheung, M., & Tsui, V. (2011). Asian Indians and depressive symptoms: Reframing mental health help-shaping behaviors. *International Journal of Social Work, 55*(1), 53–70.

Library of Congress. (2012). *Chinese immigration to the United States, 1851–1900.* Retrieved from http://www.loc.gov/teachers/classroommaterials/presentationsandactivities/presentations/timeline/riseind/chinimms/

McBride, M. (2012). *Health and health care of Filipino American elders.* Retrieved from http://www.stanford.edu/group/ethnoger/filipino.html

McLaughlin, L., & Braun, K. (1998). Asian and Pacific Islander cultural values: Considerations for health care decision-making. *Health and Social Work, 23*(2), 116–126.

Medical News Today. (2009). *What is acupuncture? What are the benefits of acupuncture?* Retrieved from http://www.medicalnewstoday.com/articles/156488.php

Nash, A. (2012). *Countries and their cultures: Korean Americans.* Retrieved from http://www.everyculture.com/multi/Ha-La/Korean-Americans.html

National Center for Complementary and Alternative Medicine. (2011). *What is complementary and alternative medicine?* Retrieved from http://nccam.nih.gov/health/whatiscam

National Center for Health Statistics. (2001). *Health, United States, 2001 urban and rural health chartbook.* Retrieved from http://www.cdc.gov/nchs/data/hus/hus01cht.pdf

NationsOnline.org. (2012). *History of the Phillipines.* Retrieved from http://www.nationsonline.org/oneworld/History/Philippines-history.htm

Northern California Cancer Center. (1993a). *Average annual age-adjusted incidence rates for selected sites, 1986–1990, for men in the San Francisco Bay Area* [Unpublished paper]. Union City, CA: Author.

Northern California Cancer Center. (1993b). *Average annual age-adjusted incidence rates for selected sites, 1986–1990, for women in the San Francisco Bay Area* [Unpublished paper]. Union City, CA: Author.

Office of Management and Budget. (1997). *Revisions to the standards for the classification of federal data on race and ethnicity.* Retrieved from http://www.whitehouse.gov/omb/fedreg_1997standards

Overfield, T. (1995). *Biologic variation in health and illness.* Reading, MA: Addison-Wesley.

Pavri, T. (2000). Asian Indian Americans. *Gale encyclopedia of multicultural America.* New York, NY: Gale Group.

Reference for Business. (2012). *Minority owned businesses.* Retrieved from http://www.referenceforbusiness.com/small/Mail-Op/Minority-Owned-Businesses.html

Rossbach, S. (2000). *Feng Shui: The Chinese art of placement.* New York, NY: Penguin.

Shin, K., Shin, C., & Blanchette, P. L. (2012). *Health and health care of Korean American elders.* Retrieved from http://www.stanford.edu/group/ethnoger/korean.html

Sophia, F. (2003). *Birthdays, those important dates.* Retrieved from http://www.newsfinder.org/site/more/birthdays_those_important_dates/

Stanford.edu. (2012). Religion. Retrieved from http://geriatrics.stanford.edu/ethnomed/filipino/introduction/religion.html

Stockton, P. (2001). *Nutrition and fasting in Cambodian culture.* Retrieved from http://ethnomed.org/clinical/nutrition/nutrition-and-fasting-in-cambodian-culture

Szczepanski, K. (2012). People's Republic of China: Facts and history. Retrieved from http://asianhistory.about.com/od/china/p/ChinaProfile.htm

Terrazas, A. (2008). *Filipino immigrants in the United States.* Retrieved from http://www.migrationinformation.org/usfocus/display.cfm?ID=694

Terrazas. A. (2009). *Korean immigrants in the United States.* Retrieved from http://www.migrationinformation.org/usfocus/display.cfm?ID=716

University of North Carolina. (2012). *Koreans*. Retrieved from http://cnnc.uncg .edu/wp-content/uploads/2012/08/koreans.pdf

U.S. Census Bureau. (2010a). *The Asian Population, 2010: 2010 Census briefs*. Retrieved from http://www.census.gov/prod/cen2010/briefs/c2010br-11.pdf

U.S. Census Bureau. (2010b). Overall census data from 2010 report. Retrieved from http://2010.census.gov/2010census/data/

U.S. Census Bureau. (2010c). Table QT-P8. Retrieved from http://factfinder2.census.gov/ bkmk/table/1.0/en/DEC/10_SF1/QTP8

U.S. Census Bureau. (2012). Updated with 2010 census data. Retrieved from http://www. census.gov/prod/cen2010/briefs/c2010br-12.pdf

U.S. Department of Health and Human Services. (1998). *Tobacco use among US racial/ethnic minority groups—African Americans, American Indians and Alaska Natives, Asian Americans and Pacific Islanders, and Hispanics: A report of the surgeon general*. Atlanta, GA: U.S. Department of Health and Human Services, Centers for Disease Control and Prevention, National Center for Chronic Disease Prevention and Health Promotion, Office on Smoking and Health.

U.S. Department of State, Office of the Historian. (2012). *Milestones: 1945–1952*. Retrieved from http://history.state.gov/milestones/1945-1952/ImmigrationAct

U.S. News and World Report. (2012). The People's vote. 100 documents that shaped America. The Chinese exclusion act. Retrieved from http://www.usnews.com/usnews/documents/ docpages/document_page47.htm

Varner, G. (2008). *The history and use of amulets, charms and talismans*. Raleigh, NC: Lulu Press.

Wang, Y., Tao, Y. Hyman, M. E., Li, J., & Chen, Y. (2009). Osteoporosis in China. *Osteoporosis International, 20*(10), 1651–1662.

Weiss, T. C. (2010). *Overview of disability in China*. Retrieved from http://www.disabled-world .com/news/asia/china/disability-china.php

Wong, C. (2012). *What you need to know about moxibustion*. Retrieved from http://alt medicine.about.com/od/chinesemedicinetcm/a/moxibustion.htm

Xinnong, C. (1987). *Chinese acupuncture and moxibustion*. Beijing, China: Foreign Languages Press.

For a full suite of assignments and additional learning activities, see the access code at the front of your book.

CHAPTER 8

Native Americans

CHAPTER OBJECTIVES

Upon completion of this chapter, the nurse will be able to:

- Describe the traditional health beliefs of Native Americans.
- Develop a plan of care that incorporates those traditional health beliefs within the American healthcare delivery system.
- Be familiar with the history of Native Americans in relation to its impact on the current health status of Native Americans.

© Comstock/Thinkstock

INTRODUCTION

There are at least two ways of learning about Native American culture. The first would be to commit to learning everything about one or two different tribes. This will limit the nurse's knowledge to only those tribes, and the nurse must understand that he or she cannot transfer that knowledge and apply it to another tribe. The second option, and the strategy employed in this chapter, is to learn general aspects of Native American culture that apply to more than one tribe's culture, with the understanding that the knowledge possessed will only be at a very superficial level. The degree of acculturation into the dominant American society and its culture will also impact each individual Native American. There will be numerous exceptions to this knowledge from one Native American culture to another.

HISTORICAL BACKGROUND

Native Americans had lived throughout the North American continent for thousands of years before European settlers came to America in the 15th century. Although still theoretical, most scientists agree that North America was populated by travelers who crossed a land bridge (Beringia) that once spanned the Bering Sea and connected Northeastern Asia to North America (Vergano, 2012). The reasons and motivations for the migration are not known. The first travelers are believed to have arrived over 10,000 years ago, just prior to the last Ice Age. Other scholars, as well as some Native Americans, believe that the ancestors of Native Americans originated in the Americas. This belief is based on oral history that has been passed down through the ages and some gaps found in archaeological records. More recently, a study published in the journal *Nature* has found DNA evidence to support that Native Americans entered America in three distinct waves that began over 15,000 years ago (Reich et al., 2012). The first arrival was the "First American" (Vergano, 2012).

What is not under dispute is the amazing ability of Native Americans to adapt to the climates and terrains of America, and their ability to utilize natural resources. Over many thousands of years, many languages and cultures from the early immigrants' descendents from Asia have developed and spread across North America and, later, South America (Vergano, 2012). According to Reich et al. (2012), most of these descendents came from a single Asian stream that is called First American. The first migration stream was halted by the Ice Age. The second and third migration streams came from Siberia. The Alaska Natives who located in the Arctic and speak the Eskimo–Aleut languages inherited approximately half of their ancestry from the second migration stream. The Na-Dene-speaking Chipewyan, who reside in Canada, inheried approximately one-tenth of their ancestry from the third and final migration stream (Reich et al., 2012).

Culture development and practices were suited to the local environment associated with the distinct geographic region. Each geographic region is made up of climate, landforms, and natural resources. In the Northeast, Native Americans used the forests to build houses, canoes, and tools. Those living in the Pacific Northwest relied on the abundance of fish and other sea life for food. In the desert of the southwest United States, corn was grown and housing developed from adobe (sun-dried brick). In the bitter arctic, adaptation continued and many survived by developing skills in hunting and fishing.

There were several hundred different Native American groups that settled in North America, many of whom still exist and have maintained their distinct culture. Each group has its own unique political structure, social systems, clothing styles, types of shelter and foods, art and musical style, language, education, and spiritual and philosophical beliefs. There are also many similarities, including a strong tie and connection to the Earth and nature.

There is a clear distinction between American Indians and Alaska Natives. The term *Native American* is intended to apply to tribes residing in the continental United States (and does not include Canadian tribes such as the Inuit). One should not believe that all American Indians reside on reservations in rural areas, as this is not correct. According to 2010 U.S. census data there are 2.9 million Americans who identify as Native American or Alaskan Native only. There was a 1.1 million increase in the American Native/Alaska Native population between the 2000 and 2010 census (U.S. Census Bureau, 2011). The majority live in California, followed by Oklahoma and Arizona (U.S. Census Bureau, 2011). There are 15 states that have a population of 100,000 or more Native Americans/Alaska Natives. According to 2010 census data, there are 334 federal- and state-recognized American Indian reservations, excluding Hawaii (U.S. Census Bureau, 2011).

Seventy-eight percent of Native Americans do not live on a reservation; 22% live on federal- or state-designated reservations or off-reservation land trusts (U.S. Census Bureau, 2011).

It is believed by many that the term *Indian* resulted from the belief by the early settlers, under Christopher Columbus, that they were in Asia. *Asia* in Spanish is "the Indies," and the native people were called *indios*, which meant "people of the Indies." Later, that was translated to *Indian*. Others believe the early natives were called "in Dios," which means "of God." The term *Native American* became popular in the 1960s, but critics feel that it really is too broad a term as it could also pertain to Hawaiians, descendents of immigrants, or to anyone born in America.

In many ways, the history of health disparities in the Native American population follows that found in the Black American population. The arrival of European settlers to the New World resulted in many consequences (Lake Champlain Maritime Museum [LCMM] & Wiseman, 2012). The Native American population was drastically reduced due to a wide range of communicable diseases that were brought to America from the crowded European cities of the settlers. Because the Native Americans had no immunity, the diseases spread quickly and lethally. The spread of infection (i.e., measles, smallpox, typhoid) was so profound that infection could spread to a Native American and annihilate an entire Native American community before they had even seen a European settler. Once the European settlers had contact with the natives, sexually transmitted infections also became a large problem. From the 16th century and up to the 20th century, epidemics and pandemics decimated the Native American population (LCMM & Wiseman, 2012).

Other consequences of European settlement were warfare, relocation, and removal of Native Americans from their homeland, and the destruction of traditional Native American ways of life (LCMM & Wiseman, 2012). Barriers to access to their land for hunting and farming resulted in starvation and malnutrition, which increased the likelihood of infections becoming lethal because of a greater susceptibility to disease. Relocation often resulted in the placement of one tribe on the land of another and hostilities often broke out.

Although Native Americans have not suffered the ignominy of slavery, there have been abuses leveled against them by our government. In 1830, America passed the Indian Removal Act (Satz, 2002). This act permitted the forcible removal of Native Americans from their homelands in Florida, Mississippi, Georgia, and Alabama to reservations in the Oklahoma territory. The trail that these native Americans were forced to travel is referred to as the "Trail of Tears" (Satz, 2002). Thousands of Cherokee Indians were killed on the Trail of Tears while being forced westward. After many battles, the Indians were finally forced, on January 31, 1876, onto reservations. Today, many Native Americans continue to live on reservations, although many others do not. There are currently 563 reservations, most of them located in the western states. The reservations are exempt from U.S. laws.

Some natives learned to live together with the European settlers by setting up trade and adopting some European ways. Many more faced turmoil and upheaval that lasted for many generations as Europeans and, later, Americans and Canadians took the land and attempted to extinguish their way of life. During the 20th century and beyond, many Native American tribes started to regain control and are experiencing a cultural resurgence. The population levels also began to increase. It is felt that the population increase is caused by decreased mortality rates, declining disease rates, improved fertility, and more people who are self-identifying as Native American on census forms.

Over the years, many treaties that promised education and healthcare services were signed between the Native Americans and the U.S. government. Provision of health care originally fell to the U.S. Army, which was not equipped to handle this responsibility. In 1955, the Indian Health Service was established (Kuschell-Haworth, 1999).

The Indian Health Service falls under the jurisdiction of the U.S. Department of Health and Human Services and coordinates federally mandated health-related services for Native Americans and Alaska Natives. The 1975 Indian Self-Determination Act allows tribes to manage health services independently if desired (Kuschell-Haworth, 1999).

Two of the most important cultural values that have been identified in Native Americans are resiliency and collaboration. Collaboration provides a force to work with or against the White non-native populations. Native Americans have proven the ability to work with and reside in different environments and with different people. This ability permitted them to learn the ways of the settlers (White people) so they could use this knowledge to guide their interactions. Resiliency is evidenced by, for example, clinging to their native language to overcome linguistic oppression.

Despite these strengths of resiliency and collaboration, today, Native Americans are the poorest, least educated, and most neglected minority group in the United States. By any mathematical standard, reservation-dwelling Native Americans are on the lowest socioeconomic rung in the United States. At least half of reservation dwellers fall under the federal poverty level and continue to survive only through the utilization of government programs, such as food stamps, welfare, and Medicaid. How desperate are the economic circumstances? According to the U.S. Census Bureau (2011), the median household income for Native Americans in 2010 was $35,062, compared with a median household income of $50,046 for the nation as a whole (U.S. Census Bureau, 2011). More alarmingly, the percentage of Native Americans who lack health insurance is 29.2% (compared to 15.5% for the nation as a whole).

Throughout the United States, numerous reservations have turned to gaming operations as a source of economic opportunity. In 1988, the U.S. Congress passed the Indian Gaming Regulatory Act, which permitted tribes to negotiate with individual states to set up casinos. By 2001, approximately one-third of federally recognized tribes owned a total of about 300 casinos in 29 states. Only an estimated 25% of gaming industry jobs are held by Native Americans. Much of the revenue and the jobs go to non-Indian investors, overhead, and taxes, so despite the generation of revenue in the billions, only a few Native American communities have seen large profits, and the economic situation continues to be bleak for many Native Americans.

STATISTICS

We must begin by stating that proper terminology usage is difficult with regard to this cultural group, as there is no consensus. Even the definition of what constitutes an Indian is subject to debate. Should the label be *Indian* or *Native American*? Many older American Indians prefer the term *Indian* to *Native American*, believing that anyone born in the United States is a "Native American," and that the term *Indian* reflects the language used in treaties with the federal government (Stanford.edu, 2012). There is no one legal definition for the term *Indian*. This lack of consensus has resulted in the courts establishing the following two-part definition: (1) the person must have some identifiable Indian ancestry, and (2) that the Indian community must recognize this person as an Indian (Pevar, 1992). At the tribal level, each tribe determines the criteria for enrollment. This is further complicated with intermarriage. For purposes of the 2010 census, the Office of Management and Budget (OMB) used the following to define *American Indian* or *Alaska Native*: "a person having origins in any of the original peoples of North and South America (including Central America) and who maintains tribal affiliation or community attachment" (Centers for Disease Control and Prevention [CDC], 2011).

Another determinant used is the amount of "Indian blood" possessed by the individual. Tribes have varying measures that must be met for tribe inclusion and enrollment (e.g., one-half, one-quarter, or one-eighth Indian blood). Finally, the Cherokee Nation accepts anyone whose ancestor's name appears on any one of several rolls, including the Dawes Roll. The Dawes Roll is a list that was drawn up by the federal government during the Allotment Era, during which Indians received a 160-acre allotment of land as their portion of the Indian Territory in Oklahoma. Part of the OMB requirement was for tribal affiliation and/or community attachment. Tribal affiliation may be Navajo, Blackfeet, Inupiat, Yup'ik, or Central American Indian groups or South American Indian groups. There were some changes made prior to the 2010 census for tribal groupings. The changes were made by the federal government after input from tribal leaders, among others.

Unfortunately, these changes in labels makes it impossible for comparisons to be made between 2000 and 2010 census data for many of the tribal groupings.

According to the 2010 census, 5.2 million people identified as American Indian and Alaska Native, either alone or in combination with one or more races. 2.9 million people self-identified as American Indian and Alaska Native alone (1.7% of all people in the United States) (U.S. Census Bureau, 2011). The American Indian population is confined to 26 states, according to census data, with the vast majority residing in the western part of the country, due to the forced westward migration of the tribes by the government.

Most Native Americans prefer to be identified by their tribal affiliation, and the most common collective terms used are *Native American* or *American Indian*. The Navajo nation had the largest American Indian and Alaska Native population (174,000 total population) of all of the American Indian reservations. The second largest reservation with regard to total population was the Osage reservation— however a large majority (38,000 out of 47,000) of residents did not identify as American Indian or Alaska Native alone or in combination (U.S. Census Bureau, 2010). The Pine Ridge reservation (17,000 residents) was the second largest reservation, with residents identifying as American Indian or Alaska Native alone or in combination with another race.

According to 2010 census data, the 10 largest American Indian nations were Cherokee (819,000), Navajo (332,129), Choctaw (195,764), Mexican American Indian (175,4940), Chippewa (170,742), Sioux (170,110), Apache (111,810), Blackfeet (105,304), Creek (88,332), and Iroquois (81,002). The percentage grouping of the largest Alaska Native tribal groups was Yup'ik (33,889), Inupiat (33,360), Tlingit-Haida (26,080), Alaskan Athabascan (22,484), Aleut (19,282), and Tsimshian (3,755) (U.S. Census Bureau, 2010).

VARIABLES IMPACTING DEGREE OF ACCULTURATION

There are many variables that impact the degree of acculturation of a Native American patient (Literacynet.org, 2012). Some of the most important variables are life experience such as geographic area of birth (on-reservation versus off-reservation or urban versus rural), previous exposure to traditional Native American health beliefs, military service, intertribal marriage, and presence or absence of health benefits, as well as the types of health benefits possessed (Indian Health Service, Medicaid, tribal contract/compact, health maintenance organization, etc.) (Literacynet.org, 2012).

DEFINITIONS OF HEALTH AND ILLNESS

Although it would be impossible to include information on each and every one of the hundreds of Indian tribes in the United States, there are common themes regarding health and illness that provide general beliefs and practices that the nurse can become familiar with in order to deliver culturally appropriate care to Native American patients. Many Native Americans consider illness a result from an imbalance in mind, body, and spirit (Hendrix, 2002).

Unlike other minority groups, the federal government is required by law and by treaty to provide healthcare services through the Indian Health Service (Pevar, 1992). Conflict can occur because in Western medicine, the provider often asks the patient for his or her impression of what may be wrong. Asking this question of Native Americans may result in them thinking the provider is ignorant, not only of their culture, but also of how to care for them as a patient. Support of the "sick role" in this culture is also not acceptable. Instead, support is directed at assisting the person to regain harmony with nature and with others. It is felt that people with illness have done something to place themselves out of harmony or have had a curse placed on them. This is especially the view with regard to mental illness or mental disorders. Mental illness is viewed as resulting from witching (the placing of a curse) on a person (Purnell, 2013). Treatment requires the expertise of a specialized Native American healer. The degree of nonacceptance of the sick role, for any disorder, is so strong that even a seriously ill elderly Native American will continue to work, even if that will result in further illness or a poor outcome. A great deal of encouragement for the patient to rest will be required, without guarantee of success.

SPECIFIC NURSING CONSIDERATIONS

It is important for the nurse to approach patient care with an appreciation and basic understanding of common factors that have been associated with Native American patients that may impact the clinical domain. Self-disclosure and the sharing of information may be a difficult hurdle for the Native American patient. The nurse should not be too aggressive in attempting to get the patient to share some health history information that may be guarded by the patient. Being too aggressive may cause irreparable damage to the nurse–patient relationship. The nurse should also avoid a problem-focused approach, such as asking, "What is your problem?" Relying on a problem-oriented framework is not recommend-ed, as Native American patients (especially if they are older) may be offended, because focusing on a problem places a power differential between the patient with the problem and the nurse who has the answer to the problem (Hendrix, 2002). This may be difficult to remember or to do because many documentation systems are established around a problem-focused framework.

Food is an important part of Native American culture, and the traditional foods are very healthy (Purnell, 2013). In recent years, because of poverty on many reservations, a reliance on foods that can be unhealthy if relied on to excess, such as cheese, lard, sugar, and white flour, has resulted. The nurse should provide nutrition guidance but be aware that the teaching must include the culturally appropriate foods of the patient's ancestors (squash, melon, corn, etc.), portions, timing of meals, and food-related rituals. Food is a part of social activity, and the sharing of food is an important part of the culture. The nurse should not be surprised to see a Native American patient sharing a meal tray with a visitor. It is culturally appropriate for the patient to offer the food to the visitor, and it would be rude for the visitor to refuse such an offer. Visitors may also bring in inappropriate foods for the patient. To avoid problems with not enough food because of sharing or access to inappropriate foods, it may be best for the nurse to encourage visiting time that avoids meal time if possible, so that the patient will have access to all of the food required for the day while hospitalized.

Request permission prior to touching the patient, as touching is viewed as inappropriate in some tribal cultures (Sanchez, Plawecki, & Plawecki, 1996). Modesty and privacy are highly valued, and the utmost effort should be attempted by the nurse to ensure that this is provided and not violated in any way (Giger, 2013). The removal of clothing should only be requested if absolutely essential, and if an accommodation can be made, the nurse should provide that accommodation. At a minimum, the patient should be draped if clothing must be removed. Speak quietly to avoid appearing rude, and also to maintain patient confidentiality.

If you suspect that you may be dealing with a mental health issue of some type, proceed with caution and sensitivity. Depression, or any other mental health complaint, may not be verbalized as the chief complaint. The nurse should be on guard for somatic complaints (fatigue, tiredness), minimization of symptoms as just being a part of life, or symptoms that may be expressed as a metaphor such as "I have a heavy heart" or "I am having an issue with my esteem." The bottom line is that symptoms of this type will be minimized by both the patient and family and, often, help will not be sought out until the physical symptoms are severe. The nurse must remember that there are vast differences in beliefs, terminology, or labels utilized, as well as other language differences that exist among various tribes (Sanchez, 1996).

Ensuring effective communication as well as providing effective patient education should also be an important focus of the nurse. According to the Agency for Healthcare Research and Quality (AHRQ, 2010) survey, compared with Whites, all minority groups reported poor communication with nurses. When providing patient education, the nurse should include demonstration whenever possible. Native Americans prefer one-on-one education rather than printed materials. Pictures and demonstrations are more effective than describing, as the traditional way of teaching in Native American culture is "doing" over "talking."

TRADITIONAL HEALTH BELIEFS

Providing culturally appropriate interventions requires that the nurse assess the Native American's degree of tribal affiliation, the level or importance given to traditional health beliefs, and the degree of acceptance or acculturation to the Western Biomedical Model of the patient. The nurse should also keep in mind that many Native Americans have had exposure to medical care through the Indian Health Service, clinics, or from military or veteran settings, which will have an impact on care expectations and comfort level. There is also the possibility that the patient may be distrustful of the healthcare system because of past abuses, as well as the belief that this system is based on money and greed and is not patient centered.

Traditional Native American views of healing and wellness emphasize seeking harmony within oneself, with others, and with one's surroundings. In the traditional Native American way, medicine can consist of physical remedies, but medicine is also much more than a pill you take to cure illness or correct a physiological malfunction. Medicine is everywhere; it is the essence of their inner being that gives inner power (Garrett, 1999). The traditional Indian belief about health is that it reflects living in total harmony with nature and being able to survive even in difficult circumstances. Native Americans highly value traditional beliefs concerning relation, harmony, balance, spirituality, and wellness; as part of valuing "relation," all these beliefs are interrelated (Tsai & Alanis, 2004). This may be an oversimplification; when discussing Native Americans, we are dealing with a multiplicity of cultures, so there cannot be only one belief.

Traditional healers are capable of understanding illness from a perspective that includes spirituality and symptom etiology relative to the patient's unique culture. Depending on the patient's degree of acculturation, the use of pharmacologic interventions may be culturally congruent, while with some patients, they will only respond to or permit traditional healing interventions/strategies. The degree of acceptance of Western medicine is variable. The goal is to address the patient's health concerns in a culturally appropriate manner. This is often best achieved when they are treated by both traditional and Western healers.

Native American patients may request Native American Healing (NAH). NAH has been practiced in North America for over 10,000 years. NAH is a broad term that includes healing beliefs and practices of hundreds of indigenous tribes of North America (American Cancer Society [ACS], 2008). It combines religion, spirituality, herbal medicine, and rituals that are used to treat people with medical and emotional conditions. The following concepts are associated with NAH: it takes a lot of time for healing to occur, healing takes place within the context of a relationship, achieving an energy of activation is necessary, biologic systems behave similarly across hierarchic levels, the distractions of modern life "inactivate" catalysts for change, modern culture systematically teaches us to ignore emotions and to maintain a low level of emotional awareness, physiologic change often requires a break in usual daily rhythms, and the importance of ceremony as a means of accessing help from the spiritual dimension for healing (ACS, 2008).

From the Native American perspective, medicine is more about healing the person than curing a disease (ACS, 2008). Traditional healers aim to "make whole" by restoring well-being and harmonious relationships with the community and the spirit of nature, which is sometimes called God or the Great Mystery (Tsai & Alanis, 2004). NAH is based on the belief that everyone and everything on Earth is interconnected, and every person, animal, and plant has a spirit or essence (ACS, 2008). Even an object, such as a river or rock, and even the earth itself, may be considered to have this kind of spirit.

Native Americans traditionally believe that illness stems from spiritual problems (ACS, 2008). They traditionally do not ascribe to germ theory as they see illness as a result from a cause-and-effect (not germ-related) event in the past or a future event yet to pass. They also say that diseases are more likely to invade the body of a person who is imbalanced, has negative thinking, or lives an unhealthy lifestyle. Some Native American healers believe that inherited conditions, such as birth defects, are caused by the parents' immoral lifestyles and are not easily treated. Others believe that such conditions reflect a touch from the Creator and may consider them a kind of gift. NAH practices aim to find and restore balance and wholeness in a person to restore them to a healthy and spiritually pure state.

There are many types of NAH practices, and they are promoted to help with a variety of ills. Some of the most common aspects of NAH include the use of herbal remedies, purifying rituals, shamanism, and symbolic healing rituals to treat illnesses of both the body and spirit (ACS, 2008). Herbal remedies are used to treat many physical conditions. Practitioners use purifying rituals to cleanse the body and prepare the person for healing. Shamanism is based on the idea that spirits cause illness, and a Native American healer called a "shaman" focuses on using spiritual healing powers to treat people. Symbolic healing rituals, which can involve family and friends of the sick person, are used to invoke the spirits to help heal the sick person.

Healers may include shamans as described above, but also herbalists, spiritual healers, and medicine men or women (ACS, 2008). Many Native Americans see their healers for spiritual reasons, such as to seek guidance, truth, balance, reassurance, and spiritual well-being, while still using conventional medicine to deal with "White man's illness." However, they believe that the spirit is an inseparable element of healing.

Healing beliefs and rituals vary a great deal because there are such a large number of tribes (over 500) (ACS, 2008). Adding to this complexity is the fact that many healing rituals and beliefs are kept secret, passed along from one healer to the next. Secrecy is considered essential because the sharing of healing information is felt to exploit the culture and weaken the healer's ability to heal. This secrecy has significantly limited the amount of information that is known about these practices. Another barrier to widespread knowledge of these practices is that some of the practices were driven underground or lost completely because they were banned or illegal in parts of the United States until 1978, when the American Indian Religious Freedom Act was passed.

The American Indian Religious Freedom Act has two sections (National Park Service, 1978). The first section defines the policy of the United States to protect and preserve for American Indians their inherent right of freedom to believe, express, and exercise the traditional religions of the American Indian, Eskimo, Aleut, and Native Hawaiians, including but not limited to access to sites, use, and possession of sacred objects, and the freedom to worship through ceremonials and traditional rituals. The second section permits the president of the United States to direct federal departments and agencies to evaluate all policies and procedures (in concert with native traditional religious leaders) to determine appropriate changes necessary to protect and preserve Native American religious cultural rights and practices (National Park Service, 1978).

One of the most common forms of NAH involves the use of herbal remedies, which can include teas, tinctures, and salves. For example, one remedy for pain uses bark from a willow tree, which contains acetylsalicylic acid (aspirin) (ACS, 2008).

Purifying and cleansing the body is also an important technique used in NAH. Sweat lodges (special, darkened enclosures heated with stones from a fire) or special teas that induce vomiting may be used by the healer for this purpose (ACS, 2008).

A practice called smudging, which involves cleansing a place or person with the smoke of sacred plants, can be used to bring about an altered state of consciousness and sensitivity, making a person more open to the healing techniques. Because some illnesses are believed to come from angry spirits, healers may also invoke the healing powers of spirits. They may also use special rituals to try to appease the angered spirits (ACS, 2008).

Another practice of NAH, symbolic healing rituals, can involve the whole community. These rituals use ceremonies that can include chanting, singing, body painting, dancing, exorcisms, sand paintings, and even limited use of mind-altering substances (such as peyote) to persuade the spirits to heal the sick person. Rituals can last hours or even weeks. These ceremonies are a way of asking for help from the spiritual dimension (ACS, 2008). Prayer is also an essential part of all NAH techniques.

Native American treatment is usually a slow process, spread over a period of days or weeks. It may involve taking time from one's daily activities for reflection, emotional awareness, and meditation. Speech should be slow, as silence is valued; long periods of silence during communication is common (Hendrix, 2002). The healer may spend a great deal of time with the person seeking help. Healing is said to take place within the context of the relationship with the healer.

Preservation of the body is an important cultural consideration (Hendrix, 2002). The nurse should be aware that it is not unusual for a Native American patient to request that any removed body tissue (such as organs removed during surgery and even trimmed nail clippings or hair) be returned to the patient for fear that the removed body products can be used to harm the patient or family (such as via spells, which is a common belief among the Navajo) (Hendrix, 2002). Autopsy is also frowned upon because of the cultural belief that the body must be whole in order to be able to cross over into the spirit world.

CULTURAL AMPLIFIERS

There are factors that have been identified by the National Native American AIDS Prevention Center (2002) that can worsen the difficulties faced by Native Americans living with a chronic illness or disease, such as HIV/AIDs. These factors are called cultural amplifiers. The identified cultural amplifiers are circular migration, holistic approach to health, traditional healing, distrust of authority, fear of breach of confidentiality, communication style, modesty, language and culture, family and community role, orientation to the present, mortality, and sexual orientation. The term *circular migration* is used to describe the movement associated with the Native American population—some by choice and some by necessity. Many Native Americans live on a reservation and need to leave to seek services, while others may not live on a reservation but they may wish to visit. The circular migration that is common with Native American people makes them vulnerable to infectious diseases (such as HIV or TB, both of which are highly prevalent in this population) (Sequist, Cullen, & Acton, 2011). Transmission easily occurs with the frequent migration from urban areas to the reservations, and this results in a tremendous potential for the outbreak of epidemics in the Native American population.

Holistic health is an extremely important health concept to Native Americans. It can only result with the existence of true harmony of the mind, body, and spirit with nature. While each tribe has its own unique healing methods and beliefs, there is tremendous overlap and consistency among tribes. The use of traditional healing methods can result in tremendous empowerment in the follower (Hendrix, 2002).

Distrust of authority is an extremely prevalent cultural concept. There is, of course, significant historical precedent for Native Americans to mistrust the government and other authorities, such as healthcare providers. There have been many episodes of ethical breaches in healthcare settings on reservations and in research, which has resulted in a fear of further breaches among many Native Americans (Marshall, 2001).

Lack of confidentiality, especially when dealing with a shame-inducing or stigma-associated illness such as HIV/AIDs, can lead to shame and isolation within the patient's community (Rowell & Bouey, 2002). There is tremendous fear in the Native American community regarding the ability of the Indian Health Service to maintain patient confidentiality and records. Communication may be a barrier due to the cultural practice of exercising caution when sharing private, family information (Rowell & Bouey, 2002).

Modesty is highly valued in the Native American culture. The nurse must strive to overcome this by learning how to discuss the body, sex, and sexuality with the patient in a nonthreatening, nonoffensive manner (Hendrix, 2002).

Language may also present unique communication barriers. Every Native language contains the key to that tribe's view of the universe. Even if a non-Native learned the language, some of the cultural elements would be lost in the translation. Therefore demonstration, with an emphasis on doing, is preferred over talking when providing patient education (Hendrix, 2002).

Another cultural amplifier that may impact the nurse is the way the family unit may be organized. Members of the same clan, or even related clans, may consider themselves to be relatives. This means that an aunt may be considered a mother, or a cousin could be considered a brother. Some native children are informally adopted, which can make navigation of the family unit by the nurse difficult.

A present time orientation also is a factor and can be problematic because the focus of the patient is often on immediate gratification and not on potential future long-term gains from health promotion and prevention behaviors (Hendrix, 2002).

Mortality factors vary by tribe and ethnicity with overall higher mortality rates associated with this population (CDC, 2011).

The final cultural amplifier, sexual orientation, can be very complex among Native Americans of differing tribes. Some tribes have maintained their recorded history from prior to the development of European settlements/colonization in the United States. These tribes were accepting of alternative gender roles and sexuality. The European settlers brought Christianity to the New World, which not only did not share those beliefs, but desired to extinguish them and to even erase them from history. In some cases, tribal records were lost or destroyed. This is why different tribes today may have varying responses to the issues of homosexuality and sexually transmitted diseases. Some Native American gay, lesbian, bisexual, and transgendered people identify as "two spirit." The term *two spirit* is a fairly new term that originated from the organizing efforts of gay, lesbian, bisexual, and transgendered Native Americans to distinguish themselves from mainstream gay and lesbian culture. The term attempts to reclaim and honor the historical roles and traditions of individuals within many tribes that were at one time inclusive of alternative gender roles and sexualities (National Native American AIDS Prevention Center, 2002).

The nurse needs to get to know the Native American patient as an individual. The nurse should learn about the Native American community so that he or she may serve by becoming aware of important aspects of the tribe's history and any and all cultural amplifiers of factors that may impact the ability to form a therapeutic relationship with the Native American patient.

Ask the patient if they use traditional healing methods in a nonjudgmental manner, educate the patient regarding any and all appropriate Western medicines. It is important to emphasize to the patient that Western and traditional medicines are more effective when used together rather than in isolation. Provide encouragement and validation if the Native American patient shares the intent to use or access tribe-specific interventions or resources. Involve the patient in the planning for care delivery every step of the way. The Native American patient may have difficulty navigating the healthcare delivery system, especially if their only previous access to health care was through the Indian Health Service. Inform the patient about the healthcare system (roles of providers, directory of services, need for referrals, etc.). Encourage your patient to ask questions and to advocate for him or herself as needed.

IMPACT OF COMMUNICATION

Traditionally, Native American languages have been passed down by tribe elders to the young. As Native American communities have been dispersed and moved to reservations, many languages have been lost. Some tribes have thousands of people who speak the tribal language, while others may have only a few, who will often be the elders of the tribe (Crawford, 1995). The reality is that the Native American languages are highly endangered, as young Native Americans are taught and choose to speak only English (Crawford, 1995). Some of the most common Native American languages are the Navajo, Cherokee, and Choctaw. Many Native Americans today are trying to revive their native language before all of the fluent elders pass away. It is felt that failing to preserve the unique language utilized during religious ceremonies will negatively impact the ability of children to speak with their elders, as well as their ability to pray.

A barrier to cross-cultural communication with Native Americans is the fact that even a minor variation in pronunciation may change the entire meaning of the message being received or sent (Hendrix, 2002). Although the dominant languages differ greatly from tribe to tribe, other forms of communication (both verbal and nonverbal) are similar across tribes. This congruence is true regarding eye contact. Most Native Americans do not maintain steady eye contact. Direct eye contact is considered disrespectful and, for elders, may even be perceived as threatening (Hendrix, 2002). The degree of acculturation that has taken place will determine the amount of eye contact offered during an encounter as well as the amount, if any, English that is spoken. Today, many Native Americans, especially the elderly, live in homes where no English is spoken at all. It is interesting when similarities in language are discovered. It has been noted that the language spoken by an Eskimo from Alaska can be understood by an Eskimo in Greenland (Crawford, 1995).

The Native American communication style tends to be circular, as opposed to the dominant American culture's linear style. This may lead to difficulties if an educator or teacher is speaking in a linear style and the Native American is used to a circular style (Tsai & Alanis, 2004). In addition, some Native Americans utilize a reserved manner when communicating. This may be interpreted by the nurse as being unfriendly. This perception may be further enhanced by the tendency of the Native American to look down or to avoid eye contact to defer to the nurse's authority or to avoid being disrespectful. The nurse should reciprocate eye contact and nonverbal cues from the patient during an encounter. Native Americans may also speak slowly and deliberately, which may be incorrectly interpreted by the nurse as a language barrier or lack of intelligence or education. For some Native Americans, English may be a second language. They may be slow (or unwilling entirely) to disclose personal information (this may also be due to the cultural amplifiers of mistrust and fear of breach of confidentiality). Native Americans, as a group, tend to be careful and thorough listeners and perceptive observers of nonverbal communication (National Native American AIDS Prevention Center, 2002). The nurse should strive to establish a trusting relationship that may ultimately enhance the communication process and the delivery of patient education and effective nursing care.

Inform the patient of the need for you to utilize direct communication when providing nursing care. The use of direct communication is not comfortable for the Native American. Explain that you may need to ask direct questions in order to provide safe and comprehensive nursing care and share that your intent is to do only that and not to be insensitive or offensive with your questioning. Make sure the patient understands that it is fine for them to ask direct questions of you in return. Remember, establishing a nurse–patient relationship that is based on trust and that utilizes direct communication will enhance patient adherence to the treatment plan and will result in improved patient outcomes.

The nurse must recognize that the Native American patient's cultural beliefs, history, and life experiences may negatively impact adherence with the treatment plan. Native Americans are often faced with death, which can result in feelings of fear and hopelessness—even resignation. They may turn to substances (such as alcohol or drugs) to help them cope with a chronic disease or life threatening diagnosis, and this may further impact adherence. Be sure to incorporate a holistic approach—an approach that will be appreciated and valued by the Native American patient. Encourage the patient to utilize traditional healers to help maintain their physical, emotional, mental, and spiritual well-being and, most importantly, to keep hope alive. If at all possible, advocate for the involvement of a Native American healthcare team member in the patient's interdisciplinary team.

Finally, do not be offended if the patient is not willing to share details regarding traditional healthcare services they may be receiving. In an effort to protect and preserve these practices, they may not be allowed to share details with you. Refrain from asking for details or offering judgments. Your genuine interest and support of the patient will not only strengthen the nurse–patient relationship, but it will also improve patient adherence, which ultimately may result in positive patient outcomes.

Native American languages do not make clear distinctions between objects and actions, and North American Native American languages often collapse objects and actions into single words, such as the Eskimo word *anerquwaatit*, which means, "he begs you to go out." This type of language, in which elements are added to nouns to form new nouns, is called an agglutinative language (Councellor, 2010). When verbs are collapsed with nouns, it suggests that the culture does not think of actions as independent from the object doing the action. European languages invoke a worldview in which action can be considered a separate entity from objects.

Always ask the patient for permission to remove their clothing or to touch them for any purpose or reason. Modesty is an important consideration. Most Native Americans will find it uncomfortable to discuss their bodies (or to perform self-examinations) and may be reluctant to discuss normal body functioning (especially sexual functioning). The nurse should strive to discuss the body and how to perform self-examination in a nonoffensive and nonthreatening manner. The National Native American AIDS Prevention Center (2002) recommends advising the patient to perform a self-examination while showering; because a shower requires touching of the body, the patient may feel more comfortable with this approach.

Formality when addressing the patient is recommended, as most Native Americans follow the tradition of having a first, middle, and last name (i.e., the patient should be called Miss, Mister, or Missus as appropriate, followed by the last name) (Hendrix, 2002).

Many Native American languages do not have words or concepts equivalent to English words or concepts, especially in the case of medical jargon. The nurse can impact the meaning of the communication through voice inflection, so consideration of this should be made. In some Native American cultures, death and dying is not discussed because of the perceived cultural link between words and action (speaking a negative outcome can cause it to occur) (Hendrix, 2002). In Navajo culture, speaking the name of the dead can delay the spirit's journey to the next world or keep the spirit in limbo (Hendrix, 2002).

The nurse should provide ample consideration time once a patient has been provided with information and expect that consultation may occur with others in the Native American community prior to any medical decisions being made.

The nurse should not rely on nonverbal cues to determine if the Native American patient is in pain. Many Native Americans were taught and socialized to withstand pain as a survival skill (Hendrix, 2002). The overt expression of pain (both verbal and nonverbal) is considered unacceptable, and for these reasons, the

Native American patient may be extremely unlikely to request pain medication and may instead rely on internal resources when coping with pain. If a request is made for a pain intervention, the nurse should respond immediately as it is not likely to be repeated. Also, the request may not come from the patient but from a family member instead. The nurse must recognize that pain is undertreated and strive to help the patient manage their pain in a culturally appropriate manner.

IMPACT OF TIME AND SPACE

The Native American concept of time is intuitive and flexible (Hendrix, 2002). There is a strong belief in cause and effect, a present time orientation, and the belief that space has no boundaries. Most Native Americans are oriented to living in the present rather than focusing on the future. The focus is on living each day as it comes, with the emphasis on immediate gratification. This orientation can impact adherence with the treatment plan, and especially drug therapy. When they feel well they may not take their prescribed medication, while on "bad days," adherence may not be a factor. This potential lack of adherence can have severe consequences when managing a life-threatening illness such as HIV/AIDs or cancer (ACS, 2008). Time is a strong factor in beliefs regarding illness, as illness is viewed as being a result of something that either happened in the past or something that will happen in the future—indeed, it is viewed as the price to be paid.

Time is linked to naturally occurring phenomena such as cycles, moons, and seasons. Very little, if any, focus is placed on the future. This is a result of the belief that many things are outside of a person's control. Time starts when the group gathers, and an event does not usually begin at a designated time. The nurse should recognize that medical appointments may not be kept, especially if something else comes up that is felt takes priority, such as helping a family member or friend.

IMPACT OF SOCIAL ORGANIZATION

The family structure varies from tribe to tribe, including gender roles; some tribes are matriarchal like the Navajo (Giger, 2013), while the majority of tribes are patriarchal. Despite this diversity, there are common core values and beliefs of traditional Native American culture that carry across tribal groups and geographic regions. These core values will be described here. Historically, most men went to war or hunted while the women stayed home cooking and caring for the children.

Most Native American social structure is based on kinship (Gilio-Whitaker, 2012). How highly organized each culture may be around this concept will vary, but it appears to be a universal theme to Native American cultures. Kinship-based societies are organized based on biologic relationships. There are two lines of descent: vertical and horizontal. The vertical lines of descent link the relationships between ancestors and descendants (this is a very important concept). Horizontal lines describe one's connection to others in one's community who are not ancestors or descendants (such as siblings or spouse). The extended family is also an important concept to Native Americans. Members of the same clan or related clans may be considered relatives. The community is a valuable resource, and an individual may turn to it for financial, emotional, or spiritual support (Gilio-Whitaker, 2012). The individual may support the community (or some of its members) in the same ways.

Native American family life is usually structured one of two ways. The first is the nuclear family, which is made up of the husband and wife and their descendants. The second is the extended family, which is the most common type of family found in Native American culture, and is made up of families of two or more generations who live together as a family.

Native Americans tend to view the entire world within the context of the relationship between the divine and human worlds, as a mother to her children (in a matriarchal society) or a father to his children (in a patriarchal society). This worldview is an important concept to know when attempting to understand Native American culture.

The most common political concept in Native American culture is chieftaincies. A chieftaincy included more than one kinship group and often more than one local settlement or clan. The principal role of the chief was to resolve conflicts among groups; beneath the chief an entire hierarchy of decision making has developed. The roles of the chief varied tremendously from society to society. In some, he was the chief arbiter of disputes and nothing more. In others, he was a military leader and nothing more. In others, he was a religious leader. Authority was vested in a chief either through a descent line or through individual achievements. Some societies allowed for several chiefs of equal authority, others limited the chieftaincy to only a single individual.

BIOLOGIC VARIATIONS

Although the Native American population is younger than the general population in the United States, it has a lower life expectancy (U.S. Commission on Civil Rights, 2004). This is due to the high morbidity and mortality rates that are a result of a wide variety of diseases and other causes. According to the CDC

(2011) some examples of important health disparities in 2006 were infant deaths (1.7 times the rate for all populations), chronic liver disease and cirrhosis (more than 2.5 times higher than for all populations), unintentional injuries (1.8 times more likely to die from a motor vehicle accident), gonorrhea (more than 5.5 times higher than the rate for Asia Americans and Pacific Islanders, who have the lowest incidence of gonorrhea), and AIDS (the third highest rate of diagnosis among all minority groups). Native Americans continue to experience significant rates of diabetes, mental health disorders, cardiovascular disease, pneumonia, influenza, and injuries (U.S. Commission on Civil Rights, 2004).

Diabetes is a major health problem for Native Americans. Much work is being done in this area because of the explosion in the numbers of patients diagnosed with type 2 diabetes mellitus (DM). The rate of DM in the Native American population has the highest prevalence in the world and it is continuing to spiral out of control (U.S. Commission on Civil Rights, 2004). One explanation focuses on genetics and is known as the thrifty gene hypothesis (Neel, 1962). This theory provides an explanation as to why the prevalence of DM is higher in some ethic groups such as Native Americans, Australian Aborigines, and Pacific Islanders. It is thought that evolutionary pressure selected for hunter–gatherers with efficient fuel storage during times of famine. When food becomes more plentiful and exercise less plentiful, this trait becomes a liability. It is felt that in earlier times, people were much more physically active and ate a diet high in protein with periods of intermittent starvation. This stress resulted in genetic selection to occur to allow for improved metabolic efficiency ("thrifty genes"). Over time, as society began and continues to modernize, changes occurred in human diet and activity level. People are ingesting more calories, increasing dietary fat intake, and decreasing physical activity. This has resulted in obesity, insulin resistance, and type 2 DM (Neel, 1962; Tsunehara, Leonetti, & Fujimoto, 1990).

Cardiovascular disease (CVD) mortality varies among tribes, but is increasing overall. American Indian and Alaska Native adults are 1.2 times more likely to suffer from heart disease than the general population. The Strong Heart Study (National Institutes of Health, 2001) integrated data on 13 different American Indian tribes (N = 4,549), with male and female subjects ages 45 to 74 from American Indian communities from three different centers (Arizona, Oklahoma, and South Dakota/North Dakota). The increasing incidence of CVD among American Indians found by the Strong Heart Study is of great concern because rates of CVD are decreasing in other groups in the United States. More intensive programs to reduce CVD risk factors are needed in American Indian communities. Because the risk factors vary by tribal groups, these programs need to be tailored to each community/tribe. DM was found to be the most important contributing factor for CVD. Prevention needs to address the modifiable risk factors of DM, which are increasing physical activity and decreasing weight to an acceptable body mass index. Lipid management and smoking cessation are also important preventive topics for this population. Blood pressure control in this study was found to be comparable or better than that of the general hypertensive population. Reduction of excessive alcohol use is also a strategy that was advocated by the authors of the Strong Heart Study (National Institutes of Health, 2001).

Alcohol abuse is a big problem in this population and its excess usage has caused a corresponding problem with fetal alcohol syndrome and domestic violence (Lobo, Talbot, & Morris, 2009). Alcohol is metabolized differently in various ethnic groups, including Native Americans (U.S. Department of Health and Human Services [USDHHS], 2007). This variability causes vasomotor symptoms, such as facial flushing and palpitations, that are not seen in other ethnic groups. It is hypothesized (and currently under further study) that the reason for these differences is caused by variations in alcohol metabolism between these groups. In Whites, alcohol is metabolized by the liver enzyme alcohol dehydrogenase at a level that is deemed "fairly efficient." Native Americans metabolize alcohol by acetaldehyde dehydrogenase, a "faster" metabolism, which is the reason for the vasomotor symptoms seen in the Native Americans (USDHHS, 2007).

Alcoholism has had a tremendous impact on mortality rates. Native people die from alcoholism at a rate 510% higher than other Americans (Lobo et al., 2009). The important issue of alcohol abuse is being addressed by legislation and federal government involvement. On July 29, 2010, President Obama signed into law the Tribal Law and Order Act. The purpose of the new legislation was to repurpose the preexisting Indian Alcohol and Substance Abuse Prevention and Treatment Act. The change was made in response to the recognition that the prevention and treatment of alcohol and drug abuse is much harder and less effective in this population. Effective measures must be designed to specifically address the reasons for the high rate of abuse and the need for culturally appropriate strategies. The second purpose for the new legislation was to address the higher-than-average rates of violence that exist among the Native American/Alaska Native populations in the United States.

According to Lobo et al. (2009), other health issues have a higher prevalence in the Native American/Alaska Native population. This includes: mental health issues and suicide, obesity, substance abuse, sudden infant death syndrome (SIDS), teenage pregnancy, liver disease, and stroke. There is a 30% higher HIV/AIDs rate compared to the general population. Overall, life expectancy is lower and the infant mortality rate is higher. Life expectancy was 2.4 years less in this group than for all other races from 1999 to 2001. The life expectancy has improved recently; however, this is still an increase of four years from the 1996 to 1998 rates. Native infants die at a rate of 8.5 per 1,000 live births, compared to 6.8 per 1,000 live births for all U.S. races (2000–2002 rates).

IMPACT OF FAITH AND SPIRITUALITY

Central to Native American spiritual traditions is the importance of *relation* as a way of existing in the world. The power of relation is symbolized by the circle of life, represented throughout the traditions, customs, and art forms of Native American people. This circle of life is believed, in many tribal traditions, to consist of the basic elements of life: fire, earth, water, and wind. Also life, from a traditional Native American perspective, is viewed as a series of concentric circles. The first circle is the inner circle, representing our spirit. The next circle is family/ clan. The third circle is the natural environment and all our relations. The fourth circle consists of the spirit world. Considering the power of relation, all life exists in an involved system of interdependence in a dynamic state of harmony and balance (Garrett & Carroll, 2000).

Among the many aspects of Native American culture is the emphasis on unity through seeking harmony and balance both inwardly and outwardly (Tsai & Alanis, 2004). Generally, Native American traditional values reflect the importance placed upon community contribution, sharing, cooperation, being, noninterference, community and extended family, harmony with nature, a time orientation toward living in the present, preference for explanation of natural phenomena according to the spiritual, and a deep respect for elders (Tsai & Alanis, 2004).

Although there is no written sacred religious book in Native American culture comparable to the Bible, some Native Americans of North America have kept written records, with sacred symbols written on wooden sticks or woven into wampum belts (Waldman, 2006). Religious stories and ceremonies have been transmitted through stories that have been passed down. Native American storytellers have kept alive both cultural and spiritual traditions by sharing stories about creation, morals, laws, and even survival skills.

Religion is a way of life. In many Native American languages, there is no word for *religion* because spiritual practices are believed to be an integral part of every aspect of daily life; spirituality is necessary for the harmony and balance, or wellness, of the individual, family, clan, and community (Waldman, 2006).

Northeast Indians believe in a spirit world that interacts with the physical or natural world. They believe in a primary spirit that pervades all existence. This

Great Spirit has different names depending on the tribe's language or dialect. Algonquians call it *Kitche Manitou*, which means *Great Spirit*; Iroquoians call it *Orenda*; and the Siouans refer to it as *Wakan* or *Wakanda*. The Great Spirit has many manifestations, as it is considered present in all things, even sickness. Shamans are believed to be capable of controlling spirits, including the Great Spirit (Waldman, 2006).

Burial is also a sacred and religious enterprise. In the United States in the past, tribes had been outraged by the desecration of their sacred burial grounds, which had been ransacked for skeletal remains and burial items. The fight for the return of these items was furious and long lasting. Finally, in 1990, the U.S. government passed the Native American Graves Protection and Repatriation Act (NAGPRA; National Park Service, 1990). NAGPRA protects Indian gravesites from looting and sets up legal procedures for Indians to reclaim artifacts of religious or ceremonial importance. Reclaiming skeletal bones, totem poles, masks, wampum belts, medicine bundles (collections of objects believed to heal disease and ward off ghosts), and other objects from museums has inspired tribes to revive old ceremonies and tribal traditions.

For thousands of years, many Native Americans, including the Navajo, have worshipped while under the influence of peyote (from the peyote cactus) (Waldman, 2006). They have a polytheistic religion with one main god (or spirit) and several smaller gods. The Peyote religion, now organized as the Native American Church, is a nativistic religion that began among the Kiowa and Comanche tribes during the second half of the 19th century. The religion is acceptable to many because it does not introduce new beliefs and because it incorporates the traditional native beliefs.

Finally, some Native Americans are Christians. Many missionaries have lived on reservations spreading the Christian religions, which has resulted in many conversions to Christianity (Giger, 2013).

NAVAJOS

The largest of the American Indian tribes today are the Navajos with 308,013 members according to the 2010 census (U.S. Census Bureau, 2011). The first written history regarding the Navajo dates back to the 1600s. Based on archaeological evidence, it is believed that the Navajos settled in northwestern New Mexico by the late 1400s or early 1500s. By the early 1600s, they had migrated into northern Arizona. The proximity to Mexico and the Pueblo peoples exerted a tremendous influence on the cultural development of the Navajo despite the fact that during periods of time, the Pueblos and Navajos were enemies (Giger, 2013). They were allies (especially against the Spanish) for much longer than the time spent as enemies or in hostility. The Navajo adopted a matrilineal clan system from the Pueblo that is still in effect today. A matrilineal lineage means that the Navajo inherits the clan from the mother and each member of the clan is considered to be a relative, each holding and carrying out unique responsibilities to each other and to the clan. Trades were also learned by the Navajo that caused the reliance on a nomadic hunting existence to become less significant. Some of the trades developed included weaving, pottery making, agriculture, and silversmithing. In fact, adopting and expanding from other cultures is considered one of the Navajos' strengths.

The Navajo people have strived to stay on the sacred land of their ancestors. The Navajo nation extends into the states of Utah, Arizona, Colorado, and New Mexico and covers over 27,000 square miles (Navajo Nation Government, 2009). This land is located between four mountains, each of which represents the four cardinal directions of east, south, west, and north, and it is believed it was granted to them by the creator. The four mountains are Mount Blanca in Colorado, Mount Taylor in New Mexico, San Francisco Peak in Arizona, and Mount Hesperus in Colorado. Historians state that to fully understand the Navajo, it is important to know that the four mountains provide the boundaries for the Navajo nation. It is believed, even today, that the mountains are sacred and were a gift to the Navajo. They are extremely important in Navajo mythology and thus the mountains are celebrated in prayers and songs (Navajo Nation Government, 2009).

In 1923, a tribal government was established in response to the desire of oil companies to lease Navajo land for exploration. In 1991, the government was reorganized to follow a three-branch organizational structure: executive, legislative, and judiciary. Government sessions are conducted in the traditional Navajo language. It is believed that the Navajo tribal government has evolved today into the largest of all forms of American Indian government (Navajo Nation Government, 2009).

A unique difference of the Navajo tribe is that, unlike many other Native Americans, they have been able to stay on their original tribal land. This is considered a great blessing as their sacred land was a gift for them to possess and protect for the Holy Ones who came down from the sky, as mentioned above. It is felt that as long as the Navajos stay on their land, the Holy Ones will take care of them.

The Creator of the universe, it is believed, provided the Navajo with all they need to live and be happy between the four sacred mountains (Beck, 2003). The Creator gave Father Sun for light and energy and Mother Earth, who provides all things that nurture and all things that can heal. The Navajo way of life focuses on the natural spirituality of the Earth intertwined with its physical attributes (i.e., the spiritual world is infused with the natural world that breathes life into every living thing on Earth). The Navajo take honor and delight in their ability to heal and care for Mother Earth, which they recognize is being damaged by some. It is stated that the Navajo believe that someday the people of the Earth will come to the Navajo for lessons on how to care for Earth and when that day comes, they will be ready (Beck, 2003).

Language is a specific talent that the Navajo possess. During World War II, there were Navajo code breakers who were essential in helping the United States transmit classified information. A secret code was developed from the Navajo language that was used to transmit messages—this secret code was considered unbreakable (Historynet.com, 2006). Today, most elderly Navajo speak only their native language and few are literate. Younger Navajo are usually bilingual and speak the tribal language in their home. There is some similarity of dialect between the Navajo and the Apache and there can therefore be some limited understanding between these tribes when communicating with each other. Regional accents and the use of slang terms can hamper this, because even a minor variation in pronunciation can change the meaning of a word or an entire sentence.

Ceremonies hold a special place in Navajo culture. There are ceremonies for many things, and they are seen as providing a link to Navajo history and to the responsibilities that the Navajo need to carry out. During ceremonies, conversations are held with the Holy Ones and the Creator, and are used to bless the sick and the body. Corn is very important to Navajo culture; it is a symbol of fertility and it serves as a food source. During a Navajo wedding ceremony, the couple eats mixed white (male) and yellow (female) corn topped with corn pollen to ensure a fertile marriage (Del Carlo, 2007).

Family is very important to Navajo culture. Navajo culture is matriarchal, and it is built on the belief that a goddess created the universe. Men and women are viewed as complementary equals, as one needs the other to survive. But in reality, the woman is the decision maker, especially in regard to health decisions. Traditional Navajos must obtain the permission of the leading female elder before entering a hospital or undergoing surgery (Diversity Resources, Inc., 2001). Beyond the immediate family is the extended family. The extended family is broken into clans that were created by the Holy Ones. The extended family can also be divided into a camp that consists of the senior married couple, their unmarried children, their married daughters, and the daughters' husbands (Diversity Resources, Inc., 2001).

Today, there are 130 Navajo clans, which have developed from the four original clans: Towering House, Bitterwater, Big Water, and One-Who-Walks-Around.

The Navajo are interested in sharing their culture and ways with the non-Navajo as they feel that the knowledge and skills they possess are a gift from the Holy Ones and are for the benefit of all human beings.

ALASKA NATIVES/AMERICAN ESKIMOS

Not surprisingly, the 2010 census revealed that Alaska had the highest percentage of American Indian/Alaska natives at 19.6% (U.S. Census Bureau, 2011). It is a relatively young population, and most live in small villages (Glanz, 2003). Many of these villages are extremely isolated by both distance and extreme weather. The largest group of Alaska Natives is Eskimos. Eskimos can be divided into three linguistic and geographic subgroups. The two main groups are the Inuit of northern Alaska, Canada, and Greenland, and the Yup'ik from southern Alaska and Russia. The third group is the Pacific (living along the northern Gulf of Alaska). The population defined as "Alaska Native" includes three distinct ethnic and linguistic groups: the Eskimos, the Indians (which can be further divided into three Southeast Coast tribes: Haida, Tlingit and Tsimshian), and the Aleut (11 Athabascan groups scattered across the interior of Alaska) (Glanz, 2003). All Alaska Natives share many cultural traits, but there are significant differences that have developed over the years as well (Glanz, 2003).

Terminology is problematic as the term *Eskimo* is not acceptable to those from Canada and Greenland, who prefer *Inuit*; however, *Inuit* is not appropriate for the Yup'ik, whose language and ethnicity is distinct from the Inuit. For purposes of this chapter, the terms *Alaska Natives* and *American Eskimos* will be used.

It is believed that the ancestors of American Eskimos came across the Bering Strait from Asia more than 30,000 years ago. It is important to note that many Alaska Natives and Native Americans do not accept this theory of the arrival of the first Americans. According to their oral histories and traditions, they have always been present in the Americas. In fact, some Alaska Natives and Native Americans find this theory to be highly offensive (Robinson, 2002).

The purchase of Alaska from Russia is considered by historians to be a good one and it has resulted in the Americanization of Alaska (Barker, 2009). Unfortunately, the consequences of this mixing of peoples and cultures were similar to those experienced by Native Americans. Epidemics broke out, killing thousands, as the natives lacked immunity to diseases such as smallpox and measles (Berg, 2012).

The plentitude of natural resources in Alaska spurred rapid settlement as miners, transportation workers, oil and gas workers, and even the military flooded into Alaska, which has caused the population of Alaska to become more diverse. According to U.S. census data (U.S. Census Bureau, 2010), only 14.8% of the population in Alaska is made up of Alaska Natives or American Indians. The indigenous populations are referred to as *Alaska Natives*. Alaska Natives can be divided into five major cultural groupings: Interior Indians (Athapascans), Aleuts, Southeast Coastal Indians (Tlingit and Haida), Northern Eskimos (Inupiat), and Southern Eskimos (Yup'ik). These groups have traditionally been enemies, despite sharing some similarities of custom and tradition. The animosity is especially prevalent between the American Eskimo and the Indians, as some American Eskimo elders caution their children to be afraid and cautious around the Indians.

The preservation of American Eskimo culture has been complicated because of acculturation into dominant American culture and the loss of young American Eskimos who leave the village to attend school, some never to return. Because the area where the American Eskimos settled is harsh and frigid, the American Eskimos are not able to rely on agriculture for survival. Instead, American Eskimos hunt, fish, trap, and gather food, which restricts the traditional diet to wild meat (caribou, seafood, and even reindeer, which was imported from Scandinavia and Russia to improve the meat supply).

Impact of Communication

According to the Encyclopedia Brittanica, Eskimoan is a difficult language to master and comprehend. Originally, the language had no written form (all American Eskimo history is recounted through storytelling, dance, and art). More recently, a written form of the American Eskimo language was developed by missionaries and is based on phonetics and is still being refined. Other complications associated with the use of the American Eskimo language is the reliance on the third person (a patient will refer to themselves in the third person, for example, as "someone"), all language is present oriented (there are no future tenses), and one word can express an entire sentence. If a word represents an extremely important concept to the American Eskimo, it may have many different word forms to provide a more thorough description (e.g., a different word to differentiate drifting snow from falling snow). Inuit in America and Canada typically speak English.

The American Eskimos also tolerate silence and may wait for several minutes before replying to even a simple statement or greeting. If the American Eskimo were to sense some intolerance from the nurse toward the use of silence, they may feel dominated and inferior, so the nurse should be cautious and not try to fill any silences.

The nurse should also be aware of the importance of nonverbal communication to this cultural group. This is helpful since American Eskimos will seldom disagree in public with others. If the nurse is not certain whether an American Eskimo patient is being polite or sincere, looking for nonverbal cues may be quite helpful. Look for raised eyebrows to indicate "yes" or a wrinkled nose to indicate "no." Agreement is indicated by action, not words.

Impact of Touch

Older American Eskimos are more likely to believe in the healing touch or powers of shamans (Hata, 2012). Although the belief in shamanism exists among some American Eskimos, it is not openly discussed and it would be extremely rare for any discussion of it to occur with or around non-Eskimos. A little is known about the practice, however. The Inuit practice a form of shamanism based on animist principles. The foundation of the belief is that all things (including humans) have a spirit, and the spirit can be influenced by supernatural entities that can be appeased through the use of animals or inanimate objects (Lyons, 2012). The member of the Inuit community who serves as a healer is the *angakkug*. The *angakkug* tends wounds and offers advice and also invokes spirits to provide assistance. They are not formally trained and are not the leader of the community. Their role is simply to invoke spirits, to assist people, and to interpret the subtle and unseen. An *angakkug* is believed to be born with their ability; they are recognized by the community as having the ability, and therefore declared an *angakkug*, as they approach adulthood.

Nursing Considerations

American Eskimos have retained many traditional beliefs despite exposure to modern American society through interaction with many settlers, missionaries, and public health workers who have come to Alaska throughout the years. Understanding that cultural differences persist will permit the nurse to provide care that is culturally responsive. Many of the adaptations that have arisen from the exposure to American culture have caused serious health consequences to the American Eskimo people (La Veist, 2005). American Eskimos are developing obesity and diabetes because of a change in diet (from wild meat to mainly car-bohydrates) and a change from a physically active lifestyle to a much more sed-entary lifestyle (Boyer et al., 2007). Alcoholism and tobacco abuse (smoking and chewing) have increased because of improved access and they have been used as a coping strategy for the stress of acculturation. New mothers often bottle feed instead of breastfeed their babies. There has also been an increase in suicide, espe-cially among Eskimo teens. It is felt this may be due to the struggle for identity as the old and new generations adapt to a more modern world. The generations have been forced to assimilate as they are exposed to modern culture and its services. This exposure to more modern societal norms that are different from their traditional heritage has caused an identity crisis in many teenagers who have responded tragically by committing suicide. Clearly, today's Alaska Natives are suffering from the undermining or outright disappearance of many traditional activities and beliefs. The accompanying despair associated with the loss of self-esteem and the disruption of the family and the community and the resultant coping mechanisms, which includes unhealthy behaviors (such as poor diet and alcohol use), is negatively impacting physical, mental, emotional, and spiritual health of the Eskimos.

Impact of Social Organization

Traditional American Eskimos lived in small bands, in voluntary association un-der a leader recognized for his ability to provide for the group (AncientWorlds .net, 2005). Social status and earning a leadership position were the results of the ability to be a successful provider of food and animal skins. Kinship was para-mount to the survival of the group in such a harsh environment. The emphasis was on group survival, not the individual. Today, strong family ties prevail. The marital customs of the Inuit are not strictly monogamous, as polygamy and open marriages can occur (Zeitzen, 2008). Marriage may also be arranged. Typically, the female can be married upon entering puberty, whereas the man is considered ready when he is an established, productive hunter. Family structure can be flex-ible, including just the nuclear family (husband, wife, and any children), or a much larger group including in-laws, siblings, and adopted children. There is a strong bond of community and a willingness to share goods within the family and the community. Traditionally, only the most personal property was consid-ered private; any unused equipment was reverted to those who had need for it. Honesty and sharing are highly valued traits. In the traditional American Eskimo economy, the division of labor between the sexes was strict; men constructed homes and hunted, and women took care of the homes.

Biologic Variations

The appearance and pigmentation of American Eskimos vary. Some are tall and slim, whereas others are short and stocky. The facial bone structure is similar to American Indians, with eye folds similar to Asians. Pigmentation depends on the amount of ancestral sun exposure (Belanger, 2004).

Disease patterns among Alaska Natives are strongly associated with the adverse consequences of poverty, limited access to health services, and cultural dislocation (Richmond & Ross, 2009). Inadequate education, high rates of unemployment, discrimination, and cultural differences all contribute to unhealthy lifestyles and disparities in access to health care for many American Indian and Alaska Native people. American Indian and Alaska Native children and youth are more than twice as likely to die by the age of 24 years (American Academy of Pediatrics, 2004). This group has the second highest infant mortality rate, after Blacks at 9.22%, based on 2007 data (Mathews & McDorman, 2011). Alaska Natives as a group have a higher risk of accidents than the general population. They also experience high rates of diabetes, liver disease/cirrhosis, and heart disease (La Veist, 2005).

Impact of Faith and Spirituality

There is no question that spiritual beliefs are an important part of Indian culture. Although there is great variability in beliefs, there are core similarities such as the interconnectedness of all things, which leads to a relationship among man, Creator/God, fellow man, and nature. In many traditions, healing, spiritual belief, and community are not separated. Often the entire community is involved in healing ceremonies and in maintaining the power of Indian medicine (Hendrix, 2002).

Traditional American Eskimo religion relied on magic to drive evil away, and it was felt there was a special magical connection among all things (Wolfson, 2001). Reincarnation was a part of the belief system, and all babies were thought to be reincarnations of recently deceased relatives. The afterlife as such was a vague concept. With the migration of Christian missionaries into Alaska, many American Eskimos converted to Christianity, leaving these traditional beliefs behind. Most American Eskimos adopted a Christianity that included some of their traditional beliefs (spirits and monsters) with peaceful behavior being rewarded with a positive and achievable afterlife. The major negative from the conversion was the loss of the art of dancing, which apparently was suppressed by the missionaries working in Alaska. The different Christian religions established strongholds in different parts of Alaska (Catholics in the Yukon River area, Presbyterians in the North Coast, and the Moravians in the Bethel region), but despite this, Christian religious practices were fairly uniform throughout Alaska (Burch, 2004). Today, churchgoing is mainly an activity valued by the middle aged; church attendance by the young and the elderly is at a much lesser level.

In traditional Inuit culture, the *angakut* (or shaman) is the spiritual leader of the tribe. The *angakut* determines the reason for the sickness or illness, determines if there is personal or family responsibility, and isolates the identified broken taboo. The *angakut* goes into a trance in order for his soul to leave his body to travel long distances, so that the cause of the illness and other community problems can be discovered.

Age of the American Eskimo seems to be the key variable related to degree of acculturation into the dominant American society. The older the American Eskimo, the more likely he or she will be to be wearing animal-skin clothing, eat seafood or caribou, speak an American Eskimo language, and believe in spirits and ghosts. The younger the American Eskimo, the more likely he or she will be a representative of the contemporary American culture.

SUMMARY

In spite of the enormous diversity in tribal cultures, languages, and religious beliefs, there are some shared beliefs among American Indian and Alaska Native tribes, especially related to health, illness, and disease prevention. A summary of shared cultural values is in **Table 8–1**. All things begin with the Creator, Supreme Creator, or Great Spirit. Illness presents an opportunity to purify the soul. Disease does not just impact the patient but also the family. Health is maintained by preserving harmony among the body, mind, spirit, and the soul. Because of the interconnectedness of all of these components, spirituality and emotions are viewed as just as important as the body and mind. The spirit world exists alongside and intermingles with the physical world, and this is why death is not viewed as an enemy but as a natural part of life. It is believed that the spirit existed before it entered the physical body and that the spirit will continue on after the physical body is gone.

A reliance on traditional health beliefs seems to be more rigid when dealing with what are perceived as "Indian" problems (such as pain, dysfunctional family relationships, or any sickness of the spirit such as alcoholism or mental illness). It is believed that these Indian problems should be treated with Indian medicine,

Table 8–1 Cultural Values

Cooperation	Silence—ability to listen and wait is valued	Present time orientation; indifference toward future planning as the future, if it comes, it will take care of itself	Extended family orientation
Group harmony	Emotional control; contemplation	Work is only done if absolutely necessary, not for work's sake	Cultural pluralism· with a resistance to assimilation; desire to retain Indian heritage
Modesty and humility	Patience; group decision by discussion and consensus	Time is flexible and nonlinear	Strong relationship with nature; love the Creator and love the land
Noninterference	Sharing and generosity; upward mobility in non-Indian society is not sought	Strong relationship with nature	Spirituality and religion; no belief in original sin or damnation; responsible for their own path

Disclaimer: This chart comprises the more commonly held values in Native American culture and as such is not comprehensive or representative of all Native Americans. Although many Native Americans have been taught these values, not all will exhibit or practice these values as there are many variables to consider such as tribe variation, individual experience, level of acculturation into the dominant American society, and the particular situation.

Source: Hendrix, L. R. (2002). *Health and health care of American Indian and Alaska Native elders.* Retrieved from http://www.stanford.edu/group/ethnoger/americanindian.html

whereas "White man's diseases" (such as DM and cancer) should be treated with "White man's medicine" (Alvord & Van Pelt, 1999). Cultural considerations for the nurse and nurse practitioner are included in **Table 8–2**.

Native North American peoples have survived an onslaught of government policies and wars dedicated to destroying them. What sustained them were traditional family and clan relationships, kinship with homelands, religious ceremonies, ancient stories connecting older and younger generations, and shared traditions that maintained each tribe's uniqueness. This should illustrate to the nurse the value that Native American culture holds for its people. Despite economic

Table 8-2 Cultural Considerations for Nurses

Establishing Respect and Rapport	Culturally Appropriate Verbal and Nonverbal Communication	Language Assessment/Literacy Considerations
Placing an emphasis on listening versus talking may be appreciated by the Native American patient. Calmness and humility are also traits that are highly valued.	Adapt your questions to the patient's level of acculturation into the dominant culture.	Consider that your Native American patient may be monolingual (only fluent in a tribal language and not English).
Try to involve elders in all discussions.	Speak slowly—especially when communicating with the elderly.	Always assess the patient's literacy level prior to giving the patient forms for completion of patient education paperwork.
Keep in mind that personal information will not be readily shared—it will take a little time.	The patient will select their words very carefully and deliberately.	If you need to utilize an interpreter, an adult interpreter of the same gender is preferred.
Ideas/feelings are often conveyed through behavior rather than words.	Questions should be framed within a caring framework and not a "prying" one.	Be careful when providing patient education to avoid probability statements as problems with translation have frequently been noted. The probability statements often do not translate properly because of grammatical differences, which causes a probability to translate into a fact.
Be on the lookout for indirect criticism (such as from a family member) to let you know that the patient may have an issue with you or your care. The delivery of direct criticism is considered rude and disrespectful and will be avoided by the Native American patient. This may also be evident with requests. Be on the alert for requests to be given to the nurse by indirect routes (such as an indirect suggestion or a suggestion that comes from a family member).	Native American languages have some of the longest pause times compared to other languages and especially English. Elders frequently complain that English speakers "talk too fast." Silence is valued; long periods of silence between speakers are commonly seen. Interruption of the person who is speaking is considered extremely rude, especially if that person is older than you.	Keep in mind that negative information may be culturally inappropriate as it may be felt that speaking of the negative may cause it to occur.

There may be a reliance on withdrawal as a form of communicating displeasure or disapproval with the situation. This is referred to as "voting with the feet."

Keep body movements to a minimum and do not touch the patient beyond an introductory handshake unless absolutely necessary (and never without permission). The handshake should not be too firm. If it is a female patient, she may only touch the fingertips when returning the handshake.

Maintaining a physical distance of several feet is customary. Eye contact is usually not direct or only briefly direct as a sign of respect. You may note that the Native American patient is directing their gaze over your shoulder.

There is a reliance on the spoken word (word of mouth) so the use of the Internet or other media for patient education would not be an effective intervention with this patient population.

If utilizing Language Line Services for translation, the service may not be proficient in all Indian languages as there are more than 150 Indian languages still spoken in the United States.

Depending on the age of the patient, and perhaps some other variables such as educational level, consider that the Native American patient may have to translate the concepts the nurse has presented into his native language to consider his response, and then back into English to provide his response to the nurse. This may take time. Try not to hurry the encounter to ensure that the message you have sent is the one received and the response sent back to you is the one that the patient intended.

Source: Hendrix, L. R. (2002). *Health and health care of American Indian and Alaska Native elders.* Retrieved from http://www.stanford.edu/group/ethnoger/americanindian.html

hardship and political oppression, Native Americans continue to survive and to preserve their unique and valuable culture.

CASE STUDY 8–1

Kai is a 58-year-old Navajo (Native American) who has been severely immobile since suffering from a cerebral vascular accident nine months ago. She is cared for on a daily basis by a home health aide and is seen by the visiting nurse on a regular schedule. Kai has many other medical problems including some rather serious comorbidities, such as brittle DM and obesity. The nurse noticed that Kai was developing some contractures and arranged for a visiting physical therapist to come out to evaluate Kai.

When the visiting nurse returned for her next scheduled visit, Kai was not in her usual mood. When the nurse asked Kai what was wrong, she was surprised to hear that the physical therapist had mentioned hospice care as a possibility for Kai's treatment plan. Kai told the nurse that she was extremely upset by this and that she "never wants to see that physical therapist again."

REVIEW QUESTIONS

1. If you were that visiting nurse, how would you respond?
2. In your response, make sure that you demonstrate your understanding of Navajo culture.

Rationale: This case demonstrates the importance that all healthcare team members have knowledge of cultural beliefs of the patients for whom they provide care. The nurse should acknowledge the PT's lack of knowledge of the patient's cultural beliefs and the nurse's intention of advocating for the patient. The nurse should reach out to the PT to share the patient's concerns and to share the nurse's knowledge of cultural competency with the other healthcare team member.

CASE STUDY 8–2

Akule is a 24-year-old Native American male who identifies as "two spirit." He was diagnosed with HIV three years ago. Due to a lack of tolerance on his reservation regarding his sexual orientation, which resulted in harassment and even physical attacks, he moved to the city of Phoenix at age 19 years. He returns home from time to time and seeks medical care at a clinic in Phoenix. He was hospitalized six months ago with a bacterial lung infection and has been abusing alcohol heavily to "cope with his diagnosis." The use of alcohol has caused interruptions in his HIV therapy. Recently, Akule's mother and grandmother have asked for him to return to the reservation so they can help to care for him. They believe that his antiretroviral therapy is making him more ill and they would like him to stop taking it. Akule's grandmother would like him to participate in a healing ceremony instead.

REVIEW QUESTION

1. How would you plan to care for Akule during this period?

Rationale: As the nurse who is caring for Akule, your goal is to support the Western medicine treatment for HIV (antiretroviral therapy), the use of traditional healing methods (including the healing ceremony), encourage adherence to all treatments (Western and traditional), and instill a sense of hope while maintaining confidentiality and trust.

Pertinent Research Studies
#1

A study of Yup'ik Eskimos in Alaska, who on average consume 20 times more omega-3 fats from fish than people in the lower 48 states, suggests that a high intake of these fats helps prevent obesity-related chronic diseases such as diabetes and heart disease. Researchers analyzed data from a community-based study of 330 people living in the Yukon Kuskokwim Delta region of southwest Alaska, 70% of who were overweight or obese. As expected, the researchers found that in participants with low blood levels of DHA and EPA, obesity strongly increased both blood triglycerides (a blood lipid abnormality) and C-reactive protein, or CRP (a measure of overall body inflammation). Elevated levels of triglycerides and CRP increase the risk of heart disease and, possibly, diabetes. Before making a public health recommendation, the researchers said that a randomized clinical trial is needed to test whether increasing omega-3 fat intake significantly reduces the effects of obesity on inflammation and blood triglycerides.

Source: Makhoul, Z., Kristal, A. R., Gulati, R., Luick, B., Bersamin, A., O'Brien, D., . . . Boyer, B. (2011). Associations of obesity with triglycerides and C-reactive protein are attenuated in adults with high red blood cell eicosapentaenoic and docosahexaenoic acids. *European Journal of Clinical Nutrition, 65*(7), 808–817. doi: 10.1038/ejcn.2011.39

#2

Peyote, a hallucinogenic drug derived from the cactus plant and believed by members of the Native American Church to promote spiritual and physical healing, is typically used once a month—and sometimes more frequently—as a religious sacrament. The use of peyote for religious purposes is legal. A study was conducted to determine the safety and the effects of the chronic use of peyote. The researchers found that Navajo Indians who regularly used peyote during religious ceremonies were no more likely to have cognitive or psychological deficits than those who do not use the drug. The authors also stated that the study findings of psychological and cognitive safety may not generalize to illicit (or nonreligious) hallucinogen users.

Source: Halpern, J. H., Sherwood, A. R., Hudson, J. I., Yurgelun-Todd, D., & Pope, H. G. (2005). Psychological and cognitive effects of long-term peyote use among Native Americans. *Biological Psychiatry, 58*(8), 624–631.

REFERENCES

Agency for Healthcare Research and Quality (AHRQ). (2010). Patient centeredness. In *National healthcare disparities report, 2010* (Ch. 5). Retrieved from http://www.ahrq.gov/qual/nhdr10/Chap5.htm

Alvord, L. A., & Van Pelt, E. C. (1999). *The scalpel and the silver bear: The first Navajo woman surgeon combines Western medicine and traditional healing.* New York, NY: Bantam.

American Academy of Pediatrics. (2004). Committee on Native American child health. *Pediatrics, 113*, 148–151.

American Cancer Society. (2008). *Native American healing.* Retrieved from http://www.cancer.org/treatment/treatmentsandsideeffects/complementaryandalternativemedicine/mindbodyandspirit/native-american-healing

Ancientworlds.net. (2005). *History of the Eskimos.* Retrieved from http://www.ancientworlds.net/aw/Journals/Journal/528859&caldate=2012-11-07

Barker, D. (2009). *Was the Alaska purchase a good deal?* Retrieved from http://www.news-releases.uiowa.edu/2009/november/David%20Barker-Alaska.pdf

Beck, J. (2003). *Native American spirituality.* Retrieved from http://www.myhero.com/go/hero.asp?hero=native_am

Belanger, C. (2004). Anatomy of Indians and Inuit. Retrieved from http://faculty.marianopolis.edu/c.belanger/quebechistory/encyclopedia/anatomy.htm

Berg, P. (2012). *Historical basis of the crisis in rural Alaska.* Retrieved from http://m.juneauempire.com/opinion/2012-03-01/historical-basis-crisis-rural-alaska

Boyer, B., Mohatt, G. V., Plaetke, R., Herron, J., Stanhope, K. L., Stephensen, C., . . . The CANHR Project Team. (2007). Metabolic syndrome in Eskimos: The Center for Alaska Native Health Research Study. Retrieved from http://www.nature.com/oby/journal/v15/n11/full/oby2007302a.html

Burch, E. S. (2004). *The Inupiat and the Christization of Arctic Alaska.* Retrieved from http://www.alaskool.org/native_ed/research_reports/christianization/burch.htm

Centers for Disease Control and Prevention (CDC) (2011). Observances—November: American Indian Alaska Native Heritage Month. Retrieved from http://www.cdc.gov/minority-health/observances/AIAN.html

Councellor, A. G. L. (2010). We are making new words: A community philosophy of language revitalization. [Dissertation] Retrieved from http://www.ankn.uaf.edu/curriculum/PhD_Projects/AprilCounceller/CouncellerDissertation.pdf

Crawford, J. (1995). Endangered Native American languages: What is to be done and why? *The Bilingual Research Journal, 19*(1), 17–38.

Del Carlo, L. (2007). Between the sacred mountains: A cultural history of the Dineh. *ESSAI, 5*, Article 15. Retrieved from http://dc.cod.edu/essai/vol5/iss1/15

Diversity Resources, Inc. (2001). *Culture sensitive health care: American Indian.* Blacksburg, VA: Virginia Tech, Office of Multicultural Affairs, Diversity and Work/Life Resource Center. Retrieved from http://erc.msh.org/provider/informatic/AIAN_Disparities_History.pdf

Eskimo-Aleut languages. (2012). In *Encyclopædia Britannica.* Retrieved from http://www.britannica.com/EBchecked/topic/192563/Eskimo-Aleut-languages

Garrett, M. T. (1999). Understanding the "medicine" of Native American traditional values: An integrative review. *Counseling and Values, 43*(2), 84–98.

Garrett, M. T., & Carroll, J. J. (2000). Mending the broken circle: Treatment of substance dependence among Native Americans. *Journal of Counseling & Development, 78*(4), 379–388.

Giger, J. N. (2013). *Transcultural nursing: Assessment and intervention* (6th ed.). Philadelphia, PA: Elsevier.

Gilio-Whitaker, D. (2012). What are the kinship lines of many Native Americans? Retrieved from http://www.ehow.com/info_8444491_kinship-lines-many-native-americans.html

Glanz, K. (2003). *Cancer in women of color monograph.* Bethesda, MD: U.S. Department of Health and Human Services, National Cancer Institute. Retrieved from http://dccps.nci.nih.gov/od/hd-overview.html

Halpern, J. H., Sherwood, A. R., Hudson, J. I., Yurgelun-Todd, D., & Pope, H. G. (2005). Psychological and cognitive effects of long-term peyote use among Native Americans. *Biological Psychiatry, 58*(8), 624–631.

Hata, K. (2012). *Inuit/Eskimo society.* Retrieved from http://www.astronomy.pomona.edu/archeo/alaska/eskimo.html

Hendrix, L. R. (2002). *Health and health care of American Indian and Alaska Native elders.* Stanford, CA: Stanford University. Retrieved from http://www.stanford.edu/group/ethnoger/americanindian.html

Historynet.com. (2006). *World War 2 Navajo code talkers.* Retrieved from http://www.historynet.com/world-war-ii-navajo-code-talkers.htm

Kuschell-Haworth, H. T. (1999). Jumping through hoops: Traditional healers and the Indian Health Care Improvement Act. *DePaul Journal of Health Care Law,* 843–860.

La Veist, T. A. (2005). *Minority populations and health: An introduction to health disparities in the United States.* San Francisco, CA: Jossey-Bass.

Lake Champlain Maritime Museum (LCMM), & Wiseman, F. (2012). *Europeans and Native Americans: A lasting impact.* Retrieved from http://www.lcmm.org/navigating/Quad Curriculum_LastingImpact.pdf

Literarynet.org. (2012). *Understanding Native Americans and acculturation.* Retrieved from http://www.literacynet.org/lp/namericans/understanding.html

Lobo, S., Talbot, S., & Morris, T. L. (2009). *Native American voices* (3rd ed.). London, UK: Pearson.

Lyons, A. S. (2012). *Primitive medicine.* Retrieved from http://www.healthguidance.org/entry/6306/1/Primitive-Medicine.html

Makhoul, Z., Kristal, A. R., Gulati, R., Luick, B., Bersamin, A., O'Brien, D., . . . Boyer, B. (2011). Associations of obesity with triglycerides and C-reactive protein are attenuated in adults with high red blood cell eicosapentaenoic and docosahexaenoic acids. *European Journal of Clinical Nutrition, 65*(7), 808–817. doi: 10.1038/ejcn.2011.39

Mathews, T. J., & McDorman, M. F. (2011). *National mortality statistics from the 2007 period.* Retrieved from http://www.cdc.gov/nchs/data/nvsr/nvsr59/nvsr59_06.pdf

National Institutes of Health. (2001). *Strong Heart Study data book: A report to American Indian communities.* Retrieved from http://www.nhlbi.nih.gov/resources/docs/shs_db.pdf

National Native American AIDS Prevention Center. (2002). *Clinician's guide: Working with Native Americans living with HIV.* Retrieved from http://www.ihs.gov/hivaids/docs/Cliniciansguide.pdf

National Park Service. (1978). *American Indian Religious Freedom Act, Title 42, USC §1996.* Retrieved from http://www.nps.gov/history/local-law/FHPL_IndianRelFreAct.pdf

National Park Service. (1990). *The Native American Graves Protection Repatriation Act (NAGPRA).* Retrieved from http://www.nps.gov/history/nagpra

Navajo Nation Government. (2009). *The Navajo nation.* Retrieved from http://www.navajo-nsn.gov

Neel, J. V. (1962). Diabetes mellitus: A "thrifty" genotype rendered detrimental by "progress"? *American Journal of Human Genetics, 14,* 353–362.

Pevar, S. L. (1992). *The Rights of Indians and tribes: The basic American Civil Liberties Union guide to Indian and tribal rights.* New York, NY: NYU Press.

Purnell, L. D. (2013). *Transcultural health care: A culturally competent approach* (4th ed.). Philadelphia, PA: F.A. Davis.

Reich, D., Patterson, N., Campbell, D., Tandon, A., Mazieres, S., Ray, N., . . . Ruiz-Linares, A. (2012). Reconstructing Native American population history. *Nature, 488,* 370–374.

Richmond, C. A. M., & Ross, N. A. (2009). The determinants of First Nation and Inuit health: A critical population health approach. *Health and Place, 15*(2), 403–411.

Robinson, B. A. (2002). *Native American spirituality.* Ontario, CA: Consultants on Religious Tolerance. Retrieved from http://www.religioustolerance.org/nataspir.htm

Rowell, R., & Bouey, P. (2002). *What are American Indian/Alaska Natives' HIV prevention needs?* San Francisco: University of California at San Francisco, Center for AIDS Prevention Studies, AIDS Research Institute. http://www.caps.ucsf.edu/nativamerican.html

Sanchez, T. R., Plawecki, J. A., & Plawecki, H. M. (1996). The delivery of culturally sensitive health care to Native Americans. *Journal of Holistic Nursing, 14,* 295–307.

Satz, R. N. (2002). *American Indian policy in the Jacksonian era.* Norman, OK: University of Oklahoma Press.

Stanford.edu. (2012). American Indian. Retrieved from http://geriatrics.stanford.edu/ethnomed/american_indian/introduction/definitions.html

Tsai, G., & Alanis, L. (2004). Journey to thinking multiculturally. The Native American culture: A historical and reflective perspective. *NASP Communique, 32*(8). Retrieved from http://www.nasponline.org/publications/cq/cq328native.aspx

Tsunehara, C. H., Leonetti, D. L., & Fujimoto, W.Y. (1990). Diet of second-generation Japanese-American men with and without non-insulin-dependent diabetes. *American Journal of Clinical Nutrition, 52*(4), 731–738.

U.S. Census Bureau. (2010). *The American Indian and Alaska Native population: 2010 (2010 Census brief).* Washington, DC: U.S. Government Printing Office.

U.S. Census Bureau. (2011). *American Indian and Alaska Native National Heritage Month: November 2011.* Retrieved from https://www.census.gov/newsroom/releases/archives/facts_for_features_special_editions/cb11-ff22.html

U.S. Commission on Civil Rights. (2004). *Native American health disparities briefing.*

U.S. Department of Health and Human Services [USDHHS]. (2007). *Alcohol metabolism: An update.* Retrieved from http://pubs.niaaa.nih.gov/publications/AA72/AA72.htm

Vergano, D. (2012). *Three waves of Native American immigration.* Retrieved from http://usatoday30.usatoday.com/tech/science/story/2012-07-11/native-american-origins/56148248/1

Waldman, C. (2006). *Encyclopedia of Native American tribes* (3rd ed.). Retrieved from http://www.scribd.com/doc/21410381/Native-American-Tribes

Wolfson, M. (2001). *Inuit mythology.* Berkeley Heights, NJ: Enslow.

Zeitzen, M. K. (2008). *Polygamy: A cross-cultural analysis.* New York, NY: Berg.

For a full suite of assignments and additional learning activities, see the access code at the front of your book.

Whites (Non-Hispanic)

CHAPTER OBJECTIVES

Upon completion of this chapter, the nurse will be able to:

- Identify traditional health beliefs of Whites (non-Hispanics) with a European heritage.
- Describe potential cultural phenomena affecting health care among Whites (non-Hispanics).
- Plan for nursing care delivery that considers the potential cultural beliefs of White (non-Hispanic) patients.

© Monkey Business Images/ShutterStock, Inc.

INTRODUCTION

There are vast differences among all people. Certain cultural characteristics will be described herein that may or may not be associated with individual patients. The intent is not to be stereotypical but instead to provide the nurse with essential generalized cultural knowledge to provide a starting point to ensure nursing care delivery that meets the patient's unique, individual needs.

Relying on stereotypes is an ending point because no further effort will be made to determine if it is appropriate to apply the information to the individual in question. A generalization, on the other hand, serves as a starting point. Having knowledge of evidence-based generalizations regarding cultural customs and beliefs can help avoid misunderstandings and enable nurses and nurse practitioners to provide better care.

HISTORICAL BACKGROUND

Throughout the history of the United States, tens of millions of immigrants have come to the "New World" to begin a new life. The constant wave of immigration contributed to the growth and development of the United States during its evolution from emerging nation to what it is today—a world power (Diner, 2008). Although most Americans view the United States as a White European nation, the result of continuous European migration since the 17th century, we now understand that European immigration was only one component in populating the American continent. From the 1820s through the 1990s, two-thirds of the nearly 65 million immigrants to the United States came from Europe. By 1965, however, less than half of the immigrants came from Europe; by the 1990s, it was less than 10% (Katzman, 2000). In 2010, European immigrants only numbered 88,730 (a small fraction when compared to the 1,042,625 total number of immigrants from all countries combined) (U.S. Department of Homeland Security, 2010). Europeans make up a small percentage of naturalized citizens as well. According to the U.S. Department of Homeland Security (2011), only 82,209 Europeans became naturalized citizens (total number of naturalized citizens was 694,193) (U.S. Department of Homeland Security, 2011).

The United States was a settler society and required large waves of immigrants to settle into large areas that were undeveloped. The establishment of a settler society is not unusual as it is associated with Canada, Australia, and New Zealand, among other countries (Diner, 2008). These settler societies had significant natural resources, such as land and capital to tap into, but lacked sufficient manpower. In the United States, the reliance on the use of Native Americans, and later on the African slaves who were brought here against their will, was not enough to meet the growing labor demands, and the call for immigration was launched. Immigration not only led to the development of the country but also shaped our society and national culture.

During the period when European immigration dominated, the source of immigrants changed. In the first two-thirds of the 19th century, most immigrants came from Ireland, Germany, and Great Britain. In the 1880s, a permanent shift occurred. In 1882, the peak year of the "old immigration," 87% of the immigrants came from Ireland, Germany, Great Britain, Scandinavia, Switzerland, and Holland. In 1907, the peak year of the "new immigrants," 81% of immigrants came from Italy, Russia, Austria-Hungary, Greece, Romania, and Turkey. From the 1820s to World War II, Germany provided 16% of immigrants, Ireland 12%, Italy 12%, Austria-Hungary 12%, Great Britain 11%, Russia 10%, and Scandinavia 5% (Katzman, 2000).

Historians have divided immigration to the United States into distinct time periods, each of which is associated with varying rates of immigration from differing areas of the world. All immigration, however, has contributed to shaping our national psyche.

SETTLERS OF THE NEW WORLD

The first and longest of the five historical time periods for immigration extended from the 17th century through the early 19th century. Although immigrants from this time came from a variety of places, the largest volume by far came from the British Isles (England, Scotland, Wales, and Ireland). Others came from southwest Germany (Palatinate), France, and the Netherlands, as well as Jews from Poland and the Netherlands (Diner, 2008). The common denominator among these immigrants from Western and Northern Europe was the lack of ability to take advantage of the modernization of their home countries' economies and the promise of cheap land in America. Reasons for leaving their homeland included desire for personal or religious freedom, crop failure, land and job shortages, famine, and rising taxes. The goal was to come to a land of economic opportunity. Because of the high travel costs associated with the journey to the United States, many of the settlers of the New World were able to come here by becoming indentured servants. A contract was signed and, in exchange for a commitment of a specific amount of time spent in hard labor, they would receive transport and, at the end of the contract, ownership of a small piece of land. The vast majority of the early immigrants were farmers who were lured here by the call of cheap land. European immigrants entered the United States through East Coast ports. More than 70% entered through New York City. Although many immigrants stayed close to the port of entry, some did find their way inland. Many under-populated states would actively recruit for immigrant settlers by offering jobs or land for farming.

MASS MIGRATION OF THE 1820s TO THE 1880s

During the years of 1820 to 1880, 15 million immigrants came to the United States (Diner, 2008). As the United States moved toward industrialization, some of the immigrants took work as migrant workers. One of the largest immigrant groups to enter the United States during this time was Irish Catholics. Unfortunately, like the Chinese, they were met with discrimination from a *nativist* movement (those immigrants who had come to the United States earlier, in this case between 1600 and 1800). In addition to the large number of Irish immigrants, a small number of Chinese also came to the United States during this time. Neither group was warmly greeted, and they were faced with hatred and violence from the earlier European arrivals. Although many of the European immigrants came to farm in the Midwest and the Northeast, a large number chose to settle in cities like New York, Philadelphia, and Boston. The opening of the Erie Canal in 1825 permitted the development of the Midwest for farming and agriculture, and industrial development led to the need for many textile workers in the cities.

European conditions influenced the stream of migrants. Poor harvests and famine sent millions of Irish, Swedes, and some Germans to the United States in the 1830s and later (Katzman, 2000). In the 1840s, political upheaval sent more Germans across the ocean, and a steady flow of religious dissenters came at all times. Limited economic opportunities in Europe sent tens of millions of peasants, small farmers, craftsmen, and unskilled workers, men and women alike, both as individuals and families, to America (Katzman, 2000). Ethnic and religious minorities including Jews from Eastern Europe, Poles and Germans from Russia, Macedonians from the Balkans, and Czechs and Bohemians from Austria-Hungary found freedom in the United States and formed settlements in areas of the country such as Kansas (Katzman, 2000).

Young men from France, newly freed from the military after the fall of Napoleon, came to the United States, as did others from England, Scandinavia, and central Europe in response to the changes in their home economies that resulted in great difficulty in making a living in their country of origin's new order (Diner, 2008).

Upon arrival to the United States, the immigrants tended to cluster together in homogenous groupings. The Midwest was populated with immigrants from Sweden, Norway, and Denmark, and from many regions of what would later become the country of Germany. The vast majority of these immigrants were Protestants, but during this time the first large-scale wave of Irish Catholics came to the United States. The arrival of Catholics was met with hostility and a wave of nativism—a fear of Catholicism and of the Irish (Perea, 1996). The nativism movement was so sweeping that it even gave birth to a political party (the Know Nothings) that made anti-immigration and anti-Catholicism its purpose (Perea, 1996).

An explosion of immigration was facilitated by improvements in technology and transportation (Sage, 2005). Ocean travel advanced from sail to motor power. The ships also became much larger, permitting 25 million European immigrants to make the transatlantic crossing during this period. Immigrants came from Italy, Greece, Hungary, and Poland. Approximately 3 million of these immigrants were Jewish. This wave of immigrants gravitated toward the cities and sought jobs in the industrial labor pool (steel, coal, garment production, and automobiles) (Sage, 2005). This influx of labor resulted in America becoming an economic strength, but also triggered a second wave of nativism. By the 1890s, immigration was viewed as posing a serious threat to our nation's health and security. In 1893, the Immigration Restriction League was formed and lobbying of Congress began in earnest to restrict future immigration into the United States. Several pieces of legislation were passed over the ensuing years. In 1924, Congress passed the final version of the National Origins Act. The act essentially gave preference to immigrants from Northern and Western Europe, severely limited the numbers from Eastern and Southern Europe, and declared all potential immigrants from Asia to be unworthy of entry into the United States. Because the act did not apply to countries in the Western Hemisphere, immigration from Western Hemisphere countries exploded in the 1920s. Historians consider the 1920s the penultimate era in U.S. immigration history (Martin & Midgley, 2003). Immigrants came to America from Mexico; various countries in the Caribbean such as Haiti, Jamaica, and Barbados; and from Central and South America. The 1924 legislation was enforced until 1965. During that 40-year period, exceptions were made on a case-by-case basis for refugees (Jewish refugees from World War II, Cubans fleeing communism and Fidel Castro, and defectors from behind the Iron Curtain), but the law remained intact and enforced.

A consequence of the civil rights revolution in the United States during the 1960s was the passage of the Hart–Cellar Act in 1965, which eliminated the racially-based quota system (Kutler, 2003). Preference was given to potential immigrants with family already in the United States and to the applicants who had skills or occupations that were deemed critical by the U.S. Department of Labor. Immigrants came from Europe but also from Korea, China, India, the Philippines, Pakistan, and from some African countries. By the year 2000, immigration had returned to the levels of 1900 (Martin & Midgley, 2003).

No matter where they come from or the timing of when they come, immigrants bring languages, cultures, and religions to the United States that contribute over time to the nation as a whole. European immigrants have a positive and negative legacy. On the negative side, there has been little respect shown for the indigenous population of the United States (Native Americans), with a history of ethnic and religious intolerance (Katzman, 2000). The positive contributions include language from the English, personalized politics from the Irish, and contributions to the culture of U.S. cities from the Germans (Katzman, 2000). The United States has thus evolved into an industrial, modern, and multicultural nation.

PROJECTIONS

In the history of the United States, the majority population has been White (non-Hispanic). Although this majority status is still true with Whites making up 72.4% of the U.S. population, the numbers are declining (U.S. Census Bureau, 2011). It is projected that by the 2030s, White deaths will begin to outpace White births (U.S. Census Bureau, 2008a), and the White population will continue its decline by about 6% between the years 2000 to 2050 (Ortman & Guarneri, 2009). By the year 2042, a White majority will no longer be a reality in the United States (U.S. Census Bureau, 2008a). This population decline is more apparent in some states than in others. Between the years 2000 and 2010, 15 states (6 of them in the Northeast) saw their White populations decline. This is significantly different than the population changes associated with the Black, Hispanic/Latino, and Asian populations. During the same 10-year time period (2000–2010) the Black population declined in only 2 states, while the Hispanic/Latino and Asian populations grew in each and every state (The Center for Public Education, 2010).

This change will occur even sooner with the younger White population. By the year 2023, more than half of the country's children will be present-day minorities. By the midcentury mark, the United States is projected to have a total population of 439 million people, but the majority, or 54% of the population, will consist of present-day racial minorities. Whites will be outnumbered by Hispanics/Latinos, Blacks Americans, Asians, American Indians, Native Hawaiians, and Pacific Islanders. In some geographic areas (such as New York, Los Angeles, Chicago, Houston, Philadelphia, and Detroit, as well as the states of California and Texas), the change in status for Whites to a minority group has already occurred (U.S. Census Bureau, 2008b). The timeline for when this change in majority to minority status for Whites will occur has been moved up from the earlier prediction of 2050. The overall population decline of Whites is due to declining birth rates and declining immigration rates from European countries to the United States.

In the year 2005, 15.7% of immigrants entering the United States self-identified as being from Europe. See **Table 9–1** for a listing provided by the Office of Homeland Security identifying the top 20 countries of birth for immigrants admitted into the United States in the year 2005. The first European country on the listing is Ukraine, in tenth place (U.S. Department of Homeland Security, 2006). By the year 2010, there were no European countries in the top twenty listing (U.S. Department of Homeland Security, 2010).

STATISTICS

The most recent U.S. census data (2010) reveals the following information: the White non-Hispanic population of the United States was 223.6 million (72.4% of the total population). The median age of Whites for both genders was 41 years of age. The national median age reveals the widening racial age gap that is continuing to grow. The overall median age was 36.8 years (as a basis of comparison, the median age for Blacks was 32 and for Asians was 31.6 years of age). The majority of Whites were female (50.8%) (U.S. Census Bureau, 2010).

Beginning in 1980, the U.S. census began to include a question regarding a person's ancestry self-identification. Ancestry is a broad concept that can mean different things to different people. The U.S. Census Bureau defines ancestry as a person's ethnic origin, heritage, descent, or "roots," which may reflect their place of birth, place of birth of parents or ancestors, and ethnic identities that have evolved within the United States. The top 10 most common self-identified ancestries listed in descending order from the 2000 census were German, Irish, African American, English, American, Mexican, Italian, Polish, French, and American Indian.

Ancestry data was not collected during the 2010 census. Ancestry data is now collected by the American Community Survey and reported by the U.S. Census Bureau. In 2010, 12.5% of respondents selected Europe as their world region of

Table 9–1 Immigrants Admitted by Region and Top 20 Countries of Birth for the Year 2005

Region of Birth	Number	Percentage
Africa	85,102	7.6
Asia	400,135	35.7
Europe	176,569	15.7
North America	345,575	30.8
Caribbean	108,598	9.7
Central America	53,470	4.8
Other North America	183,507	16.3
Oceania	6546	0.6
South America	103,143	9.2
Unknown Country	5303	0.5
Country of Birth		
1. Mexico	161,445	14.4
2. India	84,681	7.5
3. China, People's Republic	69,967	6.2
4. Philippines	60,748	5.4
5. Cuba	36,261	3.2
6. Vietnam	32,784	2.9
7. Dominican Republic	27,504	2.5
8. Korea	26,562	2.4
9. Colombia	25,571	2.3
10. Ukraine	22,761	2.0
11. Canada	21,878	1.9
12. El Salvador	21,359	1.9
13. United Kingdom	19,800	1.8
14. Jamaica	18,346	1.6
15. Russia	18,083	1.6
16. Guatemala	16,825	1.5
17. Brazil	16,664	1.5
18. Peru	15,676	1.4
19. Poland	15,352	1.4
20. Pakistan	14,926	1.3
Other	**395,180**	**35.2**
All countries	**1,122,373**	**100.0**

Source: U.S. Department of Homeland Security. (2005). *2005 yearbook of immigration statistics.* Washington, DC: U.S. Department of Homeland Security: Office of Immigration Statistics.

Table 9–2 Ten Leading Countries by Rank for Immigration in 2009

Country	Number
Mexico	11,478,234
Philippines	1,733,864
India	1,665,055
China	1,425,814
El Salvador	1,157,217
Vietnam	1,149,355
Korea	1,012,911
Cuba	982,862
Canada	814,122
Dominican Republic	791,593

Source: Patten, E. (2012). *Statistical portrait of the foreign-born population in the United States, 2009, Table 5, country of birth: 2009.* Pew Hispanic Center. Retrieved from the Pew Hispanic Center website: http://www.pewhispanic.org/2012/02/21/statistical-portrait-of-the-foreign-born-population-in -the-united-states-2010/

birth (U.S. Census Bureau, 2010). See **Table 9–3** for the top 10 self-identified European-only ancestries from the 2000 census. See **Table 9–4** for the top 10 countries of birth of the foreign-born population for the years of 1850 to 2000 from the U.S. Census Bureau.

Table 9–3 Top 10 Most Common Self-Identified European Ancestries from the 2000 U.S. Census

2000 Ranking Among All Ancestries	European Ancestry Group	Number	Percentage
1	German	42,841,569	15.2
2	Irish	30,524,799	10.8
3	English	24,509,692	8.7
4	Italian	15,638,348	5.6
5	Polish	8,977,235	3.2
6	French	8,309,666	3.0
7	Scottish	4,890,581	1.7
8	Dutch	4,541,770	1.6
9	Norwegian	4,477,725	1.6
10	Scotch–Irish	4,319,232	1.5

The ancestry groups listed on this table were self-identified. Many respondents listed more than one area of ancestry. Overall, about 500 different ancestries were reported during the 2000 census.

Source: U.S. Census Bureau. (2004). *Ancestry 2000.* Retrieved from http://www.census.gov/ prod/2004pubs/c2kbr-35.pdf

Several White ethnic groups will be described in this chapter with a focus on common cultural beliefs related to traditional health beliefs, disease management, and interactions with the healthcare delivery system to help the nurse plan for and deliver culturally appropriate care.

Table 9–4 Top 10 Countries of Birth of the Foreign-Born Population of the United States, 1850–2000

Ten Leading Countries by Rank*	1850	1880	1900	1930	1960
1.	Ireland 962,000	Germany 1,967,000	Germany 2,663,000	Italy 1,790,000	Italy 1,257,000
2.	Germany 584,000	Ireland 1,855,000	Ireland 1,615,000	Germany 1,609,000	Germany 990,000
3.	Great Britain 379,000	Great Britain 918,000	Canada 1,180,000	United Kingdom 1,403,000	Canada 953,000
4.	Canada 148,000	Canada 717,000	Great Britain 1,168,000	Canada 1,310,000	United Kingdom 833,000
5.	France 54,000	Sweden 194,000	Sweden 582,000	Poland 1,269,000	Poland 748,000
6.	Switzerland 13,000	Norway 182,000	Italy 484,000	Soviet Union 1,154,000	Soviet Union 691,000
7.	Mexico 13,000	France 107,000	Russia 424,000	Ireland 745,000	Mexico 576,000
8.	Norway 13,000	China 104,000	Poland 383,000	Mexico 641,000	Ireland 339,000
9.	Holland 10,000	Switzerland 89,000	Norway 336,000	Sweden 595,000	Austria 305,000
10.	Italy 4,000	Bohemia 85,000	Austria 276,000	Czechoslovakia 492,000	Hungary 245,000

Ten Leading Countries by Rank*	1970	1980	1990	2000
1.	Italy 1,009,000	Mexico 2,199,000	Mexico 4,298,000	Mexico 7,841,000
2.	Germany 833,000	Germany 849,000	China 921,000	China 1,391,000
3.	Canada 812,000	Canada 843,000	Philippines 913,000	Philippines 1,222,000
4.	Mexico 760,000	Italy 832,000	Canada 745,000	India 1,007,000
5.	United Kingdom 686,000	United Kingdom 669,000	Cuba 737,000	Cuba 952,000
6.	Poland 548,000	Cuba 608,000	Germany 712,000	Vietnam 863,000
7.	Soviet Union 463,000	Philippines 501,000	United Kingdom 640,000	El Salvador 765,000
8.	Cuba 439,000	Poland 418,000	Italy 581,000	Korea 701,000
9.	Ireland 251,000	Soviet Union 406,000	Korea 568,000	Dominican Republic 692,000
10.	Austria 214,000	Korea 290,000	Vietnam 543,000	Canada 678,000

*Data are not totally comparable over time because of changes in boundaries for some countries. Great Britain excludes Ireland. United Kingdom includes Northern Ireland. China in 1990 includes Hong Kong and Taiwan.

Source: U.S. Census Bureau. (2001). *Profile of the foreign-born population in the United States: 2000.* Retrieved from http://www.census.gov/prod/2002pubs/p23-206.pdf

IRISH AMERICANS

Historical Background

Ireland comprises 26 counties and became a free state in 1921 (Central Intelligence Agency [CIA], 2012). The Republic of Ireland was proclaimed in 1948, when Ireland withdrew from the British Commonwealth. The British government reasserted its claim to Northern Ireland, a claim that was not recognized by the Republic of Ireland. Since that time, warfare has been present with repeated on and off cease-fires negotiated. Today, the unrest continues and many Irish Americans send money to support the Irish Republican Army. According to the CIA (2012), a peace settlement with Northern Ireland is gradually being negotiated despite difficulties. In 2012, the population of Ireland was estimated to be 4.7 million (CIA, 2012). Ireland is bordered on the northeast by Northern Ireland (province of Ulster), which remains a part of the United Kingdom. It is bordered by the Atlantic Ocean to the south and west. The ocean separates Ireland from Great Britain by an average of 50 miles. Ireland was colonized by European settlers from Great Britain with the Celtic influence remaining dominant today.

Throughout the history of the United States, immigrants have made their way from Ireland (Martin & Midgley, 2003). During colonial times, the early Irish immigrants were Presbyterian Protestants from Ulster, now known as Northern Ireland. The motivation to come to America was to seek financial gain and a better life. The majority of the Ulster-born Irish immigrants were tenant farmers or skilled artisans. The Irish who came later were motivated not to seek a better life but to simply survive. The famine in Ireland, a result of a blight that struck the potato crop between the years 1845 and 1854, left death and destruction in its wake. Tenant farmers were left with no crop and therefore no money. Although some landlords were initially compassionate, the passage of the Poor Law Extension Act of 1847 by Parliament changed that. Because of that law, a landlord became financially responsible for the cost of care for their tenants—an expense that many landlords were not financially able to handle, so evictions became extremely common. Once evicted, the tenant farmer was left with few options: move into a disease-infested workhouse or starve while searching for food and shelter. Many chose to flee their native land and come to America, with the goal and hope of survival. These Irish immigrants were different than the Ulster Irish in many ways. The Ulster Irish were Protestant and the newer Irish immigrants were Catholics. The penal laws in Ireland had long placed Irish Catholics at a distinct disadvantage. They were poor farmers who were uneducated and totally dependent on their rocky plot of land (that was owned by the landlord) for survival. The potato crop was the sole food source. They came from large families with a lifestyle that favored close social interaction. Although they possessed little, they shared readily and enjoyed celebrating their beliefs with tradition, song, dance, and religious rituals. When their land was lost, they felt there was no place left for them in Ireland. Between 1840 and 1860, more than 1.5 million Irish came to the United States. Where they settled was determined by their financial situation. Although a large contingent settled in New Orleans and other cities, the Irish who immigrated to escape the famine stayed in the eastern port cities of New York or Boston simply because they had no money or marketable skills to move on. Some were forced to move westward to Chicago in search of employment. The vast majority were poor and Catholic and were the first wave of non-Anglo-Saxon immigrants to the United States, and because of this difference, they were often met with hostility. Another unique difference was that many of the immigrants were unaccompanied women. Many women took jobs as domestic servants in the homes of the wealthy. The uneducated men took jobs of hard labor, digging ditches or building canals or bridges. Both men and women worked and saved with the goal to bring additional family members to America. Although they were on the lowest rung of American society, over time they began to dare to dream their own version of the American dream.

Today, approximately 36.9 million people of Irish descent live in the United States (American Community Survey, 2009). This number is almost eight times larger than the current population of the country of Ireland. Irish ranks as the second largest ancestry group in the United States, second only to German.

Table 9–5 Cultural Values of Euro-Americans (White Non-Hispanics)

Competition	Strong Expression of Opinion	Saving for the Future (Retirement)	Mastery over Nature
Individual achievement	Action valued over inaction; direct confrontation	Puritan work ethic; work for work's sake Rigid schedule	Judeo-Christian beliefs; emphasis on a second coming and the need for salvation
Overt identification of accomplishments; pride	Rapid responses and decision making valued	Euro-centric obsession with money (i.e., time is money)	Nuclear family orientation; measure of successful child rearing is the child being able to leave home and thrive
Advice giving, directness	Individual ownership; upward social mobility	Future orientation; ability to delay gratification to the future	Follow the rules of dominant society, which is to work to get ahead; one who has developed social and economic mobility

Source: Hendrix, L. R. (2002). *Health and health care of American Indian and Alaska Native elders.* Retrieved from http://www.stanford.edu/group/ethnoger/americanindian.html

Table 9–6 Nursing Considerations for the White Non-Hispanic Patient (Euro-American)

Appropriate Ways to Show Respect and Establish Rapport	Culturally Appropriate Verbal and Nonverbal Communication	Language Assessment/ Literacy Level
Utilize a firm handshake as it denotes power and authority. Self-disclosure is valued. Strive for an open and honest communication style. Expect directness in all patient interactions: direct criticism will be utilized to alter behavior; disapproval will be directly expressed; and requests will be made directly.	Use direct eye contact as it is viewed as a sign of honesty and sincerity. Rely on the verbal expression of ideas/feelings (the speech is more important than the behavior). Speaking is emphasized over listening; the expression of one's opinion is highly valued. Verbal and written communication are valued over nonverbal communication.	Consider the use of alternative methods for patient education such as media and internet, as this type of information passing is culturally appropriate.

Source: Hendrix, L. R. (2002). *Health and health care of American Indian and Alaska Native elders.* Retrieved from http://www.stanford.edu/group/ethnoger/americanindian.html

Traditional Health Beliefs

Traditional health beliefs and practices among different ethnic or cultural groups are divided into three groups: beliefs that result in no harm, beliefs that may produce beneficial health outcomes, and beliefs that may have serious or harmful outcomes (Gale Encyclopedia of Public Health, 2002). Harmless beliefs should not be discouraged by the nurse because the patient having faith in his or her beliefs may actually result in a positive patient outcome. On the other hand, traditional health beliefs that can have serious or harmful outcomes (such as female genital mutilation) must be discouraged by the nurse.

Some Irish Americans still follow folk medicine beliefs. These beliefs have not totally died out in Ireland. In fact, some aspects have seen a resurgence due to an interest in natural treatments and holistic medicine. These remedies originally grew out of a belief that injuries and illnesses were the result of unkindness or disrespect directed toward faerie folk (Preet, 2008). Further it was believed that any cures or treatments in the possession of doctors or other healers were provided by faeries (Preet, 2008). Until the 19th century, folk remedies were the preferred treatment for most maladies. After the 19th century, traditional medicine became more popular. Although out of mainstream favor, if a patient wishes to utilize folk medicine, such treatments are considered to be neutral (do not cause benefit or harm) (Giger, 2013). These activities include blessing of the throat, tying a bag of camphor around the neck to prevent flu, keeping closet doors closed to block evil spirits, not looking in a mirror at night, boiling sheep droppings in milk to cure whooping cough, keeping a strong and loving family, and the wearing of holy medals.

Irish Americans often have a reactive rather than a proactive approach to illness as they often delay seeking medical attention until the situation is quite serious. The first line of treatment will often be home remedies. Some folk medicine practices are deemed beneficial: getting plenty of rest, maintaining a positive attitude, eating a balanced diet, and taking vitamins (Spector, 2008).

Impact of Communication

The official languages of Ireland are Irish (Irish Gaelic) and English. English is universally spoken in Ireland while Irish Gaelic is mainly spoken along the western coast of the country (CIA, 2012). An understanding of this Celtic language is necessary. The Irish language was initially an oral one, so the culture was passed on orally, most notably through poetry. Although a modern day Irish language persists today, it was almost wiped out because of the onslaught of the English language in the 19th century. Because many Irish immigrants arriving in the United States spoke English, they had an easier time with assimilation into the dominant American society than other immigrants (Martin & Midgley, 2003).

The development of a therapeutic relationship is essential for effective nursing care delivery. When dealing with the Irish American, the nurse should consider maintaining a friendly distance initially. The first step for the nurse is to determine the level of cultural identification the Irish American has to Ireland. Patients of Irish descent may range from those who uphold many if not all of the traditional health beliefs to others who may have little or no knowledge of Ireland or its culture. Patients who live in community settings that are made up of many other Irish would be more likely to have a strong attachment to their Irish identity and its associated cultural beliefs. Irish Americans who are more likely to uphold traditional cultural beliefs are usually older and are usually reluctant to share their feelings. The nurse should avoid exploring the patient's feelings and instead focus on a more logical approach—appealing to the Irish Americans' strong sense of responsibility. This is an especially effective strategy when providing patient education. The Irish tend to find indirect communication more natural than the specific and direct approach utilized by nurses and other healthcare providers. Directness can be perceived as rudeness. In addition, the use of constant eye contact by the nurse will be viewed as disrespectful by the patient. It can be a challenge for the

nurse to rely on a more indirect approach, but doing so will improve the therapeutic relationship that can develop.

The nurse should also be aware of the tendency of Irish Americans to under-
state—especially their emotional state or pain level. Any complaint of emotional
or physical pain should be explored by the nurse and not minimized in any way,
because it is likely the pain is more severe than being acknowledged by the Irish
American patient.

Finally, the choice of words by the nurse is an extremely important consideration. There is a strong cultural theme that discourages discussing problems for
fear that they will become worse. This belief often results in the avoidance of
certain words (such as cancer) that are replaced with the use of less threatening
euphemisms. For this same reason, therapy is frowned upon as it is felt to have
little value. In fact, "paying to talk" is very troublesome to the traditional Irish.

Impact of Time and Space

The use of time and space are also important considerations when providing
nursing care to the Irish American patient. As every nurse knows, time is of extreme importance in healthcare delivery. It is important to avoid rushing the Irish
American patient if at all possible. Rushing is viewed as extremely impolite and
the patient may internalize this as a reflection of their unimportance. The nurse
should strive to make the patient feel that they are the priority. An appreciation
of patient boundaries by the nurse will make the patient feel more respected.
This can best be achieved through the use of a casual and more physically distant
approach by the nurse.

Impact of Social Organization

The parish church was the center of social activity. Because many of these Irish
immigrants were viewed as different because they were Catholic, they faced hostility in society. The result was the formation of tightly knit social circle. As time
passed, the children of these immigrants began to see possibilities for a better
future because of their large numbers and ambition. They began to explore politics, which was a natural progression from the organizational structure of the
parish system (Bankston & Hidalgo, 2006). In many cities, precinct by precinct,
the Irish began to embrace the political system of the United States as not only
a tool to improve their personal situation, but as an outlet for social change
(Bankston & Hidalgo, 2006). The Irish political machine was particularly powerful and effective in New York (where Alfred E. "Al" Smith became governor of
New York in 1918), Kansas City, and Chicago. Political expansion was difficult

outside of these strong enclaves due to fear and distrust of the Irish, and the fear of involvement or interference of the Pope in government, which existed within the larger American society. These factors contributed to the defeat of governor Smith when he ran for president of the United States in 1928. These factors were not overcome until the election of President John F. Kennedy (a descendant of peasant Irish Catholic stock) in 1960—a feat that has not been repeated to date.

Labor unions were also a social organizing force for Irish Americans. Political activity and the church were seen as the best means for upward mobility. The Catholic Church also established Catholic universities such as Notre Dame, Fordham, and Boston College to provide higher education opportunities for Irish Americans.

The family unit is extremely significant to Irish Americans. The nurse should include the family when planning care, for it is felt that nursing interventions will only be successful if the family is included. This may not be true of the male patient, however. The nurse should be aware that male Irish American patients may resist family involvement in their care due to a strong desire to handle things on their own. The nurse should determine the patient preference on family involvement prior to involving the family in the plan of care.

Family roles tend to be gender-based, with the Irish American woman viewing her role as primary caretaker. If the primary caretaker is ill, the nurse must help the family cope with the role strain and help the family develop strategies to meet the family's needs in the absence of the caretaker.

Impact of Faith and Spirituality

The Ulster Irish were Protestant, and the majority of famine Irish were Catholic. As noted previously, the Irish Catholics were isolated by their religious beliefs and set up parishes within their neighborhoods. The Catholic parishes evolved into social and educational centers for the community. The parish priest served as a role model and counselor for the community. The church cared for the immigrants' spiritual, social, educational, medical, and emotional needs. As the number of immigrants increased, parishes and religious orders built schools, hospitals, and orphanages to meet the needs of the communities (Bankston & Hidalgo, 2006).

Biologic Variations

Some genetic variations have been identified in Irish Americans. Some are only associated with some identified Irish subgroups such as the Travellers of Ireland. These genetic variations include neural tube defects, sarcoidosis, cystic fibrosis, Tay-Sachs disease, bimaxillary dental protrusion, abdominal aortic aneurysm, and alcoholism.

Among all American ethnic groups, Irish Americans have either been ranked the highest or near highest for alcoholism rates (Butler, 1996). Although the prevalence of alcohol use and abuse is high in the Irish, if the situation is handled with cultural sensitivity by the nurse and other healthcare professionals, the Irish American will embrace abstinence more easily than members of other ethnic groups. The nurse should remember that for Irish Americans, alcoholism is influenced by a variety of factors, including patterns and characteristics of the family, social and economic conditions, and psychological orientation, rather than a biologic variation. Because some Irish drink for reassurance and to escape what is perceived as an intolerable burden, the nurse must develop strategies to teach such individuals more positive ways to alleviate stress and tension. Such individuals should be taught to verbally communicate feelings and anxiety rather than repressing or denying such feelings. The client must be taught the value of verbal expression to communicate needs. In addition, it is important to assist these clients in developing positive outlooks on life that may be perceived as positive coping strategies. The nurse also must remember the value of working not only with the client but also with the family because of the perception of family relationships as being paramount to a healthful existence.

CASE STUDY 9–1   `www`

Irish American Case Study

This case demonstrates what can occur during a cross-cultural encounter (the culture of the patient and the provider are different).

A middle-aged Irish woman was hospitalized and scheduled to have bowel resection surgery once her condition stabilized. After a few days, the patient suddenly started complaining of severe abdominal pain to her family but said nothing to her physician. Her physician was unaware of the cultural manifestations of pain in Irish Americans; that is, the Irish, as a group, tend to minimize expressions of pain. When the patient's family spoke to the physician about the patient's pain, the physician expressed little concern because in the physician's country, women having serious pain are much more vocal than this patient was. The physician did not listen to the patient's family and also did not follow up with the patient to see if the pain complaint was legitimate. The physician ignored the family's request that the surgery be done sooner, deeming it unnecessary. The surgeon had placed his cultural beliefs onto the patient, which impacted his medical judgment.

By the time the patient went to surgery, her condition had worsened, and she died from the surgery. The family felt that had the surgeon operated when they first complained about the patient's pain, she might have lived, and they filed a malpractice case against the surgeon.

REVIEW QUESTIONS

1. What is the nurse's role/responsibility during a cross-cultural surgical case encounter?

Rationale: In this case, the surgeon made the mistake of stereotyping the patient—she was a woman, and in the physician's experience, women complained loudly when in pain. Therefore, the physician exercised poor and negligent medical judgment when he failed to reexamine the patient. If the physician had been aware of the generalization about Irish people in pain, the patient's complaints may have been taken more seriously, which may have led to an earlier surgical intervention.

Source: Galanti, G. A. (2000). An introduction to cultural differences. *Western Journal of Medicine, 172*(5), 335–336.

ITALIAN AMERICANS

Historical Background

Italian Americans are immigrants or descendants of immigrants from mainland Italy, Sicily, Sardinia, and other Mediterranean islands that make up Italy. Most of these immigrants came to the United States during the "great migration" between 1880 and 1922 (Martin & Midgley, 2003). Today, the descendants of those early immigrants number nearly 17.3 million, making them the sixth largest European ethnic group in the United States (U.S. Census Bureau, 2010). The frequency of intermarriage has resulted in the number of Americans who have at least one Italian grandparent to be estimated at 26 million. Because there is no one common identity for Italian Americans, they are considered to be one of the most diverse of all of the ethnic or cultural groups. Most have assumed a mainstream American cultural identity. Therefore, the nurse must proceed with extreme caution to avoid stereotyping when interacting with an Italian American patient. There still is the likelihood of a strong attachment to some if not all aspects of Italian culture, especially in the areas of food, drink, and art, as well as a strong commitment to family.

Traditional Health Beliefs

Italian Americans have several traditional health beliefs that may still be of importance to some, especially older, Italian American patients (Lassiter, 1995).

Some may believe that the cause of illness is a result of a contagion or contamination. Contamination can be a result of the supernatural or from a human cause. Wind currents or drafts can bring disease as well (Lassiter, 1995). Older and first-generation immigrants are more likely to ascribe to these traditional health beliefs. There is no objection to the use of traditional Western medicines; there may be the desire to supplement this with their own home remedies.

It is important to make the distinction between "fresh air" and drafts. Fresh air is considered healthy and vital for health maintenance while drafts, on the other hand, are a cause of illness (Lassiter, 1995). Ventilation of the home and workplace is valued, but avoidance of drafts is essential.

Supernatural causes of illness include the "evil eye" (*malocchio*) and curses (*castiga*) (Lassiter, 1995). The severity of the illness is related to the supernatural causes, with curses resulting in the most serious, or even fatal, medical problems. Curses are from God or are sent by an evil person, and they may be seen as a punishment for sinning or other bad behavior. A belief in supernatural causes is more prevalent in immigrants and their descendants from rural areas in Italy.

Coining may be practiced by older Italian Americans (Migrant Resource Center, 2008). Coining can be used for a wide variety of ailments. Coining is usually performed on the forehead, abdomen, base of the nose, between the eyes, on the neck, chest and/or back. The resultant bruises or marks can be, and have been, mistaken for signs of abuse. The nurse must exercise caution not to jump to this conclusion without first considering the possibility of coining.

Emotions need to be released, which is one explanation for the animation associated with the Italian culture. Keeping emotions bottled up is unhealthy, and if an outlet for release of these emotions is not found, serious consequences will result.

Impact of Communication

According to data from the 2009 American Community Survey, there were 798,801 speakers of Italian in the United States, which ranked eighth on the top 10 list of languages spoken in the home excluding English and Spanish (**Box 9–1**) (U.S. Census Bureau, 2000). Many scholars have attributed the loss of the Italian language to the treatment of Italian Americans during World War II (Del Boca & Venturini, 2003). The American government had a strong propaganda campaign telling Americans not to speak the enemy's language. Also during the war, some Italian Americans (as well as Japanese Americans) were placed in internment camps—this was more likely to occur if Italian was spoken (Fox, 2000).

The Italian language of today (what is taught in schools and colleges) is different than traditional Italian. Over 80% of Italian Americans are of Southern Italian

Box 9-1 Ten Languages Most Frequently Spoken at Home Other Than English and Spanish, 2010

Population Aged 5 Years and Older	Number in Millions
Chinese	2.46
French	1.36
Tagalog	1.44
German	1.12
Vietnamese	1.20
Korean	1.05
Russian	0.85
Italian	0.81
Arabic	0.76
Polish	0.63

Source: U.S. Census Bureau. (2010). *New Census Bureau report analyzes nation's linguistic diversity.* Retrieved from https://www.census.gov/newsroom/releases/archives/american_community_survey_acs/cb10-cn58.html

descent where the Neapolitan or Sicilian dialects were spoken. Today, this Italian is anachronistic and demonstrates Southern Italy dialects of the past and not the language of the present (Italian Standard). The language situation is even more pronounced for Italian Americans of Northern descent, as their language is even more linguistically different than Southern Italian dialects. Because of this, Italian Americans who wish to learn Italian are learning a language that does not include many of the phrases they may have learned from their families. According to the 2009 American Community Survey, Italian is not one of the top 10 languages spoken in ELL students' homes (limited English proficient students aged 5 to 18) (American Community Survey, 2009).

The nurse can face language problems when an elderly or new Italian immigrant seeks medical care. Modesty may impact the nurse's ability to get adequate or complete answers to medical questions, even when an interpreter is used. Italian Americans tend to overreport symptoms or report their symptoms in a very dramatic manner. Because of this, physicians tend to diagnose emotional problems more often for Italian American patients than for any other ethnic group (Giordano & McGoldrick, 2005).

The nurse should recognize that Italian Americans are motivated to seek full and complete explanations regarding their health status and the proposed treatment plan. If the instructions are clear, cooperation is enhanced. It is recommended to provide thorough oral patient education, followed up with written instructions to ensure safety and adherence.

Impact of Social Organization

The family is the main organizing framework in Italian American culture (Lassiter, 1995). The family provides strength, helps with coping with stresses, and provides a sense of continuity. Italian Americans take pride in their family and their home. The man is the head of the household, and the female is considered the heart of the family. The church is also an important focus of Italian American life (Lassiter, 1995). Italian feasts are commonplace and provide the opportunity for proliferation of the culture's love of food and its devotion to God and patron saints.

Often, the care of illness is managed in the home, with all family members contributing to patient care and management of household responsibilities. Intermarriage is common, with more than 80% of Italian Americans marrying people from a different ethnic group (Giordano & McGoldrick, 2005).

Italian Americans place great value on family (Lassiter, 1995). Divorce is frowned upon and often elderly family members live in the home with the younger generations. There are several organizations, including the Order Sons of Italy and the Italic Institute of America, that are working to represent and actively promote the interests of Italian Americans in the United States.

Impact of Faith and Spirituality

Most Italian Americans are Catholic, and it has been reported that many immigrants become even more devoutly Catholic once they arrive in America, although they do not demonstrate strong leadership in the church despite their large numbers (Lassiter, 1995). There are some who, despite possessing a Catholic background, have chosen to leave the church to practice Protestant Christianity for various reasons. Some worship in non-Catholic churches but continue to enroll their children in parochial schools. Some have become disenchanted with the leadership in the Catholic Church, abhor lack of agreement with certain church rituals, and believe that the Catholics have misinterpreted certain important Christian doctrines. A very small number of Italians are Jews and Muslims (approximately 2%) (Pozzetta, 2000). Overall, Italians possess a strong belief in the afterlife, where the good are rewarded, the bad are punished, and sins can be purged in purgatory (Lassiter, 1995). The deceased are spoken of in a respectful manner and are remembered. Failing to attend a wake or funeral service is a serious thing, and would only be excused for a valid reason.

Biologic Variations

There are two genetic diseases commonly seen in Italian Americans, both of which are anemia disorders (Pozzetta, 2000). The first is favism, a severe hemolytic anemia that results from a deficiency of the X-linked enzyme glucose-6-phosphate dehydrogenase (Chiarelli et al., 2006). The anemia is triggered when the patient eats fava beans. The second type of anemia disorder is the thalassemia syndrome, of which there are two subgroups. Beta-thalassemia, also referred to as Cooley's anemia or thalassemia major, is a serious form of the disease. The other subgroup is alpha-thalassemia. The thalassemias are a diverse group of hereditary blood diseases that result in reduced or flawed production of hemoglobin. Some cases of thalassemia can be quite debilitating, requiring extensive medical intervention, whereas others require little or no medical intervention.

APPALACHIANS

Historical Background

Appalachians are people who were either born in or live in the Appalachian Mountain region of the United States. It is home to over 25 million Americans (Pollard & Jacobsen, 2012). This large area crosses 13 states and is considered a rural, nonfarming area. It extends from Mississippi to New York and has 3 subregions. Although there is diversity among Appalachians, there are some commonalities. Originally the region was populated by Native Americans. Today the majority of the population is White (approximately 84%), primarily of Scottish-Irish or British descent, and predominately following the fundamentalist Protestant religion (Pollard & Jacobsen, 2012). Others trace their ancestry to Germany and France. Most Appalachians also share a genetic link to the Native Americans who lived in the area prior to European settlement. This area is historically ravaged by poverty. One in six people live below the poverty level in Appalachia (Pollard & Jacobsen, 2012). It is also plagued by low literacy rates. The ruggedness of the terrain has resulted in a loyal, family-oriented, religious, and resourceful people with a deep-rooted work ethic (Marger & Obermiller, 1987). The isolation that is provided by the mountains has helped to preserve many traditions. Despite the geographic boundaries, Appalachians have developed the ability to function biculturally. They can choose to utilize the values that give the most meaning to the immediate situation. See **Table 9–7** for the 12 identified values of Appalachians.

Table 9–7 Twelve Identified Values of Appalachians

1. Traditionalism
2. Familism
3. Individualism
4. Solidarity
5. Patriotism
6. Religion
7. Neighborliness
8. Personalism
9. Modesty
10. Love of home
11. Sense of beauty
12. Sense of humor

Source: Jones, L. (1994). *Appalachian values.* Ashland, KY: Jesse Stuart Foundation.

Traditional Health Beliefs

Appalachians have a general distrust of all outsiders, including nurses and other healthcare professionals (Russ, 2010). They accept a wide variety of healers (Cavender, 2003). Because of the isolation, these folk healers are often the primary providers of health care. One of these is the "granny midwife." Granny midwives are usually older women who may be responsible for all of the births in their region of the Appalachians (Cavender, 2003).

The traditional healer's goal is the restoration of harmony. Products from nature are utilized, including poultices and teas (Cavender, 2003). A strong belief in folk medicine is a part of the culture, and these practices are followed by all persons from all socioeconomic and educational levels (Cavender, 2003). It is essential that the nurse become familiar and knowledgeable about these herbs because their use is so prevalent. Some of the ingredients can have serious side effects and may interact with prescribed pharmacologic therapies. The nurse must ascertain if the patient intends to use folk medicines at the same time as any prescription medications so that the treatment plan can be modified and essential education imparted to the patient to prevent untoward or adverse events. See **Table 9–8** for information about herbal remedies.

Impact of Communication

Although the dominant language is English, there are some words from the 16th century Gaelic and Saxon languages that persist. Appalachians speak with a distinct dialect and the speech tends to be indirect (Russ, 2010). In addition, it is

Table 9–8 Appalachian Traditional Herbal Therapies

Medical Condition	Herbal Therapy
Arthritis	1. Ginseng tea—ingested orally or rubbed onto affected joints. Nursing implication: Ginseng can prolong bleeding; use caution with heparin, warfarin, aspirin, and nonsteroidal anti-inflammatory drugs. Interacts with monoamine oxidase inhibitors. Used in combination with stimulants (caffeine), can elevate blood pressure. Concomitant use with furosemide, nifedipine, and estrogen may increase risk of side effects. 2. Tea made from alfalfa seeds or stems, or tea from the stems of the barbell plant. 3. Drink a combination of liquor with the roots of ginseng and goldenseal, or tea from rhubarb and whiskey. 4. Drink a mixture of honey, vinegar, and liquor.
Asthma	1. Drink tea from the bark of wild yellow plum trees, mullein leaves, and alum twice a day. 2. Combine gin and the heartwood of a pine tree twice a day. 3. Drink a mixture of honey, lemon juice, and whiskey.
Boils/Sores	1. Apply a poultice of walnut leaves or the green hulls with salt. 2. Apply a poultice of the house leek plant. 3. Apply a poultice of flaxseed meal.
Fever	1. Drink water from wild ginger. Nursing implication: Ginger may inhibit platelet aggregation or decrease thromboxane production, theoretically, increasing bleeding risk. There is evidence that ginger may increase stomach acid production, which may be of significance in patients with peptic ulcer disease or who are prescribed antacids, H2 receptor antagonists, or proton pump inhibitors. Other studies indicate that ginger may act to protect the stomach. Ginger may interfere with medications affecting heart contraction (including beta-blockers and digoxin, among others). Ginger may also interact with drugs taken for nausea and vomiting, arthritis, blood disorders, high cholesterol, high or low blood pressure, allergies (antihistamines), cancer, inflammation, vasodilators, or weight loss. Caution is advised when taking ginger with drugs that weaken the immune system, because of a possible interaction. 2. Drink tea made from butterfly weed, wild horsemint, or feverwood.
Headache	1. Drink tea made of lady's slipper plants. Nursing implications: Lady's slipper contains quinines, which may have an additive effect when taken concomitantly with other quinine-containing agents, often used to treat malaria. Lady's slipper is thought to contain tannins, glycosides, resins, and quinines. Patients taking cardiac glycosides or digoxin should use with caution. Based on traditional use, lady's slipper may have additive effects when used with other sedatives. 2. Rub camphor and whiskey on the head.

(Continues)

Table 9–8 *Continued*

Medical Condition	Herbal Therapy
Hypertension	1. Drink sarsaparilla tea. 2. Drink a half cup of vinegar.
Heart Disease	1. Drink tea made from heartleaf leaves or bleeding heart. 2. Eat garlic.
Kidney Disease	1. Drink tea made from peach leaves or mullein roots. 2. Drink tea made from corn silk or arbutus leaves.
Sore Throat	1. Gargle with the sap from a red oak tree. 2. Eat honey and molasses. 3. Drink honey and whiskey. 4. Apply a poultice of cottonseed to the throat.
Warts	1. Apply milkweed juice to the affected area.

Source: Purnell, L. D. (2013). *Transcultural health care: A culturally competent approach.* (4th ed.). Philadelphia, PA: F. A. Davis, p. 109.

important to engage in small talk at the beginning of the encounter to avoid being perceived as rude (Russ, 2010). The nurse should remember these important points when conducting a patient history or during any verbal exchanges. Also, some areas have perpetuated Elizabethan English that can cause communication difficulties during health encounters if the nurse is not familiar with the characteristics of that speech. The best policy when confronted with an unfamiliar word is to request clarification from the patient.

Impact of Social Organization

The traditional Appalachian identity has been preserved through the passing down of folklore to the younger generations. Arts and crafts are valued in the culture. There is no other geographic area in the United States where so many family members live in such close proximity to their birth place. This is because an Appalachian's personal identity is dependent on his or her community and ties to his or her kinfolk (Russ, 2010). There is an extensive kinship network in Appalachia. Children learn from their family and clan, as the surname not only serves as identification of family membership but also provides a link to a network of kinfolk. The family and kin are highly valued and will be fiercely protected if needed.

The traditional household is male led, with the women responsible for childrearing (Russ, 2010). There is an emphasis on the separateness of the division of labor for the husband and the wife. Women usually marry young (by age 20), and men usually marry by the age of 28 (McNeil, 1989). Because of a loss of welfare benefits and services upon marriage, some Appalachians are deciding not to marry. Women are also relied upon for their emotional strength. Older women are responsible for perpetuating the culture and for caring for the ill through the preparation of remedies. Grandparents are often called upon to be caregivers to the children of the family. The elders are rewarded for this commitment to the family, as the physical structures of many Appalachian homes are designed to permit function in aging persons. Nursing home placement is not culturally acceptable, as it is considered the equivalent of a death sentence (Halperin, 1994). The rough mountainous terrain makes travel difficult in the Appalachians. The result of this has been the formation of informal social networks that also serve to meet the need for worship. Difficulty with travel makes attendance at organized churches difficult, although fundamentalist Protestant religion is important to the community. Difficulty with access and the lack of public transportation and insufficient and inadequate roads are responsible for the continued geographic and social isolation. Isolation has also resulted in a dichotomous population divided by educational level: poorly educated or well-educated.

Acceptance is an important characteristic of Appalachian culture (Russ, 2010). There is an emphasis on the avoidance of confrontation because it would be detrimental to community or to the group as a whole (Russ, 2010). Alternative lifestyles (divorce, homosexuality) are accepted, but not usually discussed. This acceptance is linked to the Appalachians' need for privacy and the desire not to interfere with other's lives through the avoidance of arguments and seeking common ground.

There is an overall general fear of the well-educated (which extends to all healthcare providers) and those in authority, as well a strong fear of hospitals (Behringer & Friedell, 2006). There also tends to be antagonism toward the law and government and organized religion. These fears can be a significant challenge for the nurse to overcome—especially when trying to provide services through a government-funded program.

Impact of Time and Space

The people of Appalachia have a present time orientation (Russ, 2010). The future is viewed through a fatalistic lens (Behringer & Friedell, 2006). The nurse's priority of time (and the importance of appointments) may not be shared, because the nurse may not be their priority if something more important has come up. Trust and respect must be earned. Politeness or surface friendliness does not equate with having earned trust and respect. Because trust and respect must be earned, and many Appalachians fear the well-educated, establishing a therapeutic relationship can be a significant challenge for the nurse to overcome—but it can be done if the nurse invests the time and effort and works to keep the lines of communication open.

Impact of Faith and Spirituality

Appalachians are predominately Christian with a strong evangelical Protestant influence (Russ, 2010). The key feature of religious expression is through affiliation with an autonomous regionalized subdenomination of one of the Christian religions. These regional churches are usually not connected or associated with the larger centralized religion. Denominations are not considered important, only the loyalty to Christ. The focus is on a literal interpretation of the King James Bible by the majority. Lay leadership within the church is very important as is the fostering of relationships. There is a fatalist world view that life is hard and must be accepted as it is, and to look instead for a better hereafter (Behringer & Friedell, 2006).

Biologic Variations

The Appalachians are predominately a poorer White population that has incurred little variation over time (Mather, 2004). The fastest growing Appalachian households (female headed and nonfamily households) have the highest poverty rates (Mather, 2004). Some can trace their genetic background to include a mixture of White European ancestry with either Cherokee or Apache Native American blood. This mixture has resulted in a darker pigmentation than would exist without the genetic Native American influence. There is a very small minority of Blacks who self-identify as Appalachians. There are no reported studies that have found variations in drug metabolism specific to this population.

Current Healthcare Problems Including Mortality and Morbidity

The environmental factors associated with geographic location and occupations of Appalachians have resulted in serious health problems. Appalachians are at a higher risk for respiratory diseases such as black lung disease, emphysema, and tuberculosis. Parasitic infections are common because many Appalachians live without electricity or access to plumbing. The incidence of type 2 diabetes is 400 to 600% greater than the national average (Brown & Obermiller, 1994). Cancer, myocardial infarction, cerebral vascular accident, mental illness, accidental injury, and suicide rates are significantly higher in Appalachians versus the general population, ranging from 150 to 400% greater (Brown & Obermiller, 1994; Edwards, Lenz, & East-Odom, 1993).

Impact of Nurses and Nurse Practitioners in Appalachia

Lay midwives (often referred to as granny midwives) have been practicing in Appalachia for many decades but it was not until 1927, when Mary Breckenridge founded the Frontier Nursing Service, that the people of Appalachia had access to formally trained nurse–midwives and nurses for healthcare delivery (Kentucky DocMagazine.com, 2011). Since then, access has expanded to include the provision of primary care in nurse-managed centers throughout the large geographic area making up Appalachia. Often it is a struggle to earn the trust of the community, as it is a slow process to earn the trust when viewed as an outsider. The nurse providing care in the home is usually a more successful approach. Asking the patient what they consider the problem to be prior to designing the treatment plan is also an effective strategy (Helton, Barnes, & Borman, 1994).

THE AMISH

Background

The Amish are linked to the Anabaptists of 16th century Europe. This group broke off from the Catholic Church because they felt the scriptures did not support infant baptism and that only believers should be baptized. The Anabaptists name came from the practice of adults being rebaptized. There were other differences such as a desire for separation of church and state, pacifism, and a commitment to live peaceably. The Anabaptists became a persecuted group throughout the next century in Western Europe. The Anabaptists, despite this persecution, gave birth to three religious movements that still exist today. These three groups are the Mennonites, the Hutterites, and the Swiss Brethren (Hostetler, 1993). The Amish are a branch of the Swiss Brethren. The name is derived from their leader Jakob Ammann, who was a Swiss Brethren bishop from Alsace (Christian Light Publications, Inc., n.d.; Gross, 1997). The most well-known descendants of the Anabaptists are the Mennonites and the Amish. According to Christian Light Publications, Inc. (n.d.), the Amish, a smaller body of Swiss Brethren, settled in Pennsylvania in Berks County in 1736. German migration to the American colonies was the impact of many wars on Germany and the desire for religious freedom. Taxes were high to pay for the wars, famine spread over the land, and the armies had trampled farmland and burned down farmsteads (Christian Light

Publications, Inc., n.d.). In Europe, the rulers determined the religion of the land, and many pious Germans found this difficult to accept. The American colonies and especially Pennsylvania offered the opportunity for religious freedom.

A break occurred between the Swiss Brethren and the Amish under Ammann's leadership in 1693. The Amish then refused to have anything to do with their former brethren or any excommunicated members, a tradition that is referred to as *shunning*.

Today, the Amish live in rural areas in over 28 states as well as in the province of Ontario in Canada. There are 250,000 Amish people. The states with the largest Amish populations are Ohio and Pennsylvania. The largest individual settlements are found at Holmes County, Ohio, and Lancaster County, Pennsylvania. Indiana has the third highest Amish population. Together these three states are home to roughly two-thirds of all Amish (Amish America, 2010). Recently, the Amish have been expanding their presence in search of affordable farmland in response to an increase in population. Reasons given for the increase in population include larger families, increase in marriages within the community, a lower than average child mortality rate, and longer life spans. Amish couples typically have five or more children. With more than four out of every five deciding in young adulthood to remain within the church, their population has grown steadily. More than half the population is under 21 years of age. A small portion of the increase is also caused by conversions to the faith. In Ontario, Canada, the only Amish community outside the United States is also growing. It consists of about 4,500 people, up from 2,300 in 1992 (Kraybill, Nolt, & Johnson-Weiner, 2008).

The Amish are attracted to areas with relatively cheap farms, a rural lifestyle, and nonfarming jobs such as construction or cabinetmaking that fit their values and allow them to remain independent. In some cases, they have migrated to resolve leadership problems or escape church-related disputes.

The most important concept that the nurse needs to know in an attempt to understand Amish culture is that the departure from contemporary American culture is due to the Amish people's perceived biblical mandate to live a life separated from a world they see as sinful (Kraybill, 2003; Hostetler, 1993). The old-fashioned appearance can be misunderstood. Although they eschew modern technological conveniences (e.g., reliance on horse and buggy for transportation, lack of electricity in the home), the Amish may be open to the use of state-of-the-art medical technology if it is deemed necessary. This does not mean that the Amish will agree to costly life-prolonging care. This is often viewed as both excessive and unjustified when a patient has a terminal prognosis. The Amish prefer death with dignity in end-of-life circumstances. The Amish rely on modern medicine to varying degrees.

Some will use modern medications and treatments, while others will prefer to rely on traditional remedies or natural methods (Amish America, 2010). The approach to the use of modern health care can vary by affiliation and community. Overall, however, the Amish will not seek out preventive health care and the most conservative Amish will totally avoid traditional health care.

Traditional Health Beliefs

The Amish wish to be born at home and to die at home. God's will is absolute as it determines all, and their belief is to accept God's will as it is. This belief is associated with a deep fear of disability—it is feared much more than death. If disability can result from the refusal of treatment, it is essential that the patient and family be educated about this risk. However, a child with birth defects or other disabilities is readily accepted as a child of God and the parents will not be deterred from having additional children. As stated previously, the use of modern medicine and medical technology is not forbidden. Prior to accepting medical care, the patient or family will ask for the blessing of the church. The reason for this is that the community will need to come together to help pay the medical bills as the Amish do not have medical insurance because it is viewed as a "worldly product" and therefore reflects a lack of faith in God. If deemed necessary, the Amish will permit surgery, anesthesia, dental work, and even blood transfusions and transplantation. The only exception is for heart transplantation, as the heart is viewed as the soul of the body. The Amish do not want to be seen by or have student practitioners participate in their care. Because they are paying cash for their medical care, they only want to be seen by experienced and licensed medical professionals. All medical decisions will be jointly made by both the husband and the wife because of the belief that they are true partners in family life (Lee, 2005).

The Amish are unlikely to seek medical attention for minor complaints. Instead, they are more likely to rely on folk or herbal remedies. They like to use healing aids such as vitamins, homeopathic remedies, health foods, reflexology, and chiropractors.

Traditional health beliefs are shaped by their conservative rural values, a preference for natural remedies, a lack of information, unfamiliarity with technology, difficulties with access, and a strong reliance on God with an associated willingness to suffer if it is God's will (Kraybill, 2001).

Impact of Communication

The Amish speak English and a hybrid language of German and Dutch referred to as Pennsylvania German or Pennsylvania Dutch (Johnson-Weiner, 1998). It is a Germanic language with a large amount of English mixed in. The Pennsylvania Dutch language is an oral one. Writing done by the Amish is in English. Many Amish are trilingual as they also speak "high German," which is the language of their bibles and the language used during church services.

The Amish will genuinely appreciate the nurse or physician who shows an understanding of Amish culture and health beliefs. Having proficiency or an appreciation for the Pennsylvania German (or Pennsylvania Dutch) language can help in establishing a therapeutic relationship (Amish America, 2010).

Impact of Social Organization

The social organization of the Amish is guided by the desire to avoid assimilation and acculturation into dominant American culture (Amish America, 2010). The Amish have been able to maintain a distinctive ethnic subculture by successfully resisting acculturation and assimilation. The Amish try to maintain cultural customs that preserve their identity. They have resisted assimilation into American culture by emphasizing separation from the world, rejecting higher education, selectively using technology, and restricting interaction with outsiders.

The Amish church prescribes dress regulations for its members, but the unwritten standards vary considerably by settlement. Men are expected to wear a wide brim hat and a vest when they appear in public. In winter months and at church services, they wear a black suit coat that is typically fastened with hooks and eyes rather than with buttons. Men use suspenders instead of belts.

Amish women are expected to wear a prayer covering and a bonnet when they appear in public settings. Most women wear a cape over their dresses as well as an apron. The three parts of the dress are often fastened together with straight pins. Various colors, including green, brown, blue, and lavender, are permitted for men's shirts and women's dresses, but designs and figures in the material are taboo. Although young girls do not wear a prayer covering, Amish children are typically dressed similarly to their parents.

Although some holidays are celebrated, such as Thanksgiving, Christmas, Easter, and New Year's Day, they are free from commercial trappings. The Amish, as conscientious objectors, do not celebrate holidays that are military based such as Memorial Day, Veterans Day, and the Fourth of July.

Cultural ties to the outside world are curbed by speaking the dialect, marrying within the group, spurning television, prohibiting higher education, and limiting social interaction with outsiders. Parochial schools insulate Amish youth from outside influences and threatening ideas. From birth to death, members are embedded in a web of ethnicity. These cultural defenses fortify Amish identity.

Biologic Variations

As a result of the inbreeding associated with a closed community like the Amish, genetic abnormalities are common because of the "founder effect" (Nolt, 2004). Almost all Amish are descended from about 200 founders. These genetic disorders, such as dwarfism, unusual blood typing, and metabolic disorders, are accepted as God's will.

ROMA (GYPSIES)

Historical Background

The Roma most likely originated in India more than one thousand years ago (Romaculture.com, 2010). The Roma are travelers and have settled in many different European countries since then. The population has experienced many divisions over the years, which makes the placement of the *Roma* into one ethnic group impossible. Today, there are approximately 12 million Roma living in the world, although it is difficult to determine an accurate number because this ethnic group is not listed in most censuses (Romaculture.com, 2010). The term *Roma* is preferred as the more well-known terminology of *Gypsy*, which has negative connotations. There is no census data on the Roma in the United States, but the population has been estimated as high as one million people (Webley, 2010). The influx of new Roma has been steady since the collapse of Communism in Eastern Europe in 1989. The population is thriving but is still considered to be virtually invisible to non-Roma in the United States. This may in part be due to the lack of homogeneity of the Roma. When they come to the United States they do not settle as one group; they cluster together based on language or nationality.

Traditional Health Beliefs

There is a general lack of knowledge about access to health services and how to provide these appropriately to the Roma population (Hajioff & McKee, 2000). The Roma people possess a strongly held set of health-related beliefs in which some diseases are seen as belonging to the Roma (to that group), therefore requiring treatment by their own traditional healers, whereas other diseases are seen as a result of contact with the outside world and as such require medical care from the American healthcare delivery system. The majority of Roma are governed by a series of rules about what is considered pure or impure. There are also a range of specific rituals dealing with birth, death, and caring for the ill. These beliefs and reliance on rituals can result in the Roma people accepting some aspects of medical care and rejecting other aspects. This behavior can be labeled as non-adherent by the medical establishment, and can be viewed as irresponsible for not fitting in with the norms of dominant American society.

Impact of Communication

The Roma speak many different dialects of the Roma language. Those from Western Europe and the majority in the United States speak Romany (also known as Romanes or Romani) (Matras, 2006). Romany is a Sanskrit-based language that belongs to the Indo-Aryan branch of Indo-European languages (Matras, 2006). All of the dialects have traces of other languages in them because of the influence of the many different countries in which Roma have lived. All Roma speak a second or even a third language from the countries in which they have lived or travelled. The Romany language is a principal factor of Roma ethnic identity (Matras, 2006). It is primarily a spoken rather than written language. Until recent years, most Roma were illiterate, and illiteracy rates remain very high in most Roma communities. In light of this, the nurse should not rely on written materials when providing patient education to Roma patients and families.

Impact of Social Organization

Roma families have settled throughout the United States. Generally there are four loyalties or family structures for the Roma people. The main identity group is the *Natsias* (nation), a *kumpania* (clan), family, and *vista* (Kemp, n.d.). "Family" consists of extended members or an alliance, as they may or may not be related by blood (Kemp, n.d.). The clan often live, work, and celebrate together. The elder members are the authority figures and decision makers in all situations. Clan leaders sometimes adopt the title of king or queen. These titles denote respect and not the possession of an actual political position. The nurse should always speak to the elders if any healthcare decisions are required.

Marriages are often arranged at a very young age. Until marriage (at the age of 12 or 13 for most Roma girls), strict morality is upheld through the use of chaperones. Marriage creates an alliance between families or clans. The payment of a "bride price" (dowry) is common. This payment from the groom's family is meant to compensate the bride's family for the loss of their daughter and to ensure that she will be well-treated as a member of her new family.

Disputes are settled within the community itself. An informal Romani court called the *kris* decides matters of common law and custom and determines penalty. A kris-determined penalty can be as severe as exclusion from the community.

Most Roma currently living in this country were born here and have adapted to many of the dominant American society cultural norms. This goes against traditional Roma beliefs, which include that society is "dirty" and potentially polluting. In traditional clans, as a result of this belief, children are often removed from school at puberty (Sutherland, 2004).

Today, some Roma have a less nomadic existence that is contradictory to the traditional Roma lifestyle, which holds that isolation from the dominant society is crucial to maintaining Roma culture (Rundle, Carvalho, & Robinson, 1999). There are a number of diverse Roma groups and not all of them have the same cultural practices.

Impact of Faith and Spirituality

Some Roma still practice the religion of their homelands, most commonly Christianity or Islam. Some are born-again Christians and follow the main Protestant holy days (Hancock, 1987). Many practice a religion similar to Wicca, which believes in both Satan and God, while placing an emphasis on luck and the supernatural (Rundle et al., 1999). There is resistance to the emergence of Christianity by those who seek to uphold the older traditions, including arranged marriages, dowries, and fortune telling (Hancock, 1987).

Biologic Variations

There is little research on the Roma population. There is evidence that their life expectancy is 10 years shorter than that of their non-Roma neighbors, and that infant mortality is up to 4 times higher (Braham, 1993). Two studies conducted in Spain found a high prevalence for the antibody to hepatitis A (a 9-fold greater prevalence) and for lead poisoning in children (McKee, 1997). Some Roma groups have a high incidence of inherited congenital abnormalities, which may be a result of a closed community and a reluctance to mix with outsiders.

JEWISH AMERICANS

Historical Background

The inclusion of Jewish Americans is important for a text describing the cultural impact on illness. Although being Jewish is not a racial identity, Judaism, unlike other religions, has its own unique culture and way of life (Jewish.org, 2012). Terms to describe Jewish people throughout history include *Hebrew*, *Israelite*, and *Jew*. The terms can be used interchangeably, as the people are called Jewish, the faith is Judaism, the land is Israel, and the language spoken is Hebrew. The United States is home to the second largest population of Jews in the world, after Israel. There are several different types of Judaism, ranging on a continuum from the most extreme or conservative (strict Orthodox), to the most liberal (liberal Reform). Although there is no formal social hierarchy within the Jewish American community, in the case of ultra-Orthodox followers, decisions may be made in concert with their rabbi. According to U.S. Census Bureau data (2007a), 1.7% of the adult American population is Jewish, which equals 5,128,000 people. This number is very close to the number of Jews living in Israel, which has been estimated by Israel's Central Bureau of Statistics as 5,656,300 people in 2009 (Central Bureau of Statistics, 2010). See **Box 9–2** to see how this compares to other religious organizations in the United States.

Box 9–2   Religious Composition of the United States in Descending Order

Religion	Percentage of Adult Population
Protestant—all types	51.3
Catholic	23.9
Unaffiliated (includes atheist, agnostic, and nothing in particular)	16.1
Mormon (also includes Church of Jesus Christ of Latter Day Saints)	3.3
Do not know	0.8
Jehovah's Witness	0.7
Unitarians and other liberal faiths	0.7
Buddhist	0.7
Muslim	0.6
Orthodox	0.6
Hindu	0.4
New Age (includes Wiccan, Pagan, and other New Age groups)	0.4

Source: From the Religious Landscape Survey, a survey conducted in the summer of 2007 among a representative sample of 35,556 adults (over age 18) living in the continental United States. The Pew Forum on Religion and Public Life. *Religious landscape survey*. Retrieved from http://www.census.gov/compendia/statab/tables/09s0074.pdf

The Jewish community of the United States is varied (Chanes, 2008). It consists mainly of Ashkenazi Jews who immigrated to the United States from Eastern and Central Europe and their descendants (U.S.-born citizens). There are other Jewish ethnic divisions as well, including Sephardics and Mizrahis. There are also Jewish Americans who are converts to the religion as well. This variability has resulted in a wide range of Jewish cultural traditions with an associated wide range of religious observance (from the extremely religious to those living a secular lifestyle).

Jews have been present in the United States for some time, perhaps even earlier than the 17th century (Bankston, n.d.). The early immigrants were almost exclusively Sephardic Jews of Spanish and Portuguese descent. Large-scale Jewish immigration began in earnest in the 19th century with the arrival of many secular Ashkenazi Jews from Germany.

Over 2,000,000 Jews arrived between the late 19th century and 1924, when the Immigration Act of 1924 and the National Origins Quota of 1924 restricted immigration (Bankston, n.d.). Most settled in the city of New York and its immediate surrounding areas, establishing what is today one of the world's major concentrations of the Jewish population. Today, the top three states with the highest proportion of Jews are New York, New Jersey, and Florida.

During the early 20th century, assimilation was encouraged and Jews became a part of American life. Half of all Jewish adult males aged 18 to 50 years served in World War II (500,000 men), and after the war ended, they participated in the suburban sprawl that occurred in the United States. Further assimilation and high intermarriage rates further contributed to secularization. As a group, American Jews have been very active in civil rights and fighting prejudice and discrimination. Some Jewish scholars attribute this to the history of the Jews beginning in slavery and the yearning for freedom.

Although Jewish Americans are included in this chapter on White non-Hispanic cultures, do not conclude that there are no Black American Jews. Estimates range from a low of 20,000 to a high of 200,000 Black American Jews in the United States. These Jews, who are not of European descent, are sometimes referred to as "Black Jews" to differentiate them from Jews who are directly descended from the Israelites of the Torah. Despite this distinction being made, the relations between the two groups are apparently amicable.

Traditional Health Beliefs

Jewish Americans are health conscious and believe in keeping both the mind and body healthy (Jacobs & Giarrelli, 2001). They practice preventive health care and will participate in routine screenings and complete all recommended immunizations. It is believed that illness requires early and prompt treatment. All branches of Judaism believe that religious requirements (if a conflict were to exist) may be disregarded if a life is at stake or if the person is suffering with a potentially life-threatening illness (Ehman, 2007). The value of saving a life is held in extremely high regard by the Jewish people (Ehman, 2007).

Ancient Jews followed good hygiene and sanitation practices, which have provided the basic principles for public health care. It was Lillian Wald, a Jewish nurse, who established the prototype for public health nursing when she established the Henry Street Settlement in Manhattan, New York City, in 1893. Physicians and nurses are held in high regard by Jews (Ehman, 2007). There is the belief that once standard therapy has failed and there is no further treatment available, the physician must be willing to change hats from "curer" to "carer" (Rosner, 1993).

Impact of Communication

American Jews speak English and a large number are bilingual, speaking modern Hebrew as well. Modern Hebrew is the official state language of Israel and is the language often used for prayers. Hebrew consists of a 22-letter alphabet and is read from right to left; books are opened from the opposite side of those written in English (Pelaia, 2012). Recent immigrants from Israel may only speak modern Hebrew. A number of other languages may also be spoken, depending upon the patient's type of religious observance and background. Many Hasidic Jews (of Ashkenazi descent) speak Yiddish. Yiddish was the primary language spoken by many European Jewish immigrants to the United States and is a Judeo-German dialect. Some Yiddish terms have become a part of American English (some examples are *schmuck* for fool and *nosh* for snack).

The Persian Jewish community (mainly centered in Los Angeles and Beverly Hills, California, and eastern parts of New York including Great Neck, Long Island) speak Persian during religious services and in the home, and even publish Persian language newspapers.

Russian Jews may speak Russian, often as the primary language in the home. American Bukhori Jews speak Bukhori (a Persian dialect) as well as Russian.

Although modern Hebrew is primarily spoken today, classical Hebrew is the language of Jewish religious literature including the *Tanakh* (Bible) and *Siddur* (prayer book).

There is also a contingent of Hispanic Jews who descended from immigrants from Latin America who speak Spanish in the home.

Impact of Time and Space

Jewish Americans have a time orientation that encompasses the past, the present, and the future, all at once (Jacobs & Giarelli, 2001). Although the emphasis is on living for today and planning for and worrying about tomorrow, they cannot escape the past for fear that if the past, (including the Holocaust), is forgotten, it may be repeated. This unique time orientation focus is a dominant part of the culture (Jacobs & Giarelli, 2001).

Modesty and humility are important Jewish values (Ehman, 2007). Modesty is expressed not only by dress but by actions. Jews do not like to call attention to themselves, nor do they appreciate when someone tries to call attention to himself or herself to impress others. This is tied to the belief that people are judged by their actions.

Hasidic American males consider women to be seductive and may not look directly upon a female's face or talk with them. Touching of the female is also an issue. They may even keep their hands in their pockets to avoid touching a female, as they are not permitted to touch a woman who is not their wife. The female nurse should not offer her hand in greeting to the male Hasidic Jew and if it is done, the nurse should not consider the patient rude if the patient refuses to accept the offered hand. Non-Hasidic Jews may be more informal, maintaining a shorter spatial distance during communication and may use touch. The nurse should always remember the underlying cultural importance of modesty—especially when caring for patients of a gender different from their own (Ehman, 2007)

Impact of Social Organization

The family is the heart and soul of Jewish society, with an emphasis placed on making sure all family members' needs are met and respected (Jacobs & Giarelli, 2001). Today, because of assimilation, there is little difference in gender roles between Jewish American and other White American families; both parents share the home and family responsibilities. Parents are honored, and that means the adult children will care for them in old age. Providing respect to the elderly is essential; even if the elder is senile or acts inappropriately, respect is still essential. Marriage is considered the ideal state because it is stated in the Bible that man should not be alone. Sexuality is deemed an important part of marriage; nonprocreative sexual intercourse is acceptable, but only within marriage. Premarital sexual activity goes against Jewish values.

Biologic Variations

According to Tobin, Tobin, and Rubin (2005) there is significant diversity among the American Jewish community. This is partially a result of historical antecedents and partially a result of contemporary social forces at work. The Jewish community is growing and changing through intermarriage, conversion, and adoption. Some of the individuals entering the community via these avenues are people of color (Tobin et al., 2005).

The skin complexion of a Jewish American is dependent upon the type of Jews they have descended from (Tobin et al., 2005). Ashkenazi Jews have the same skin coloring as other White Americans. Darker-complexioned Jews, similar to people from the Mediterranean areas, are descended from Sephardic Jews. There are also Jews from throughout Africa whose pigmentation of skin is considered black.

Just as skin color is dependent on the type of Jew the patient is, so are the biologic variations the nurse should consider or assess for. Most genetic conditions are seen in descendents of immigrants from Eastern Europe (Ashkenazi Jews). The majority of genetic conditions result from autosomal recessive disorders (the gene is carried by both parents), and as such most of the resulting genetic conditions result in death in infancy or early childhood. These genetic disorders include Tay-Sachs disease, Bloom's syndrome, cystic fibrosis, familial dysautonomia, and Gaucher's disease (Fares et al., 2008). With the exception of Tay-Sachs disease, there is no simple biochemical or enzymatic test to detect for carriers of these autosomal recessive disorders (Vallance & Ford, 2003). Tay-Sachs disease, arguably the most widely known of these disorders, results in progressive neurologic degeneration and has a carrier frequency of around 1 in 25 to 30 people of Ashkenazi Jewish origin. This is a likelihood of occurrence 10-fold higher than is found in other groups.

There are a few adult disorders associated with Jews of Ashkenazi descent. Kaposi sarcoma is most commonly seen in males who are over 50 years of age. The nurse should expect the manifestation to be malignant tumors of the endothelium that are slow growing and confined to the skin, and the condition should not be confused with the Kaposi tumors seen in patients with acquired immunodeficiency syndrome (AIDS). The tumors in AIDS patients are much more aggressive, and they also affect internal organs as well as the skin. In one study by Engels, Clark, Aledort, Goedert, and Whitby (2002), it was found that the Kaposi's sarcoma herpes virus seroprevalence rate (this virus is the Kaposi's sarcoma agent) in elderly U.S. Jews was 8.8% (similar to other studies rates, which ranged between 5 and 10%).

An important nursing implication is the higher incidence of a serious adverse drug reaction in persons of Ashkenazi descent with the use of clozapine (an antipsychotic drug especially used to treat schizophrenia). In the general population, the side effect rate for agranulocytosis is about 1%, but in this Jewish population the incidence significantly increases up to 20% (Rajagopal, 2005). A genetic cause has been identified to account for this difference. The nurse should remind the provider that adequate laboratory testing to monitor for agranulocytosis should be provided for the Jewish patient on clozapine, or better yet, advocate for the use of a safer antipsychotic medication.

Impact of Faith and Spirituality

Judaism is one of the world's oldest religions, formed in the Middle East and dating back more than 3,500 years (BBC.com, 2012). It is a monotheistic faith (the belief in one God as the creator of the universe) (BBC.com, 2012). The history and the laws of Judaism are chronicled and described in the Old Testament of the Bible. The first five books of the Bible are handwritten in the Hebrew language on scrolls made of parchment. This is called the Torah. The Torah is kept in a "Holy Ark: under an eternal light within each synagogue" (Project Genesis, Inc., n.d.). These are the Jewish laws, and they guide the Jews on every aspect of how they should live their lives. The spiritual leader is the Rabbi (which translates to *teacher* in English), and the Rabbi serves as the interpreter of Jewish law. It is not believed that a Rabbi is any closer to God than any other Jew, and a Jew can pray directly to God. Unlike in other religions, including different types of Christianity, the spiritual leader is not needed to intercede on the person's behalf with God, does not grant atonement, and does not hear confession. The Sabbath is the holiest day, and it begins 18 minutes before sunset on Friday and ends 42 minutes after sunset, or when 3 stars can be seen, on Saturday evening. If at all possible, elective or nonemergent procedures should not be performed on the Sabbath, but the nurse should be aware that illness is considered a valid reason to keep the Jew from the synagogue on the Sabbath.

Although there is only one Jewish religion, the religion has three main branches: Orthodox (most traditional), Conservative (less strict, as the branch makes concessions to modern life), and Reform (considered a liberal or progressive denomination). It is estimated that 13% of American Jews are Orthodox, 26% are Conservative, and 34% are Reform, while 25% identified as "just Jewish" (Jewish Federation Organization, 2001). There are also multiple smaller groups of ultra-Orthodox Jews. One of the most widely known of these are the Hasidic Jews; they wear full beards, dark clothing, and fully covered extremities. A newer denomination of Judaism is the Reconstructionists (2% of all Jews according to the Jewish Federation Organization, 2001), which is an amalgamation of the three main branches, and views the Jewish religion in evolution as its followers seek to adapt to and reside in a more modern world than is described in the Old Testament or the Torah.

The nurse should be careful not to assume that a deep faith or even a belief in God exists in all patients. This is also true of the Jewish American patient. Jewish religious practice is quite varied, ranging from the highly devout to the atheist. It appears that American Jews are more likely to be atheist or agnostic than most Americans, especially so compared with Protestants or Catholics. A 2003 Harris poll found that while 79% of Americans believe in God, only 48% of American Jews do, compared with 79% and 90% for Catholics and Protestants, respectively. While 66% of Americans said they were "absolutely certain" of God's existence, 24% of American Jews said the same. And though 9% of Americans believe there is no God (8% Catholic and 4% Protestant), 19% of American Jews believe God does not exist (Taylor, 2003).

Although the Torah is silent on the issue of an afterlife, traditional Judaism has evolved over the centuries with a few possible descriptions of the afterlife (Pelaia, 2012). Many Jews believe in an afterlife in which the soul continues to thrive. It is felt by some that in the afterlife, things that were not understood in life will become known and clear. Although not much thought is given to life after death on a daily or even regular basis, it is believed that the righteous will be rewarded with a place in the afterlife.

The nurse needs to be aware that for an actively religious Jew, the provision of active euthanasia is often forbidden (Ehman, 2007). At a minimum it is a highly debated topic in the Jewish community (Ehman, 2007). It if often helpful for the nurse to offer for the patient and his or her family to discuss this issue with their Rabbi (Ehman, 2007). For some, active euthanasia is considered murder, which is in direct violation with one of the Ten Commandments. A dying patient with a terminal prognosis is considered a living being and, as such, active euthanasia (when something is given or done to cause or have the result of death) is not permitted. Suicide is also not permitted. Suicide is so frowned upon that it is considered both a criminal act and a moral violation. It is believed that the act of suicide prevents any prospect of repentance. In cases of adult suicide, full burial rights are not provided (unless the patient is deemed mentally incompetent), the person will be buried in the outer perimeters of the Jewish cemetery, and mourning will not be conducted. Suicide in the case of children is never viewed as a voluntary act.

Passive euthanasia is a grayer area, and it may be permitted depending on the situation and interpretation of that situation (Ehman, 2007). Anything that artificially prevents death (i.e., cardiopulmonary resuscitation, mechanical ventilation) may possibly be withheld depending on the patient's and family's wishes, as well as their specific and individual religious views (Ehman, 2007). The nurse should consider this information fully prior to initiating any do not resuscitate discussions with the patient and his or her family.

RUSSIAN AMERICANS

Historical Background

The former Soviet Union was made up of 15 republics, of which Russia is the largest. Russia is also referred to as The Russian Federation. Russia is the largest country in the world; it extends to both the continents of Europe and Asia, and is approximately two times the size of the United States. There are Russian-born nonethnic Russians living inside and outside of Russia and over 100 nationalities in total from Russia; thus, it is important to distinguish their separate identities. By far, the largest numbers are Russian, at approximately 81.5% (CIA, 2009).

There is a huge unemployment problem as well as extensive poverty in Russia. Forty percent of the population of Russia falls below the poverty line. Both of these financial issues have resulted in life today in Russia being very difficult, and crime is on the rise. Health indicators in the country are very poor. Low birthrates and high death rates have contributed to a population decline of more than 500,000 people annually. Life expectancy is significantly less for males—it is believed that men die much sooner than women because of cardiovascular disease, accidents, alcoholism, and suicide (Aslund, 2001). As of 2001, life expectancy for Russians is 66 years compared to 78 years for Americans (CIA, 2012). Infectious disease also has resulted in a public health crisis. The rate of human immunodeficiency virus (HIV) is astronomical, almost double the rate in the United States (0.6% adult rate compared to 1.1% adult rate) (CIA, 2012). Access to effective treatments, including pharmaceuticals, also makes treatment difficult. Since the financial collapse of Russia in 1998, there are only a few pharmaceutical companies left. The Russian healthcare system is publicly supported but has problems with inefficiency, corruption, and very low salaries for both physicians and nurses.

All of these factors have spurred the desire to emigrate from Russia to come to the United States. A significant increase in immigration rates has been noted recently in response to these factors, but immigration to the United States has been ongoing since 1917; this coincides with the end of the Russian Revolution.

The first Russian immigrants were very well-educated and left Russia after the Russian Revolution. Conflict spurred the second wave of immigration, which occurred at the end of World War II. Anti-Semitism after World War II became a significant issue and many Russian Jews who were well-educated entered the United States as refugees. Immigration restrictions limiting U.S. immigration based on family presence has resulted in new Russian immigrants being related to earlier Russian immigrants. This has resulted in a close-knit circle grouping of Russian Americans.

During the waning years of the Soviet Union, the United States encouraged free immigration among Soviet Jews. As a direct result of a 1973 law, a large wave of Soviet Jews arrived in the United States—66,480 people in the 5-year period between 1975 and 1980. Policy in the Soviet Union during these waves of immigration was quite strict. If one family member wanted to leave (and this was usually the younger ones), the entire family also had to leave. This means that there are a significant number of Russian Americans who did not wish to emigrate and leave their homeland. The amount of time required for immigration has decreased over time. It is not uncommon to find an older immigrant who arrived in the 1980s sharing that they experienced a 10-year wait to be able to immigrate, while today the wait is often closer to 1 year in length. This has caused some frustration and bitterness between newer and older immigrants. Toward the end of the Soviet Union, the numbers of immigrants from Russia to the United States dramatically increased. In the final year of the Soviet Union, it was the foremost provider of immigrants to the United States.

Another factor impacting immigration is the rise in international adoption rates. There are a growing number of Russian children who have been adopted by citizens of the United States; in fact, the number is so significant that Russia has become the number-one source for adopted foreign children in the United States.

The nurse should recognize that he or she may be called upon to care for Russian Americans of all ages—the very young who may be newly adopted, and the elderly who may be here reluctantly. More than half of the arriving Russian immigrants are over 50 years old, which may impact assimilation. It is important to consider the reasons for immigration or presence in the United States when planning for nursing care delivery. You may encounter Russian immigrants (someone who wishes to live in another country) or Russian American Jews who are refugees. Refugees come to the United States because of declared political problems—in this case, anti-Semitism and a need for safety. Refugees are entitled to numerous services, including financial help, access to training programs, and the granting of permanent resident status, to assist with the transition.

Statistics

U.S. census figures show that there are more than 3 million people of Russian ancestry in the country, or 1% of the total population in the United States (U.S. Census Bureau, 2007b). Almost a million more (0.3% of the total U.S. population) is of Ukrainian heritage, and nearly as many others indicate Slavic origins. All of them could have recognizable ties to history and culture associated with Russian-speaking peoples.

Ukraine

After Russia, Ukraine is the second largest country in Europe. After the breakup of the Soviet Union, Ukraine got its independence in 1991. The official language is Ukrainian. Since gaining independence, the economy has been suffering a crisis in spite of Ukraine being a highly industrialized country. Agricultural issues, such as inadequate harvests and a fuel shortage, have further compounded the economic problems and many are experiencing malnourishment in Ukraine. Another complicating factor is the nuclear power plant accident that occurred at Chernobyl in 1986, which caused an explosion and contamination. Approximately 116,000 people were evacuated in the spring and summer of 1986 while another 220,000 were relocated in subsequent years (Kubiszewski & Cleveland, 2009). These factors have led many Ukrainians to leave their country of origin and immigrate to other countries, including the United States.

Traditional Health Practice

Russian immigrants frequently view the U.S. medical system with mistrust due to their previous experience in an authoritarian healthcare system in Russia (EuroMedInfo.com, n.d.). Preventive health care is practiced by Russian Americans, and health screening is seen as the key to good health; in fact, illness or disease indicate the patient did not do something right (Stratis Health, 2010). The exception to this is that routine mammograms and routine breast examinations are seen as being of little value, as are cholesterol screening tests. A criticism made by many Russian Americans is that the U.S. healthcare system does not place enough emphasis on prevention and instead relies on pharmaceuticals. Russians instead prefer to utilize alternative therapies such as cupping, massage therapy, and acupressure/acupuncture.

Some Russian immigrants, especially the elderly, like to utilize homeopathic or folk medicines (Stratis Health, 2010). Amber can be ground into a powder and, when added to hot water, becomes a medicine. Herbs are also utilized in either enema or drink form. Hot steam baths are utilized, as is drinking mineral water. Home remedies, such as oil rubs, mud, steam baths and exposure to fresh air and sunlight, are often used prior to medical care. The *bonki* is a cold and flu remedy to ease symptoms through the application of glass cups on the back and shoulders of the patient (Stratis Health, 2010).

Health is seen as a goal to strive for and a gift to possess. Illness is seen as a disharmony in the body. Spirituality holds an important place in end-of-life care. Russians do not believe that a poor prognosis should be given to a terminally ill patient because it will only result in anxiety, lessen hope, and perhaps even hasten death (Stratis Health, 2010). The preference will be for the family to be told the terminal diagnosis and then the family will decide if or how to inform the patient (Stratis Health, 2010).

Traditional Health Practices for Ukrainian Americans

In Ukraine, to some extent folk medicine retains its place in the community in both attitude and practice. Herbal and folk medicines are used along with Western pharmaceuticals. In rural areas where access is an issue, the use of folk medicines is higher. An example of a commonly used medication is *zelenka*, a mercurochrome-based green ointment for skin problems. Overall, folk medicines are believed by Ukrainians to be less harmful than pharmaceuticals, or "chemical medicine" (Bologova, 1996). Physical disease was often driven out of the body by squeezing, sucking, or frightening it away by shouting (Fedunkiw, 2012). Diseases could also be charmed away through the use of incantations and prayers (Fedunkiw, 2012). Newer traditional interventions used by Ukrainians include baths, bleeding (using leeches or cupping), and massage (Fedunkiw, 2012). All of these methods have fallen out of favor, however, as the Ukrainian has become assimilated into the dominant American culture. This assimilation is apparent by the number of Ukrainians who have entered the healthcare professions (especially in the areas of dentistry and chiropractic).

Trust is essential to the doctor–patient or nurse–patient relationship. If the Ukrainian American patient does not trust the provider, the treatment plan will not be followed (Stratis Health, 2010). Ukrainian Americans prefer value dialogue but a close one-on-one relationship from their healthcare providers (Stratis Health, 2010). There is a general belief that Western physicians rely too much on fancy diagnostics and not enough on history taking. There is also a preference for the Ukrainian view of medical care, which is to reveal the cause of the disease.

Ukrainian Americans feel that in the United States, the physician has little concern with the cause of disease and the main focus is on treatment. The nurse should be aware that it is culturally appropriate for a Ukrainian to offer a gift to ensure cooperation. This may result in an uncomfortable situation because in Ukraine it is not uncommon for people to offer their district doctor a bribe to maintain a good relationship.

Chiropractors are gaining respect within the Ukrainian American population and the use of a chiropractor in certain situations is preferred (Bologova, 1996). Chiropractic is a popular profession among Ukrainian Americans. Unfortunately, mental problems are often still considered taboo and the discussion of this does not occur even within the affected family. In Ukraine, mental illness was considered shameful, and it could even be dangerous to the family if it became known that a family member had mental health issues.

The nurse should recognize the prevalence of alternative therapy use in this population. If the use is nonharmful or neutral, the nurse should remain open to usage. The nurse should ask the patient about the use of any alternative healthcare practices as part of the initial data gathering.

Impact of Communication

Because of increased exposure to English-speaking media by most Russians, English is widely used. Some may have even studied English in school, although it is most likely British English rather than American English. Some elderly Russian Americans may also speak Yiddish. In the former Soviet Union, the speaking of Yiddish was discouraged and considered to be an antistate activity (Petersen, 2001). The official language of Russia is Russian. Russia is a Slavic language consisting of a 33-character alphabet; approximately one-sixth of the world's population speaks Russian. There are geographic variances associated with the language. Tone, inflection, speed, and pauses, as well as nonverbal cues, are important when communicating in the Russian language as it denotes the value being placed on the words that are being said. Russian Americans may use an increased voice volume when attempting to have their needs met. The nurse should not feel that the Russian American patient is being rude if even normal conversation appears to be loud and boisterous. Due to the importance of nonverbal and subtle meanings of the verbal language, it is important to use professional interpreters when working with Russian Americans who are not fluent in American English. The use of family members as interpreters is especially problematic with this population. The close-knit community of Russian Americans breeds a high level of familiarity, which can make confidentiality impossible to maintain or ensure.

Impact of Communication for Ukrainian Americans

The Ukrainian language has been different than other Slavic languages, including Russian, since the 12th or 13th century (Accredited Language Services International, 2012). The language developed independently until Russia seized Ukraine at the end of the 17th century. By the mid 17th century the language divergence of Russian and Ukrainian was so dramatic translators were needed when negotiating treaties (Accredited Language Services International, 2012). By the beginning of the 19th century, the Russian Czars banned the use of the Ukrainian language and the language fell into decay. In western Ukraine, the language absorbed influences from Polish, Hungarian, German, and Romanian. Ukrainian was restored as the official language of Ukraine in 1917.

Most Ukrainian Pentecostals (many of whom are refugees who came to the United States because of religious oppression) speak only Ukrainian, but can often understand Polish and Russian. Ukrainian Jews, on the other hand, are often bilingual and speak both Ukrainian and Russian. A few may also speak or understand Yiddish.

Impact of Time and Space

Touch is freely shared among close or intimate friends, as is closer proximity (HealthCareChaplaincy.org, 2010). Affection is readily demonstrated as women will kiss women and men will kiss men. They may also exchange three kisses on each cheek, which appears to be a cultural trait carried over from the Middle East. A handshake is particularly significant and is often viewed as more binding than a signed document. The handshake should be extremely firm while maintaining direct eye contact, when a male shakes hands with a female the handshake will be less firm (Magocsi, 2012).

In Eastern Europe, hospital gowns are not used, requiring patients to be examined in undergarments; nudity is also not considered shameful (Stratis Health, 2010).

A consequence of the many years of communist rule in Russia is that many Russian Americans still try to act in a neutral manner: avoiding eye contact, maintaining a flat affect, and having slouchy posture (Khrushcheva, 2000). Once exposed to a society that values personal freedom, such as in the United States, some will loosen up, but others may maintain the stance of neutrality. Great warmth will be expressed in private when dealing with close friends and family; unannounced or unplanned visits are common. The nurse should expect many visitors when caring for a Russian American patient.

The expectation is that the nurse will remain professional and caring at all times. A robotic approach to healthcare delivery will result in the loss of trust. Formality is also expected and the nurse should greet the patient as Mr. or Mrs. followed by the surname. To address a Russian American patient by their first name only is a major faux pas. It is also considered inappropriate to use terms of endearment in place of the patient's formal name (e.g., honey or sweetie) (Smith, 1996). It is considered appropriate for the nurse to enter the patient's personal space within a professional capacity—this space is usually reserved for the spouse and children. It would be wise for the nurse to fully communicate the need to enter the patient's personal space or if any violation of modesty is required in advance.

Russian American patients place a high premium on a nurse being very friendly, warm, and caring and to be there to help the patient and family cope with physical and psychosocial consequences of illness. The nurse can best communicate friendliness by maintaining an open body posture, smiling frequently, and speaking in a calm, pleasant tone. It has also been noted, interestingly enough, that Russian American patients prefer to be cared for by a nurse from any cultural group other than Russian. It had been reported anecdotally that for some Russian Americans, it is felt they will experience more compassion and their needs will be better met by a non-Russian provider (Lester, 1998).

Impact of Social Organization

Family is an important concept for Russian Americans and in America, as in Russia, extended family members often live together and rely on each other to make life easier (Stratis Health, 2010). If the Russian American has family still in Russia, those family members who are with the patient in the United States become even more significant to them. Within the family structure, the father exerts the greatest influence. The female role is to care for the children. Women's liberation is not a part of the traditional Russian family structure. If the wife is well-educated, her husband may consult her on some decision making. Arguments within the family, when they occur, can be quite loud and dramatic and objects may be thrown.

Social events are often framed around the arts. The arts, such as ballet, theater, music, and museums, are highly valued in Russian culture. The family often strives to keep the arts alive by exposing the children to this early in life.

The elderly, who were usually cared for in exchange for child care, may be a reminder of the old ways in the home country. It is not unusual for the elderly Russian immigrant to lose their authority and status within a short time after immigration to the United States (Casado & Leung, 2001).

Within a few years of immigration to the United States, children become completely assimilated into American culture. Children are very important in Russian culture; they are seen as symbols of innocence and the family's hopes for the future (Stratis Health, 2010). Children often grow up overprotected and cared for by elderly family members as the hope is that the child's life will be easier than that of his or her parent (CactusLanguage.com, n.d.). One-child families are very common and extended family members, such as cousins, are treated as substitute siblings. If a child becomes ill, the family will fight vehemently for the child's rights and may request unnecessary diagnostic testing or prolonged hospital stays. Russians may be accustomed to longer lengths of stay than are typical today in the United States, as the average in-patient stay in Russia is 3 weeks (Rundle et al., 1999). The nurse should assure the family that the primary concern is the child's welfare, which may ease the worry. In addition, helping both patients and families understand the differences between the Russian and U.S. healthcare systems, and how to navigate the U.S. healthcare system, is time well spent by the nurse.

Impact of Social Organization for Ukrainian Americans

Ukrainians often have very large families, and the older family members help to care for the children (CactusLanguage.com, n.d.). Because of limited housing and cost, it is not uncommon to have three generations of a Ukrainian family all living together in a small space. Pentecostal Ukrainians, by virtue of their refugee status, are able to receive refugee benefits and services from refugee organizations in their new communities.

Impact of Faith and Spirituality

In Russia, as a consequence of communism, the nonreligious may make up the majority of the population. The nonreligious constitutes anywhere between 24 and 48% of the population, according to a study by Zuckerman (2007). Russia ranks 3rd on the listing of top 20 atheist countries in the world (Zuckerman, 2007). Russian Orthodox has a following of 45% of Russians, although the vast majority do not attend church. In a poll conducted in 2007 by the Russian Public Opinion Research Center, about 75% of Russia's people affirm the Orthodox faith, and only 10% are regular churchgoers. In a post–Soviet Union Russia, Orthodoxy has become the national faith. It is difficult to gauge the actual number of followers because many Russians, although they may never attend church services, identify and consider themselves Russian Orthodox. The CIA (2006) estimated the number of practicing worshippers of Orthodoxy in Russia as being between 15 and 20%, with Muslims making up 10 to 15%, and other Christians 2%. The CIA states that post-Soviet rule, Russia was left with a large population of nonpracticing believers and nonbelievers. The remaining Russians are Tatars (an Islamic religion) and Jews. Despite these varying statistics, there can be no doubt that the fall of communism has brought a resurgence of the Christian religion in Russia.

Impact of Faith and Spirituality for Ukrainian Americans

The largest religion in Ukraine, just as in Russia, is Eastern Orthodox, a branch of Christianity. Prior to 1990, the Ukrainian Orthodox Church was forced to become part of the Russian Orthodox Church. After Ukrainian independence, the Ukrainian Orthodox Church was restored. The second largest Christian religion in Ukraine is the Greek Catholic Church. In the past, Pentecostal and Baptist churches were active in western Ukraine. Persecution resulted when Ukraine was under Russian control, prompting many Pentecostals to flee as refugees from the former Soviet Union. This is another example of people being forced to leave their homeland for the United States in search of religious freedom. Indeed, the primary reason for leaving Ukraine is religious oppression (Bologova, 1996). Ukrainian Pentecostals value hard work and the family, and they have strict rules against drugs and alcohol usage. The rejection of birth control usage, supported by the religion, often results in very large families.

Biologic Variations

There is a significant genetic mutation problem within the Russian population. It is felt that because of chronic exposure to environmental toxins from pesticides, cigarette smoking, and even the Chernobyl nuclear power plant accident, genetic mutation rates are higher, with an associated higher risk for health consequences caused by accumulated genetic damage. It has been estimated that the rate of accumulated genetic damage is 250% higher in Russians than Americans (Vadlamani et al., 2001). This genetic damage seems to be implicated in higher colorectal neoplasm rates in this population, which should highlight for the nurse the need for vigilant cancer screenings in this population.

The foods that are preferred in Russian culture have contributed to an obesity problem in this population, especially among elderly women. Many foods are high in fat and salt, which also has resulted in a significant problem with hypertension and coronary heart disease. There has been a trend in decreasing life expectancy in Russia since 1990. It is felt that this decrease is a result of a tremendous increase in coronary heart disease mortality among men, which increased by about

30% in Russia between 1990 and 2000 (Landsbergis & Klumbiene, 2003). Poor diet, excessive alcohol intake, and tobacco usage have been implicated in the high coronary heart disease numbers. Hyperlipidemia and hypercholesterolemia are also problematic in this population because most Russians, although compliant with most health screening; do not see the value or accuracy of cholesterol screening tests. Cholesterol levels among Russian Americans are generally well above normal limits (Mehler et al., 2001).

Higher rates of TB are also seen in this population. About 1.1 million people, or almost 0.6–0.7% of the population in Russia, developed TB between 1995 and 2004 (Marquez, Jakubowiak, Pashkevich, & Grechukka, 2012). The reasons for this include problems within the Russian healthcare system, a significant number of HIV/AIDS patients, an increased prison population, and indifference. The advance practice nurse should have a high index of suspicion and consider TB in this population and provide for infection control practices as needed.

Alcoholism and excessive alcohol usage is a tremendous public health issue in Russia. Alcohol consumption is nearly 3 times higher than it was 15 years ago and the country currently ranks first in alcohol sales (Mogul, 2012). The nurse should not assume that the Russian American will have an alcohol issue. Russian alcoholics have lost hope and would not be motivated to emigrate from Russia in search of a new life. Most immigrants from Russia to the United States, on the other hand, are extremely motivated to change their lives for the better and want to survive here in America. Those immigrants who are religious also will be unlikely to drink alcohol because of the religious sanctions against its use and abuse among Jewish and Pentecostal affiliates.

SUMMARY

As we have seen, the White non-Hispanic population is extremely diverse and is unified by a similarity of skin pigmentation. The White population has diverse and multiple places of origin within Europe. The majority of the American population is currently considered White non-Hispanic, and it is important to understand the differences among the various ethnic groups with regard to historical background, statistics, traditional health beliefs, and barriers to care. As with all patients, it is important to question the White American patient to determine his or her health and illness beliefs, so that a culturally competent plan of care can be developed for that unique individual.

REFERENCES

Accredited Language Services International. (2012). Ukrainian. Retrieved from http://www
.alsintl.com/resources/languages/Ukrainian/

American Community Survey. (2009). *Top ten spoken languages in ELL students' homes.* Retrieved
from http://www.migrationinformation.org/ellinfo/FactSheet_ELL3.pdf

Amish America. (2010). *Where do the Amish live?* Retrieved from http://amishamerica.com/
where-do-the-amish-live/

Aslund, A. (2001). Think again: Russia. Retrieved from https://www.foreignpolicy.com/
articles/2001/07/01/think_again_russia?page=0,5

Bankston, C. L. (n.d.). *American immigration history.* Retrieved from http://www.academia
.edu/937663/American_Immigration_History

Bankston, C. L., & Hidalgo, D. (2006). *Immigration in US history.* Pasadena, CA: Salem Press.

BBC.com. (2012). Judaism. Retrieved from http://www.bbc.co.uk/religion/religions/judaism/

Behringer, B., & Friedell, G. H. (2006). Appalachia: Where place matters in health. *Preventing
Chronic Disease, 3*(4), A 113. Retrieved from http://www.ncbi.nlm.nih.gov/pmc/articles/
PMC1779277/

Bologova, N. (1996). *Voices of the Ukrainian community.* Retrieved from http://www.xculture
.org/files/UKRAINE.pdf

Braham, M. (1993). *The untouchables: A survey of the Roma people of central and eastern Europe.*
Geneva, Switzerland: UNHCR.

Brown, M. K., & Obermiller, P. J. (1994). The health status of children living in urban Appalachian neighborhoods. In K. M. Borman & P. J. Obermiller (Eds.), *From mountains to
metropolis: Appalachian migrants in American cities* (pp. 70–82). Westport, CT: Bergin &
Garvey.

Butler, S. (1996). Substance misuse and the social work ethos. *Justice of Substance Misuse, 1*(3),
149–154.

CactusLanguage.com. (n.d.). Russian culture. Retrieved from http://www.cactuslanguage.com/
en/culturesmart/culture_russia.php

Casado, B. L., & Leung, P. (2001). Migratory grief and depression among elderly immigrants.
Social work practice with the Russian American Elderly, 36, 5–26. Binghamton, NY: The
Haworth Social Work Practice Press.

Cavender, A. (2003). *Folk Medicine in Southern Appalachia.* Chapel Hill, NC: University of
North Carolina Press.

Center for Public Education. (2010). *The United States of education: The changing demographics
of the United States and their schools.* Retrieved from http://www.centerforpubliceducation
.org/You-May-Also-Be-Interested-In-landing-page-level/Organizing-a-School-YMABI/
The-United-States-of-education-The-changing-demographics-of-the-United-States-and-
their-schools.html

Central Bureau of Statistics. (2010). Statistical abstract of Israel. Retrieved from http://www1
.cbs.gov.il/reader/shnaton/templ_shnaton_e.html?num_tab=st02_02&CYear=2010

Central Intelligence Agency (CIA). (2006). *The world factbook: Religions.* Retrieved from https://www
.cia.gov/library/publications/the-world-factbook/fields/2122.html

Central Intelligence Agency (CIA). (2009). *The world factbook: United States.* Retrieved from
https://www.cia.gov/library/publications/the-world-factbook/geos/us.html

Central Intelligence Agency (CIA). (2012). *The world factbook: Ireland.* Retrieved from https://
www.cia.gov/library/publications/the-world-factbook/geos/ei.html

Chanes, J. A. (2008). *A primer on the American Jewish community*. Retrieved from http://www.ajc.org/atf/cf/%7B42d75369-d582-4380-8395-d25925b85eaf%7D/PRIMER%20AMERICAN%20JEWISH.PDF

Chiarelli, L. R., Fermo, E., Abrusci, P., Bianchi, B., Dellacasa, C. M., Galizzi, A., ... Valentini, G. (2006). Two new mutations of the P5N-1 gene found in Italian patients with hereditary hemolytic anemia: The molecular basis of the red cell enzyme disorder. *Haemotologia, 91*(9), 1244–1247.

Christian Light Publications, Inc. (n.d.). *The Germans come to North America*. Retrieved from http://www.anabaptists.org/history/ss8001.html

Del Boca, D., & Venturini, A. (2003). *Italian migration*. Retrieved from http://ftp.iza.org/dp938.pdf

Diner, H. (2008). *Immigration and US History*. Retrieved from http://www.america.gov/st/diversityenglish/2008/February/20080307112004ebyessedo0.1716272.html

Edwards, J. B., Lenz, C. L., & East-Odom, J. C. (1993). Nurse-managed primary care: Serving a rural Appalachian population. *Family & Community Health, 16*(2), 50–56.

Ehman, J. (2007). *Religious diversity: Practical points for care providers*. Retrieved from http://www.uphs.upenn.edu/pastoral/resed/diversity_points.html

Engels, E. A., Clark, E., Aledort, L. M., Goedert, J. J., & Whitby, D. (2002). Kaposi's sarcoma-associated herpes virus infection in elderly Jews and non-Jews from New York City. *International Journal of Epidemiology, 31*(5), 946–950.

EuroMedInfo.com. (n.d.). *How culture influences health beliefs*. Retrieved from http://www.euromedinfo.eu/how-culture-influences-health-beliefs.html/

Fares, F., Badarneh, K., Abosaleh, M., Harrari-Shaham, A., Diukman, R., & David, M. (2008). Carrier frequency of autosomal-recessive disorders in the Ashkenazi Jewish population: Should the rationale for mutation choice for screening be reevaluated? *Prenatal Diagnosis, 28*(3), 236–241.

Fedunkiw, M. P. (2012). *Ukrainian Americans*. Retrieved from http://www.everyculture.com/multi/Sr-Z/Ukrainian-Americans.html

Fox, S. (2000). *Uncivil liberties*. Boca Raton, FL: Universal.

Galanti, G. A. (2000). An introduction to cultural differences. *The Western Journal of Medicine, 172*(5), 335–336.

Gale Encyclopedia of Public Health. (2002). *Traditional health beliefs*. Retrieved from http://www.answers.com/topic/traditional-health-beliefs-practices

Giger, J. N. (2013). *Transcultural nursing: Assessment and intervention* (6th ed.). St. Louis, MO: Mosby.

Giordano, J., & McGoldrick, M. (2005). Italian families. In M. McGoldrick, J. Giordano, & J. K. Pearce (Eds.), *Ethnicity and family therapy* (3rd ed.) (pp. 501–520). New York, NY: Guilford.

Gross, L. (1997). *Background dynamics of the Amish movement: The Dutch Mennonites vis-á-vis the Swiss Brethren: Pivotal individuals within the Swiss Brethren division of the 1690s, and the question of Reformed (Calvinist) influence*. Retrieved from http://www.orrar.net/amish/bdamishmovement.htm

Hajioff, S., & McKee, M. (2000). The health of the Roma people: a review of the published literature. Retrieved from http://jech.bmj.com/content/54/11/864.full

Halperin, R. H. (1994). Appalachians in cities: Issues and challenges for research. In K. M. Borman & P. J. Obermiller (Eds.), *From mountains to metropolis: Appalachian migrants in American cities* (pp. 70–82). Westport, CT: Bergin & Garvey.

Hancock, I. F. (1987). *The pariah syndrome: An account of gypsy slavery and persecution.* Ann Arbor, MI: Karoma.

HealthCareChaplaincy.org. (2010). *A dictionary of patients' spiritual and cultural values for health care professionals* (pp. 87–89). Retrieved from http://www.healthcarechaplaincy.org/userimages/Cultural%20&%20Spiritual%20Dictionary%2012-20-10.pdf

Helton, L. R., Barnes, E. C., & Borman, K. M. (1994). Urban Appalachia and professional intervention: A model for education and social service providers. In K. M. Borman & P. J. Obermiller (Eds.), *From mountains to metropolis: Appalachian migrants in American cities* (pp. 106–120). Westport, CT: Bergin & Garvey.

Hendrix, L. R. (2002). *Health and health care of American Indian and Alaska Native elders.* Retrieved from http://www.stanford.edu/group/ethnoger/americanindian.html

Hostetler, J. A. (1993). *Amish society* (4th ed.). Baltimore, MD: John Hopkins University Press.

Jacobs, L. A., & Giarelli, E. (2001). Jewish culture, health belief systems and genetic risk for cancer. *Nursing Forum, 36*(2), 5–12.

Jewish.org. (2012). Jewish identity and culture. Retrieved from http://jewish.org/

Jewish Federation Organization. (2001). *United Jewish communities report series on the national Jewish population survey 2000–2001.* Retrieved from http://www.jewishfederations.org/local_includes/downloads/7579.pdf

Johnson-Weiner, K. (1998). Community identity and language change in North American Anabaptist communities, *Journal of Sociolinguistics, 2/3,* 375–394.

Jones, L. (1994). *Appalachian values.* Ashland, KY: Jesse Stuart Foundation.

Katzman, D. M. (2000). European immigrants leave mark on continent. *The Brown Quarterly, 4*(1), 2. Retrieved from http://brownvboard.org/sites/default/files/BQ_Vol4No1.pdf

Kemp, C. (n.d.). Gypsy (Roma). Retrieved from http://www3.baylor.edu/~Charles_Kemp/gypsy_health.htm

KentuckyDocMagazine.com. (2011). Mary Breckenridge: Pioneering nurse brought health care to Appalachia. Retrieved from http://kentuckydocmagazine.com/2011/12/05/mary-breckinridge-pioneering-nurse-brought-health-care-to-appalachia/

Khrushcheva, N. L. (2000). *Cultural contradictions of post-communism: Why liberal reforms did not succeed in Russia.* Retrieved from http://www.units.muohio.edu/havighurstcenter/publications/documents/khrushcheva_000.pdf

Kraybill, D. B. (2001). *The riddle of Amish culture* (rev. ed.). Baltimore, MD: The John Hopkins University Press.

Kraybill, D. B. (2003). *The Amish and the state* (2nd ed.). Baltimore, MD: The Johns Hopkins University Press.

Kraybill, D. B., Nolt, S. M., & Johnson-Weiner, K. (2008). *The Amish in America.* New York, NY: John Hopkins University Press.

Kubiszewski, I., & Cleveland, C. (2009). Chernobyl, Ukraine. Retrieved from http://www.eoearth.org/article/Chernobyl,_Ukraine

Kutler, S. (2003). Immigration Act of 1965. *Dictionary of American History* (3rd ed.). New York, NY: Charles Scribner's Sons.

Landsbergis, P., & Klumbiene, J. (2003). Coronary heart disease mortality in Russia and Eastern Europe. *American Journal of Public Health, 93*(11), 1793.

Lassiter, S. M. (1995). *Multicultural clients: A professional handbook for health care providers and social workers.* Westport, CT: Greenwood Publishing Group.

Lee, D. (2005). *Our Amish neighbors: Providing culturally competent care* (Multicultural Health Series) [Videotape and handout]. UMHS, PMCH, Cultural Competency Division.

Lee, J. (2011). *U.S. naturalization: 2011.* U.S. Department of Homeland Security. Retrieved from http://www.dhs.gov/xlibrary/assets/statistics/publications/natz_fr_2011.pdf

Lester, N. (1998). Cultural competence: A nursing dialogue 2. *The American Journal of Nursing, 98*(9), 36–43.

Magocsi, P. R. (2012). *Russian Americans.* Retrieved from http://www.everyculture.com/multi/Pa-Sp/Russian-Americans.html

Marger, M. N., & Obermiller, P. J. (1987). Urban Appalachians and Canadian Maritime migrants: Comparative study of emergent ethnicity. In P. J. Obermiller & W. W. Philliber (Eds.), *Too few tomorrows: Urban Appalachians in the 1980s* (pp. 23–34). Boone, NC: Appalachian Consortium Press.

Marquez, P. V., Jakubowiak, W., Pashkevich, D. D., & Grechukka, V. A. (2012). *Battle against tuberculosis: Some gains in Russia.* Retrieved from http://web.worldbank.org/WBSITE/EXTERNAL/COUNTRIES/ECAEXT/0,,contentMDK:22717729~pagePK:146736~piPK:146830~theSitePK:258599,00.html

Martin, P., & Midgley, E. (2003). *Immigration: Shaping and reshaping America.* Retrieved from http://www.prb.org/Source/58.2ImmigrShapingAmerica.pdf

Mather, M. (2004). *Demographic and socioeconomic change in Appalachia.* Retrieved from http://www.arc.gov/assets/research_reports/HouseholdsandFamilies.pdf

Matras, Y. (2006). Romani. In K. Brown (Ed.), *Encyclopedia of languages and linguistics* (2nd ed.). Oxford: Elsevier.

McKee, M. (1997). The health of gypsies. *British Medical Journal, 315*(7117), 1172–1173.

McNeil, W. K. (1989). *Appalachian images in folk and popular culture.* Ann Arbor, MI: UMI Research Press.

Mehler, P. S., Scott, J. Y., Pines, I., Gifford, N., Biggerstaff, S., & Hiatt, W. R. (2001). Russian immigrant cardiovascular risk assessment. *Journal of Health Care for the Poor and Underserved, 12*(2), 224–235.

Migrant Resource Center. (2008). *Italian cultural profile.* Retrieved from http://www.miceastmelb.com.au/documents/pdaproject/CulturalProfiles/ItalianCulturalProfile2010.pdf

Nolt, S. M. (2003). *A history of the Amish.* Intercourse, PA: Good Books.

Ortman, J. M., & Guarneri, C. E. (2009). *United State population projections: 2000 to 2050.* Retrieved from http://www.census.gov/population/www/projections/analytical-document09.pdf

Patten, E. (2008). *Statistical portrait of the foreign-born population in the United States, 2009, Table 5, country of birth: 2009.* Retrieved from the Pew Hispanic Center website: http://www.pewhispanic.org/2012/02/21/statistical-portrait-of-the-foreign-born-population-in-the-united-states-2010/

Pelaia, A. (2012). *The Hebrew language.* Retrieved from http://judaism.about.com/od/jewishhistory/a/Hebrew-Language-Origins-History.htm

Perea, J. F. (Ed.). (1996). *Immigrants out! The new nativism and the anti-immigrant impulse in the United States.* New York, NY: NYU Press.

Petersen, R. D. (2001). *Resistance and rebellion: Lessons from Eastern Europe.* New York, NY: Cambridge University Press.

Pew Forum on Religion & Public Life. (2008). *Religious landscape survey.* Retrieved from http://religions.pewforum.org/pdf/report-religious-landscape-study-full.pdf

Pollard, K., & Jacobsen, L. A. (2012). The Appalachian region in 2010: A data overview from the 2006–2010 American community survey. Retrieved from http://www.arc.gov/research/researchreportdetails.asp?REPORT_ID=96

Pozzetta, G. (2000). Italian Americans. *Gale encyclopedia of multicultural affairs.* Retrieved from http://www.encyclopedia.com/topic/Italian_Americans.aspx

Preet, E. (2008, April/May). Sláinte!: A charmed life. *Irish America*. Retrieved from http://irishamerica.com/2008/04/slainte-a-charmed-life/

Project Genesis, Inc. (n.d.). Slainte!: A charmed life. Retrieved from http://www.torah.org/

Purnell, L. D. (2013). *Transcultural health care: A culturally competent approach* (4th ed.). Philadelphia, PA: F. A. Davis.

Rajagopal, S. (2005). Clozapine, agranulocytosis, and benign ethnic neutropenia. *Journal of Postgraduate Medicine, 81*(959), 545–546.

RomaCulture.com. (2010). History. Retrieved from http://romaculture.com.mk/site/history/

Rosner, F. (1993). Hospice, medical ethics and Jewish customs. *American Journal of Hospice & Palliative Care, 10*(4), 6–10.

Rundle, A. K., Carvalho, M., & Robinson, M. (1999). *Cultural competence in health care: A practical guide*. San Francisco, CA: Jossey-Bass.

Russ, K. A. (2010). Working with clients of Appalachian culture. Retrieved from http://counselingoutfitters.com/vistas/vistas10/Article_69.pdf

Russian Public Opinion Research Center. (2007). Retrieved from http://wciom.com

Sage, H. J. (2005). *American economic growth*. Retrieved from http://www.academicamerican.com/jeffersonjackson/topics/EconomicIssues.htm

Smith, L. S. (1996). New Russian immigrants: Health problems, practices and values. *Journal of Cultural Diversity, 3*(3), 68–73.

Spector, R. E. (2008). *Cultural diversity in health and illness* (7th ed.). New York, NY: Prentice-Hall.

Stratis Health. (2010). Cultural group guides: Russian. Retrieved from http://www.dimensionsofculture.com/culture-fact-sheets/

Sutherland, A. H. (2004). Roma of the United States and Europe. In C. R. Ember & M. Ember (Eds.), *Encyclopedia of medical anthropology: Health and illness in the world's cultures*. New York, NY: Kluwer Academic/Plenum.

Taylor, H (2003). *While most Americans believe in God, only 36% attend a religious service once a month or more often*. The Harris Poll #59. Retrieved from http://www.harrisinteractive.com/vault/Harris-Interactive-Poll-Research-While-Most-Americans-Believe-in-God-Only-36-pct-A-2003-10.pdf

Tobin, D. K., Tobin, G. A., & Rubin, S. (2005). *In every tongue: Ethnic and racial diversity in the Jewish Community*. San Francisco, CA: Institute for Jewish and Community Research.

U.S. Census Bureau. (2000). *United States Census 2000*. Retrieved from http://www.census.gov/main/www/cen2000.html

U.S. Census Bureau. (2001). *Profile of the foreign-born population in the United States: 2000*. Retrieved from http://www.census.gov/prod/2002pubs/p23–206.pdf

U.S. Census Bureau. (2002). *Population profiles by age, sex, race and Hispanic origin: Summary File 3*. Washington, DC: U.S. Government Printing Office.

U.S. Census Bureau. (2004). *Ancestry 2000*. Retrieved from http://www.census.gov/prod/2004pubs/c2kbr-35.pdf

U.S. Census Bureau. (2007a). *Religious composition of US population: 2007*. Retrieved from http://www.census.gov/compendia/statab/tables/09s0074.pdf

U.S. Census Bureau. (2007b). *Selected social characteristics in the United States: 2007*. Retrieved from http://factfinder2.census.gov/faces/tableservices/jsf/pages/productview.xhtml?src=bkmk

U.S. Census Bureau. (2008a). *An older and more diverse nation by midcentury*. Retrieved from https://www.census.gov/newsroom/releases/archives/population/cb08-123.html

U.S. Census Bureau. (2008b). Table 4: Annual estimates of the Black or African American alone or in combination population by sex and age for the United States: April 1, 2000, to July

1, 2007. Population Division, U.S. Census Bureau. Retrieved from http://www.census.gov/popest/data/historical/2000s/vintage_2007/index.html

U.S. Census Bureau. (2010). *Selected social characteristics in the United States, 2006–2010 American Community Survey*. Retrieved from http://factfinder2.census.gov/faces/tableservices/jsf/pages/productview.xhtml?pid=ACS_10_SF4_DP02&prodType=table

U.S. Census Bureau (2011). *2010 census shows America's diversity*. Retrieved from http://2010.census.gov/news/releases/operations/cb11-cn125.html

U.S. Department of Homeland Security. (2005). *2005 yearbook of immigration statistics*. Washington, DC: U.S. Department of Homeland Security: Office of Immigration Statistics. Retrieved from http://www.dhs.gov/xlibrary/assets/statistics/yearbook/2005/OIS_2005_Yearbook.pdf

U.S. Department of Homeland Security. (2010). *2010 yearbook of immigration statistics*. Retrieved from http://www.dhs.gov/xlibrary/assets/statistics/yearbook/2010/ois_yb_2010.pdf

Vadlamani, A., Maher, J. F., Shaete, M., Smirnoff, A., Cameron, D. G., Winkelmann, J. C., & Goldberg, S. J. (2001). Colorectal cancer in Russian-speaking Jewish emigrés: Community-based screening. *American Journal of Gastroenterology, 96*(9), 2755–2760.

Vallance, H., & Ford, J. (2003). Carrier testing for autosomal-recessive disorders. *Critical Reviews in Clinical Laboratory Sciences, 40*(4), 473–497.

Webley, K. (2010, October 13). Hounded in Europe, Roma in the US keep a low profile. *Time*. Retrieved from http://www.time.com/time/nation/article/0,8599,2025316,00.html

Zuckerman, P. (2007). Atheism: Contemporary numbers and patterns. In M. Martin (Ed.), *The Cambridge companion to atheism*. New York, NY: Cambridge University Press.

For a full suite of assignments and additional learning activities, see the access code at the front of your book.

Muslims and Hindus

© iStockphoto/Thinkstock

BACKGROUND

Muslims

Not all Muslims (believers in Islam) share all of the same health beliefs. The health beliefs, values, and practices of Muslims are influenced by geographical, cultural, and ethnic factors, in addition to the individual degree of faith and spirituality a Muslim may possess. There are differences in health belief practices among Arab, Asian, African, and Black American Muslims.

Islam is the second largest and fastest growing religion in the world. While the perception in the United States is that Islam is a Middle Eastern religion, according to PBS.org (2012) only about 12% of Muslims worldwide are Arabs, and the majority of Arab Americans are Christian. About 30% of U.S. Muslims are Black American (Ohm, 2003). Followers of Islam are known as Muslims, Moslems, or Islamic. The Arabic word *Islam* means peace, submission, and obedience. There are also sects of traditional Muslims. Sunnis represent about 90% and Shiites represent 10 to 15% of traditional Muslims. There are also several smaller sects, including Sufi, Ahmadiyya, Wahhabi, Ismaili, and Dawoodi Bohra. According to the American Religious Identification Survey (Kosmin & Keysar, 2009), which evaluated subjects' self-reported data, the followers of Islam make up 0.6% of the American population (1,349,000).

There are five pillars of Islam (BBC.com, 2009): *Shahadah*, which is the declaration of faith to the one supreme being, Allah; *Salat*, which is daily prayer five times a day; *Sawm*, which is fasting during Ramadan (for 28 days during the 9th lunar month), *Zakat*, which is giving to the poor (the systematic giving of 2.5% of one's wealth annually to benefit the poor); and lastly, *Hajj*, which is a pilgrimage to Mecca, Saudi Arabia, at least once in a lifetime (if physically and financially able). Muslims believe that the words of their sacred text, the Koran (Qur'an), were revealed to the prophet Muhammad by the angel Gabriel when Muhammad was 40 years of age.

Hindus

The Hindu religion is practiced by the vast majority of Indians as well as in Nepal. Practiced by 14% of the world's population, Hinduism is the world's third largest religion. It is estimated that there are well over one million Hindus in the United States (The Pluralism Project at Harvard University, 2010). According to the American Religious Identification Survey (Kosmin & Keysar, 2009), 0.4%, or 767,000, individuals practice Hinduism in the United States. Some of these Hindus may be immigrants from India, Nepal, Trinidad, or Africa. There is now a second generation of Hindus who have grown up entirely in the United States. Hinduism is the world's third largest religion and is often referred to as the "oldest living religion on Earth" (Levinson, 1998), as it began around 1500 BC. Its foundation is based on the principles of karma (what you do is done onto you) and living in harmony.

Hinduism varies from other monotheistic religions in that it is a religion of evolution—due to its wide variety of traditions, its followers have significant freedom of belief and practice, and this has resulted in an appreciation for religious tolerance (Levinson, 1998). Hindu followers recognize a single deity, and view other gods and goddesses as manifestations or aspects of the one supreme God. This does not provide a complete view of this complex religion as some classify it as monotheistic (one God), while others would call it polytheistic, because gods and goddesses are worshipped (although most religious scholars state this would not be accurate as three gods and goddesses are manifestations of one supreme God). Still others view it as Trinitarian—one supreme God with three personas: Brahma the Creator, who is continuing to create new realities; Vishnu or Krishna the Preserver, who preserves the new creations; and Shiva the Destroyer, who can be compassionate, erotic, and/or destructive (ReligiousTolerance.org, 2012). Finally, some religious scholars consider the religion to be henotheistic, because the earliest Hindu scriptures recognize multiple deities (both male and female) but recognize that one deity reigns supreme (ReligiousTolerance.org, 2012). Most urban Hindus follow one of the two major divisions within Hinduism: Vaishnavaism, which regards Vishnu (or Krishna) as the ultimate deity, or Shivaism, which regards Shiva as the ultimate deity (ReligiousTolerance.org, 2012).

PRINCIPLES OF THE MUSLIM FAITH

The supreme being of Islam is Allah and the religion's founder is the Prophet Muhammad (Levinson, 1998). The holy book is called the Koran or Qur'an. Daily living of Muslims is guided by the Koran and also by additional teachings from Muhammad, the Hadith, and the Sunna. Some Muslims use prayer beads and prayer rugs and may pin amulets and charms to their clothing. The use of idolatry is forbidden and the use of statues, figurines, or other likenesses that attempt to personify Allah or Muhammad are considered idol worship.

MUSLIM HEALTH BELIEFS

Muslims view illness as an atonement for sins. Illness is dealt with by both the patient and family by praying (Taheri, 2008). They are open to receiving medical treatment, but if it is felt it is time for death, they will view it as an opportunity to begin their journey to meet their Lord. The major tenet of Islam is peace and submission to the will of God (Allah). Cleanliness is an important concept to Muslims as maintaining cleanliness is viewed as being "half of the faith" (Athar, 2008). The Qur'an, the holy book, prohibits eating pork or pork products, meat of dead animals, and blood, and encourages the avoidance of all intoxicants. The practice of fasting, which occurs from dawn to dusk daily for one month a year during Ramadan, is considered restorative and is viewed as restful to the body.

IMPORTANT NURSING IMPLICATIONS

There are certain health practices that are generally acceptable and others that are not acceptable to the Muslim patient. As with any other cultural group, it is essential that the nurse question the patient to determine what beliefs and practices are of significance to him or her as an individual (Taheri, 2008). Modesty (*hijab*) is an important consideration for the female Muslim patient. The nurse should ask for permission first before exposing the female Muslim patient's body prior to providing any nursing interventions such as injections or assessments (Taheri, 2008). Once the female enters puberty it is proper to keep the head and arms covered when in public. This practice may have implications for nursing care delivery. Generally, female patients who are modest will also avoid touching or being in close proximity to males. This may be a challenge for the male nurse to perform physical assessment or to deliver some aspects of nursing care that require touching. The nurse should ensure the patient's comfort and advocate for the patient whenever the modest Muslim patient is faced with the need for a physical examination by a male provider, especially examinations that involve or include the female anatomy. Generally, the following healthcare practices are permitted by the Muslim patient: circumcision, blood transfusions (after proper screening), transplantation (with some restrictions), reproductive technology (but only within an intact marriage), living wills, and genetic engineering (but not cloning). The following healthcare practices are generally not acceptable to the Muslim patient: assisted suicide/euthanasia, autopsy (unless required by law), maintaining a terminal patient on life support for a prolonged period in a vegetative state, abortion (unless it is to save the mother's life), and cloning.

Table A–1 describes what nurses can and should do for the Muslim patient.

PRINCIPLES OF THE HINDU FAITH

Hindus believe in the repetitious transmigration of the soul, or the transfer of one's soul after death into another body. This produces a continuing cycle of

Table A–1 Cultural Implications when Providing Nursing Care to Muslim Patients

Physical Examination/ Assessment	If an examination can be performed over a gown, it should be done that way.
	Provide for modesty/privacy.
	Always examine a female patient in the presence of another female patient (this is mandatory if the nurse or physician is male). It is best to provide same sex health care if at all possible.
	Preferably no males in the delivery room during labor (except the husband).
Nutrition/Diet	Offer Muslim or Kosher meals.
	Permit the family to bring in food if there are no dietary restrictions. If restrictions are necessary, request that the dietitian work with the family to incorporate foods from home if possible.
Faith/Spirituality	Allow for uninterrupted prayer and for the patient to read the Koran.
	Allow their Imam to visit.
	Do not insist on autopsy or organ donation.
	In the event of patient death, allow the family and Imam to follow Islamic guidelines for preparing the dead body for an Islamic funeral.
	After death, the female body should be given the same respect and privacy as if she was still living.
Communication	Inform them of their patient rights and encourage living wills.
	Take time to explain diagnostic tests, treatments, and procedures. Many Muslims are new immigrants and there may be a language barrier.
	Identify the patient clearly as Muslim on the patient chart and ID bracelet.

Source: Adapted from Athar, S. (2008). *Information for health care providers when dealing with a Muslim patient.* Retrieved from http://www.islam-usa.com/index.php?option=com_content&view=article& id=169:information-for-health-care-providers-when-dealing-with-a-muslim-patient&catid =68:health—medicine&Itemid=137

birth, life, death, and rebirth through their many lifetimes (Levinson, 1998). It is called *samsara*. Karma is the accumulated sum of one's good and bad deeds. Karma determines how you will live your next life. Through pure acts, thoughts, and devotion, one can be reborn at a higher level. Eventually, one can escape *samsara* and achieve enlightenment. Bad deeds can cause a person to be reborn at a lower level, or even as an animal. The unequal distribution of wealth, prestige, and suffering are thus seen as natural consequences for one's previous acts, both in this life and in previous lives.

HINDU HEALTH BELIEFS

Hinduism is considered not only a religion but a way of life (Sukumaran, 1999). Meditation is often practiced, with yoga being the most common type. In India, many rural Hindus worship the goddess of their village or an earth goddess who rules over fertility and disease and therefore is responsible for life and death. For a Hindu, the ultimate goal of life is to achieve *moksa*, which is freedom from *samsara* upon death. This is an important concept for the nurse to keep in mind when caring for a Hindu patient. Hindus see the purpose of the body solely as transport for the soul on its journey to God. When the body has served its purpose it will be discarded and the soul will either find another body or end its journey to be with God. Hindus do believe in preserving a body to its end, so assisted suicide is not encouraged, but they also believe that the true self is immortal and it does not die with the body. There are some general health beliefs associated with Hindus (individual practices may vary). Generally, Hindus will reluctantly accept a blood transfusion. While donating and receiving organ transplants and genetic engineering for disease prevention may be allowed by the patient, there may be reluctance or even refusal, because the patient may be of the firm belief that it may not allow for the complete release of the soul of the organ donor (Sukumaran, 1999). Autopsies are permitted. Circumcision is not performed. It is not encouraged to provide extraordinary life support measures for a persistent vegetative state or therapeutic abortions, unless medically indicated.

IMPORTANT NURSING IMPLICATIONS

When caring for a Hindu patient it is essential for the nurse to provide privacy and modesty (Andrews, 2006). A female Hindu may prefer to be examined by a nurse or physician of the same sex. There is a belief that Western medicine relies on overmedication—especially in the use of antibiotics and narcotics (Sukumaran, 1999). The use of narcotics, alcohol, or caffeine is discouraged, as the only way acceptable way to achieve an elevated state is through meditation and increased awareness (Sukumaran, 1999). Hindus may appreciate a more comprehensive treatment plan that includes ayurveda and homeopathic remedies. The nurse should also avoid using his or her left hand when administering medications or foods, as the left hand is considered impure (Sukumaran, 1999).

One potentially sensitive area is institutional policy for removal of jewelry and storing of valuables. In Indian culture, a red dot or bindi on the forehead indicates that a female is married. It is also used to ward off disease or the "evil eye." Marital status may also be shown through the use of jewelry such as necklaces, bracelets, or toe rings. The married female may be reluctant to remove these items of jewelry. The nurse must take the time to explain the reason why the jewelry must be removed (if indeed it is medically necessary), as well as the policy on safe keeping of valuables within your healthcare institution.

Some male Hindu patients (over the age of 13) may be wearing the "sacred thread" over the shoulder (Sukumaran, 1999). The thread is an important part of the Upanayna ceremony, which is performed when the male is 12 or 13 years of age, and is never removed. Extremely devout Hindus (of both sexes) may have a prayer book or other aids at the bedside and may wish to listen to devotional music.

The nurse may need to work closely with the dietary staff because most Hindus are devout vegetarians (note that gelatin must be avoided, as it is derived from beef products) (Sukumaran, 1999). Extremely orthodox Hindus may also exclude onion and garlic from their diet. If there are no medically necessary dietary restrictions, the nurse should encourage the patient's family to bring in food for the patient to consume.

End-of-life issues are rare because Hindus do not believe in prolonging life. Cremation is the expectation after death and it must be performed very shortly after death, preferably no later than 24 hours after the person has died (Sukumaran, 1999).

SUMMARY

Whatever the religious beliefs of the patient (Muslim, Hindu, Christian, or other), more and more medical research is supporting the belief of the faithful that prayer has the power to heal. A meta-analysis of research studies in this area was conducted in 2012 by Dr. Harold Koenig of Duke University (NewsMaxHealth, 2012). The analysis of more than 1,500 reputable medical studies "indicates people who are more religious and pray more have better mental and physical health," Koenig says. Out of 125 studies that looked at the link between health and regular worship, 85 showed regular churchgoers live longer. Koenig (NewsMaxHealth, 2012) identified the following benefits of prayer to health: better coping with stress, a sense of greater well-being, less depression and anxiety with less episodes of suicide, a stronger immune system, lower blood pressure, and overall better cardiovascular functioning. As nurses, no matter what our spiritual beliefs, we must strive to support the spirituality and health beliefs of all of the patients for whom we provide nursing care.

REFERENCES

Andrews, C. S. (2006). Modesty and healthcare for women: Understanding cultural sensitivities. *Community Oncology, 3*(7), 443–446.

Athar, S. (2008). *Information for health care providers when dealing with a Muslim patient.* Retrieved from http://www.islam-usa.com/index.php?option=com_content&view=article&id=115:information-for-health-care-providers-when-dealing-with-a-muslim-patient&catid=60:articles&Itemid=145

BBC.com. (2009). The five pillars of Islam. Retrieved from http://www.bbc.co.uk/religion/religions/islam/practices/fivepillars.shtml

Levinson, D. (1998). *Religion: A cross-cultural dictionary.* New York, NY: Oxford Press.

NewsMaxHealth.com. (2012). *Proof of the healing power of prayer.* Retrieved from http://www.newsMaxHealth.com/headline_health/prayer_healing_power/2012/04/06/443812.html

Ohm, R. (2003). The African American experience in the Islamic faith. *Public Health Nursing, 20*(6), 478–486.

PBS.org. (2012). *Caught in the crossfire: Arab Americans.* Retrieved from http://www.pbs.org/itvs/caughtinthecrossfire/arab_americans.html

Pluralism Project at Harvard University. (2010). *Resources by tradition.* Retrieved from http://pluralism.org/resources/tradition/?trad=5

ReligiousTolerance.Org. (2012). *Hinduism: The world's third largest religion.* Retrieved from http://www.religioustolerance.org/hinduism.htm

Sukumaran, A. (1999). *Hinduism and medicine: A guide for medical professionals.* Retrieved from http://www.angelfire.com/az/ambersukumaran/medicine.html

Taheri, N. (2008). *Health care in Islamic history and experience.* Retrieved from http://ethnomed.org/cross-cultural-health/religion/health-care-in-islamic-history-and-experience

For a full suite of assignments and additional learning activities, see the access code at the front of your book.

Glossary of Additional Cultural Terms

Acculturation—becoming a competent participant in the dominant culture. In the United States, it is assumed that the usual course of acculturation takes three generations for completion (i.e., the grandchildren of an immigrant would be considered fully acculturated or Americanized) (Spector, 2004).

Assimilation—becoming in all ways like the members of the dominant culture; the process by which an individual develops a new cultural identity (Spector, 2004).

Bicultural—a person may self-identify with more than one cultural group; the bicultural person sees both sides and can function in two worlds (McGrath, 1998).

Biopsychosocial Model—incorporates social, psychological, and emotional factors in diagnosis and treatment. It recognizes that illness cannot be studied or treated in isolation from the social and cultural environment. Whereas the Biomedical Model prioritizes professional knowledge, the Biopsychosocial Model expects health caregivers and doctors to acknowledge and take into account individual patient circumstances.

Collectivism—"the subjugation of the individual to a group—whether to a race, class or state does not matter. Collectivism holds that man must be chained to collective action and collective thought for the sake of what is called 'the common good'" (Rand, 1944). "Collectivism is the political theory that states that the will of the people is omnipotent, an individual must obey; that society as a whole, not the individual, is the unit of moral value" (Bernstein, 2005).

Cultural awareness—an appreciation of the objective, external signs of diversity, such as the arts, music, dress, and physical characteristics (Lattanzi & Purnell, 2006).

Cultural competency—no single definition of cultural competency is universally accepted, yet all of the definitions share the requirement that healthcare professionals adjust and recognize their own culture in order to understand the culture of the patient (Johnson, Saha, Arbelaez, Beach, & Cooper, 2004).

Cultural diversity—interacting with persons from a culture different from your own (Purnell, 2013). It refers to diversity in race, color, ethnicity, national origin, religion, age, gender, sexual orientation, ability/disability, social and economic status or class, education, occupation, religious orientation, marital and parental status, and other related attributes of groups of people in society (Giger et al., 2007).

Cultural humility—incorporates a lifelong commitment to self-evaluation and self-critique, to redress the power imbalances in the patient–clinician dynamic, and to develop mutually beneficial and advocacy partnerships with communities on behalf of individuals and defined populations. Cultural humility is proposed as a goal in healthcare education (Tervalon & Murray-Garcia, 1998).

Cultural mismatch—when the healthcare provider has a personal style of interaction that does not match the patient's style. It is essential that this cultural mismatch be recognized, or the healthcare provider risks the consequences that result when a therapeutic alliance is not established with the patient (Leininger, 1991).

Cultural sensitivity—experienced when neutral language, both verbal and not verbal, is used in a way that reflects sensitivity and appreciation for the diversity of another. Cultural sensitivity may be conveyed through words, phrases, and categorizations that are intentionally avoided, especially when referring to any individual who may be interpreted as impolite or offensive (Giger et al., 2007).

Culturally competent care—the provision of appropriate, sensitive care to people from ethnic backgrounds different from that of the provider (Giger, 2013).

Culturally discordant care—arises from unaddressed cultural differences between healthcare providers and their patients (Assemi, Cullender, & Hudmon, 2004; Saha, Komaromy, Koepsell, & Bindman, 1999).

Culture—the totality of socially transmitted behavioral patterns, arts, beliefs, values, customs, life ways, and all other products of human work and thought characteristics of a population of people that guide their worldview and decision making (Purnell, 2013). A learned, patterned behavioral response acquired over time that includes explicit and implicit beliefs, attitudes, values, customs, norms, taboos, arts, habits, and life ways accepted by a community of individuals. Culture is primarily learned and transmitted within the family and other social organizations, is shared by the majority of the group, includes an individualized worldview, guides decision making, and facilitates self-worth and self-esteem (Giger et al., 2007). Culture influences beliefs about what causes illness and how it should be treated. These cultural beliefs may guide patient actions in health maintenance and during times of illness in patients, their families, and the community.

Diversity—the concept of diversity encompasses acceptance and respect. It means understanding that each individual is unique and recognizing our individual differences. These can be along the dimensions of race, ethnicity, gender, sexual orientation, socioeconomic status, age, physical abilities, religious beliefs, political beliefs, or other ideologies. It is the exploration of these differences in a safe, positive, and nurturing environment. It is about understanding each other and moving beyond simple tolerance to embracing and celebrating the rich dimensions of diversity contained within each individual. The range of human variation, including age, race, gender, disability, ethnicity, nationality, religious and spiritual beliefs, sexual orientation, political beliefs, economic status, native language, and geographical background.

Ethnic group—a group of people whose members have different experiences and backgrounds from the dominant culture by status, background, residence, religion, education, or other factors that functionally unify the group and act collectively on each other (Giger et al., 2007).

Ethnicity—the condition of belonging to a particular ethnic group. According to the Office of Minority Health (2001), ethnicity is a group of people that share a common and distinctive racial, national, religious, linguistic, or cultural heritage.

Ethnocentrism—the universal tendency of human beings to think that their ways of thinking, acting, and believing are the only right, proper, and natural ways; this can be a major barrier to providing culturally conscious care. Ethnocentrism perpetuates an attitude that beliefs that differ greatly from one's own are strange, bizarre, or unenlightened, and therefore wrong (Purnell, 2013). Ethnocentrism is a belief in the superiority of one's own ethnic group.

Giger and Davidhizar Transcultural Assessment Model—provides a framework to systematically assess the role of culture on health and illness and has been used extensively in a variety of settings and by diverse disciplines. The model postulates that every individual is culturally unique and should be assessed according to six phenomena (Giger, 2013). It is important to emphasize that the model does not presuppose that every person within an ethnic or cultural group will act or behave in a similar manner (Giger, 2013). In fact, Giger (2013) insists that a culturally appropriate model must recognize differences in groups while avoiding stereotypical approaches to client care.

Healing—according to Spector (2004), there are four types of healing: spiritual healing, inner healing, physical healing, and deliverance or exorcism. Healing should consider the impact of religion or spirituality to the patient. A healing focus would be on the removal of evil that has originated inside or outside the body.

Health—defined by Florence Nightingale (1860) as "being well and using one's powers to the fullest extent." It is defined by the World Health Organization (1946) as "not only the absence of infirmity and disease but also a state of physical, mental and social well-being."

Health Illness Belief Model—based on the constructs of perceived susceptibility, severity, benefits, barriers, and cues to action. The Health Belief Model suggests that patients are more likely to comply with doctors' orders when they feel susceptibility to illness, believe the illness has the potential to have serious consequences for health or daily functioning, and do not anticipate major obstacles, such as side effects or costs (Conrad, 2008).

Health disparities—differences in the incidence, prevalence, mortality, and burden of diseases and other adverse health conditions that exist among specific population groups in the United States (National Institutes of Health, 2010).

Health literacy—the degree to which individuals have the capacity to obtain, process, and understand basic health information and services needed to make appropriate health decisions (U.S. Department of Health and Human Services, 2000).

Illness—a highly personal state in which the person feels unhealthy or ill; may or may not be related to disease (Kozier, Erb, Berman, & Burke, 2000).

Interdisciplinary health care—implies the existence of a team. It is an integrated approach to patient care in which all team members actively coordinate care across all healthcare disciplines.

LEARN—a pneumonic developed to help the nurse navigate a cross-cultural encounter. L, listen to the patient's explanation of the problem; E, explain your perception of the problem; A, acknowledge similarities and differences; R, recommend, suggest an intervention or treatment; and N, negotiate to find a mutually acceptable plan (Berlin & Fowkes, 1983).

Leininger's Sunrise Model—illustrates the major components and interrelationships of Leininger's Culture Care, Diversity, and Universality Theory. Nurses can use the Sunrise Model when caring for patients to ensure that nursing actions are culture specific. The Culture Care, Diversity, and Universality Theory states that nurses must take into account the cultural beliefs, caring behaviors, and values of individuals, families, and groups to provide effective, satisfying, and culturally congruent nursing care (Leininger, 1991).

Multidisciplinary health care—involves membership in a clinical group, practicing with an awareness of and toleration for other disciplines. Groups of professionals provide discipline-specific care independently of one another. The patient's problems are subdivided and treated in parallel. Each provider conducts his or her practice in a parallel relationship with that of other group members.

National Standards for Culturally and Linguistically Appropriate Services in Health Care (CLAS)—Fourteen standards established in 1997 by the Office of Minority Health (within the Department of Health and Human Services) that must be met by most health-care-related agencies. Accreditation and credentialing agencies can access and compare providers who say they provide culturally competent services and assure quality care for diverse populations, including the Joint Commission on Accreditation of Healthcare Organizations (JCAHO), the National Committee on Quality Assurance, American Medical Association (AMA), American Nurses Association (ANA), and Peer Review Organization. (The standards are listed in Box 4–1.)

Patient-centered health care—health care the patient needs, provided when they need it and in the manner that they want. It is care that is informed by both scientific evidence and the patient's values.

Purnell Model of Cultural Competence—to provide a framework for all health-care providers to learn inherent concepts and characteristics of culture; define circumstances that affect one's cultural worldview in the context of historical perspectives; provide a model that links the most central relationships of culture; interrelate characteristics of culture to promote congruence and facilitate the delivery of consciously competent care; provide a framework that reflects human characteristics such as motivation, intentionality, and meaning; provide a structure for analyzing cultural data; and view the individual, family, or group within a unique ethnocultural environment (Purnell, 2013).

Race—a term that relates to biology but has sociologic implications. Members of a particular race share distinguishing physical features such as skin color, bone structure, or blood group. Race is a social construct, which limits or increases opportunities depending on the setting (Giger et al., 2007).

Sick role—in our society, a person is expected to have the symptoms viewed as an illness confirmed by a member of the healthcare profession. Parsons (1951) described four main components of the sick role: (1) the sick person is exempted from the performance of certain normal social obligations; (2) the sick person is also exempted from a certain type of responsibility for their own state; (3) the legitimization of the sick role is only partial; this means that the sick role is only considered acceptable if it falls within a reasonable time frame as determined by health care and society; (4) being sick, except in the mildest of cases, is being in need of help.

Stereotyping—the assumption that all people in a similar cultural, racial, or ethnic group are alike and share the same values and beliefs (Giger, 2013).

Unidisciplinary practice—care delivery where a healthcare professional functions in isolation from members of other healthcare disciplines.

U.S. Biomedical Model (Health Belief Model)—tenets are dichotomization of mind and body, the belief that individuals can control their environment, and the value of taking responsibility for one's own health (Reiser, 1985). There is a strong emphasis on disease prevention in this model, but disease prevention in many cultures is a foreign concept. This is especially so in the areas of childbirth preparation, the care of newborns, the taking of medications, and the death or dying process. Inquiring about the patient's preferences and practices with the goal to incorporate and negotiate acceptable approaches to healthcare delivery will serve the patient and provider best. How long one has been living in the United States also is an important variable as it may greatly impact a patient's attitude toward health care.

Vulnerable populations—social groups with increased relative risk (i.e., exposure to risk factors) or susceptibility to health-related problems. The vulnerability is evidenced in higher comparative mortality rates, lower life expectancy, reduced access to care, and diminished quality of life (Center for Vulnerable Populations Research, 2008).

Western Biomedical Model—the focus is on objective, measurable phenomena, and technology can be used to achieve diagnoses. Advances in medical technology led to a greater ability to localize disease processes within the body so that sites of pathology could be pinpointed with greater accuracy (Helman, 2001).

REFERENCES

Assemi, M., Cullender, C., & Hudmon, K. S. (2004). Implementation and evaluation of cultural competency training for pharmacy students. *The Annals of Pharmacotherapy, 38*(5), 781–786.

Berlin, E. A., & Fowkes, Jr., W. C. (1983). A teaching framework for cross-cultural health care: Application in family practice. *The Western Journal of Medicine, 139*(6), 934–938.

Bernstein, A. (2005). Villainy: An analysis of the nature of evil (Part 5 of 5). *Capitalism Magazine.* Retrieved from http://capitalismmagazine.com/?s=villainy+an+analysis+of+evil&submit.x=3&submit.y=5

Center for Vulnerable Populations Research, UCLA School of Nursing. (2008). Who are vulnerable populations? Retrieved from http://nursing.ucla.edu/site.cfm?id=388

Conrad, P. (2008). *The sociology of health and illness* (8th ed.). New York, NY: Worth.

Giger, J. N. (2013). *Transcultural nursing: Assessment and intervention* (6th ed.). St. Louis, MO: Mosby.

Giger, J., Davidhizar, R. E., Purnell, L., Harden, J. T., Phillips, J., & Strickland, O. (2007). American Academy of Nursing Expert Panel report: Developing cultural competence to eliminate health disparities in ethnic minorities and other vulnerable populations. *Journal of Transcultural Nursing, 18*(2), 95–102.

Helman, C. G. (2001). Health beliefs about diabetes: Patients versus doctors. *The Western Journal of Medicine, 175*(5), 312–313.

Johnson, R. L., Saha, S., Arbelaez, J. J., Beach, M. C., & Cooper, L. A. (2004). Racial and ethnic differences in patient perceptions of bias and cultural competence in health care. *Journal of General Internal Medicine, 19*(2), 101–110.

Kozier, B., Erb, G., Berman, A. J., & Burke, K. (2000). *Fundamentals of nursing, concepts, process, and practice.* Upper Saddle River, NJ: Prentice-Hall Health.

Lattanzi, J. B., & Purnell, L. D. (2006). *Developing cultural competence in physical therapy practice.* Philadelphia, PA: F. A. Davis.

Leininger, M. M. (1991). *Culture care diversity and universality: A theory of nursing.* New York, NY: National League for Nursing.

McGrath, B. B. (1998). Illness as a problem of meaning: Moving culture from the classroom to the clinic. *Advances in Nursing Science, 21*(2), 17–29.

National Institutes of Health. (2010). Health disparities defined. Retrieved from http://crchd.cancer.gov/disparities/defined.html

Nightingale, F. (1860). *Notes on nursing: What it is and what it is not* (1st American ed.). New York, NY: D. Appleton and Company. Retrieved from http://digital.library.upenn.edu/women/nightingale/nursing/nursing.html

Office of Minority Health. (2001). OMB standards for data on race and ethnicity. Retrieved from http://minorityhealth.hhs.gov/templates/browse.aspx?lvl=2&lvlID=172

Parsons, T. (1951). *The social system.* Glencoe, IL: The Free Press.

Purnell, L. D. (2013). *Transcultural health care: A culturally competent approach.* (4th ed.) Philadelphia, PA: F. A. Davis.

Rand, A. (1944, January). The only path to tomorrow. *Readers Digest,* 88–90.

Reiser, S. J. (1985). Responsibility for personal health: A historical perspective. *The Journal of Medicine and Philosophy, 10*(1), 7–17.

Saha, S., Komaromy, M., Koepsell, T. D., & Bindman, A. B. (1999). Patient–physician racial concordance and the perceived quality and use of health care. *Archives of Internal Medicine, 159*(9), 997–1004.

Spector, R. E. (2004). *Cultural diversity in health and illness* (6th ed.). Upper Saddle River, NJ: Pearson-Prentice-Hall.

Tervalon, M., & Murray-Garcia, J. (1998). Cultural humility versus cultural competence: A critical distinction in defining physician training outcomes in multicultural education. *Journal of Health Care for the Poor and Underserved, 9*(2), 117–125.

U.S. Department of Health and Human Services. (2000). Quick guide to health literacy. Fact Sheet. Retrieved from http://www.health.gov/communication/literacy/quickguide/factsbasic.htm

World Health Organization. (1946). Redefining health. Retrieved from http://www.who.int/bulletin/bulletin_board/83/ustun11051/en/

Index